Frontiers in Respiratory Medicine

(Volume 1)

(Advances in Interventional Pulmonology)

Editor

Ali I. Musani

Vice Chair, Global Health, Department of Medicine,
Professor of Medicine and Surgery
Director, Ave, Complex Airway Pillar of the Comprehensive, Lungs and Breathing Program, Director, Interventional Pulmonology
Division of Pulmonary Sciences and Critical Care Medicine
University of Colorado School of Medicine, Denver, USA

&

Associate Editor

Hervé Dutau

Department of Thoracic Oncology, Pleural Diseases and Interventional Pulmonology, North University Hospital, Chemin des Bourrely, 13015, Marseille, France

Frontiers in Respiratory Medicine

Volume # 1

Advances in Interventional Pulmonology

Editor: Ali I. Musani

Associate Editor: Hervé Dutau

ISSN (Online): 2589-1855

ISSN (Print): 2589-1847

ISBN (Online): 978-1-68108-591-3

ISBN (Print): 978-1-68108-592-0

Bentham Science Publishers Ltd.
Executive Suite Y - 2
PO Box 7917, Saif Zone
Sharjah, U.A.E.
Email: subscriptions@benthamscience.org

BENTHAM SCIENCE

CONTENTS

PREFACE

The vast spectrum of Interventional Pulmonology (IP) spans from preventative to palliative medicine. Interventional Pulmonology offers cost effective, out-patient, and minimally-invasive diagnostic and therapeutic strategies for chest diseases. Examples of such interventions include lung cancer diagnosis and staging with minimally invasive approaches such as Endobronchial Ultrasound (EBUS) and navigation technologies. Similarly, from the therapeutic aspect, examples include management of complex airway strictures and stenoses with rigid bronchoscopy and airway stenting as well as treatment of severe emphysema with Bronchoscopic Lung Volume Reduction (BLVR) with novel devices such as airway valves and coils. IP also has dramatically changed how we manage complex pleural effusions in this day and age with indwelling pleural catheters and medical pleuroscopy.

The brisk progress of IP over the last 15 years has expanded its horizons beyond anyone's wildest imagination. Millions of patients with a broad spectrum of pulmonary diseases benefit from the cutting-edge diagnostic and therapeutic approaches offered by IP around the globe.

Some of the current clinical studies and device trials underway include bronchoscopic ablative therapies utilizing navigation technology and manually created tunnels through the lung parenchyma, robotic devices allowing multiple instruments to operate simultaneously in the airways, bronchoscopes with multiple working channels, and steerable and trackable instruments.

IP has already shifted decades-old diagnostic and therapeutic paradigms in many areas of pulmonary diseases. The relentless progress in technologies and skills of IP physicians undoubtedly carries the promise to revolutionize the field of pulmonary medicine.

Finally, I am incredibly thankful to my associate editor and good friend, Dr. Herve Duatau and all the contributing authors who volunteered their precious time and expertise in writing evidence-based, state of the art review articles for this edition of eBook on Interventional Pulmonology.

Ali I. Musani, MD, FCCP
Vice Chair, Global Health, Department of Medicine,
Professor of Medicine and Surgery,
Director, Complex Airway Pillar of the Comprehensive Lungs and Breathing Program,
Director, Interventional Pulmonology,
Division of Pulmonary Sciences and Critical Care Medicine,
University of Colorado School of Medicine, Denver,
USA
E-mail: Ali.Musani@ucdenver.edu

ACKNOWLEDGEMENTS

I would like to thank my wife Lubna Sorathia and our children Sara and Sef for allowing me to pursue my ambitions by sacrificing their needs. They allow me to dedicate a major portion of my life to many academic endeavors. Their support and love make it all possible.

List of Contributors

Abdul Aziz Marwan — Faculty of Medicine and Health Sciences, Universiti Sains Islam Malaysia, Negeri Sembilan, Malaysia

Ahmed Awab — University of Oklahoma Health Sciences Center, Oklahoma City, Oklahoma, USA

Akrum Al Zubaidi — Division of Pulmonary, Critical Care and Sleep Medicine, Department of Medicine, National Jewish Health, Denver, Colorado CO, Denver, CO, USA

Amit Taneja — Division of Pulmonary & Critical Care Medicine, Department of Medicine, Medical College of Wisconsin, Milwaukee, WI, USA

Benjamin Young — Department of Pulmonary Medicine, Respiratory Institute, Cleveland Clinic, Cleveland, OH, USA

David P. Breen — Department of Respiratory Medicine, Galway University Hospitals, Galway, Ireland

David Fielding — Department of Thoracic Medicine, Royal Brisbane and Women's Hospital, Herston QLD, Australia

David Hsia — Division of Respiratory and Critical Care Physiology and Medicine, Harbor-UCLA Medical Center, Torrance, CA, USA

Dhiraj Baruah — Department of Radiology, Medical College of Wisconsin, Wisconsin, USA

Donald R. Lazarus — Department of Pulmonary and Critical Care Medicine, Michael E. DeBakey VA Medical Center, Baylor College of Medicine, Houston, TX, USA

Gaurav Kumar — Department of Pulmonary & Critical Care, 9200 West Wisconsin Avenue, Specialty Clinics Building, Suite E52000, Milwaukee, WI 53226, USA

George A. Eapen — MD Anderson Cancer Center, Houston, TX, USA

Hervé Dutau — Department of Thoracic Oncology, Pleural Diseases and Interventional Pulmonology, North University Hospital, Marseille, France

Ioannis Psallidas — Oxford Centre for Respiratory Medicine and Oxford Respiratory Trials Unit, Oxford University Hospitals NHS Foundation Trust, Oxford, UK

Jamalul Azizi Abdul Rahaman — Pulmonology Unit, Department of Medicine, Serdang Hospital, Selangor, Malaysia

James H. Finigan — Division of Pulmonary Sciences and Critical Care Medicine, Department of Medicine, University of Colorado, Aurora, CO, USA
Division of Oncology, Department of Medicine, National Jewish Health, Denver, CO, USA
Division of Pulmonary and Critical Care Medicine, Department of Medicine, National Jewish Health, Denver, CO, USA

Javier Alfayate — Bronchoscopy and Interventional Pulmonology, IIS - Fundación Jiménez Díaz University Hospital –CIBERES, Madrid, Spain

Javier Flandes — Bronchoscopy and Interventional Pulmonology, IIS - Fundación Jiménez Díaz University Hospital –CIBERES, Madrid, Spain

Jeffrey A. Kern Division of Pulmonary Sciences and Critical Care Medicine, Department of Medicine, University of Colorado, Aurora, CO, USA
Division of Oncology, Department of Medicine, National Jewish Health, Denver, CO, USA
Division of Pulmonary and Critical Care Medicine, Department of Medicine, National Jewish Health, Denver, CO, USA

Juan A. Cascón Bronchoscopy and Interventional Pulmonology Unit, Hospital Universitario de Salamanca, Salamanca, Spain

Kaushik Shahir Department of Radiology, Medical College of Wisconsin, Wisconsin, WI, USA

Lakshmi Mudambi MD Anderson Cancer Center, Houston, TX, USA

Lubna T. Sorathia Division of Pulmonary and Critical Care Medicine, Medical College of Wisconsin, Wisconsin, USA

Maged Hassan Chest Diseases Department, Alexandria Faculty of Medicine, Alexandria, Egypt

Michael Machuzak Department of Pulmonary Medicine, Respiratory Institute, Cleveland Clinic, Cleveland, OH, USA

Mohammed Ahmed Department of Respiratory Medicine, Galway University Hospitals, Galway, Ireland

Muhammad Sajawal Ali Division of Pulmonary and Critical Care Medicine, Medical College of Wisconsin, Wisconsin, USA

Najib M. Rahman Oxford Centre for Respiratory Medicine and Oxford Respiratory Trials Unit, Oxford University Hospitals NHS Foundation Trust, Oxford, UK

Nathaniel R. Little Division of Pulmonary Sciences and Critical Care Medicine, Department of Medicine, University of Colorado, Aurora, CO, USA

Nishant Gupta Department of Radiology, Columbia University Medical Center, New York, NY, USA

Noriaki Kurimoto St. Marianna University, Kanagawa Prefecture, Japan

Peter Y. Hahn Metro Health-University of Michigan Health, Wyoming MI, USA

Rabih I. Bechara Cancer Treatment Centers of America, Southeastern Regional Medical Center, Newnan, GA, USA

Rahul Nanchal Division of Pulmonary and Critical Care Medicine, Medical College of Wisconsin, Wisconsin, WI, USA

Roberto F. Casal Department of Pulmonary Medicine, The University of Texas M.D. Anderson Cancer Center, Houston, TX, USA

Rosa Cordovilla Bronchoscopy and Interventional Pulmonology Unit, Hospital Universitario de Salamanca, Salamanca, Spain

Rosmadi Ismail Pulmonology Unit, Department of Medicine, Serdang Hospital, Selangor, Malaysia

Septimiu Murgu Interventional Pulmonology Fellowship Program Director, The University of Chicago Medicine, Chicago, IL, USA

Shaheen Islam Section of Interventional Pulmonology, Division of Pulmonary, Allergy, Critical Care and Sleep Medicine, Ohio State University Wexner Medical Center, Columbus, OH, USA

Sonali Sethi	Department of Pulmonary Medicine, Respiratory Institute, Cleveland Clinic, Cleveland, OH, USA
Srinivas R. Mummadi	Metro Health-University of Michigan Health, Wyoming MI, USA
Steven J. Campbell	Section of Interventional Pulmonology, Division of Pulmonary, Allergy, Critical Care and Sleep Medicine, Ohio State University Wexner Medical Center, Columbus, OH, USA
Suhaib Khan	University of Oklahoma Health Sciences Center, Oklahoma City, Oklahoma, USA
Tayfun Caliskan	Department of Pulmonology, University of Health Sciences, Istanbul, Turkey
Thomas R. Gildea	Department of Pulmonary Medicine, Respiratory Institute, Cleveland Clinic, Cleveland, OH, USA

CHAPTER 1

Flexible Bronchoscopy

Donald R. Lazarus[1] and **Roberto F. Casal**[*, 2]

[1] *Department of Pulmonary and Critical Care Medicine, Michael E. DeBakey VA Medical Center, Baylor College of Medicine, Houston, Texas, USA*

[2] *Department of Pulmonary Medicine, The University of Texas M.D. Anderson Cancer Center, 1515 Holcomb Blvd. Houston, Texas, USA*

Abstract: Since its advent in the late 1960s, flexible bronchoscopy has revolutionized pulmonary practice. It allows the pulmonologist to examine the airways to the subsegmental level while obtaining diagnostic samples using techniques such as bronchoalveolar lavage, endobronchial biopsy, cytology brushing, transbronchial lung biopsy, and transbronchial needle aspiration. Even recent advancements in bronchoscopic technology have not rendered essential bronchoscopic techniques irrelevant, and the well-trained pulmonologist must be well versed in all of these techniques to provide optimal patient care.

Keywords: Bronchoalveolar lavage, Bronchoscopy, Endobronchial biopsy, Flexible bronchoscopy, Transbronchial lung biopsy, Transbronchial needle aspiration.

INTRODUCTION

Flexible bronchoscopy is the most commonly used invasive technique for diagnosing and treating diseases of the lungs and bronchi [1, 2]. The flexible bronchoscope can be used to visually examine the airways to the subsegmental level using only moderate sedation in most cases. Various complementary techniques and instruments allow them to be used to sample the bronchi and lung parenchyma as well, and its versatility and ease of use have significantly contributed to its popularity among pulmonologists in the modern era. This chapter will briefly discuss the history and development of the flexible bronchoscope. It will also review the indications and contraindications of the procedure and discuss basic diagnostic techniques, including bronchoalveolar lavage (BAL), endobronchial biopsy (EBBX), transbronchial lung biopsy (TBLB), and transbronchial needle aspiration (TBNA). More advanced diagnostic

* **Corresponding author Roberto F. Casal:** Department of Pulmonary Medicine, The University of Texas M.D. Anderson Cancer Center, 1515 Holcomb Blvd. Houston, Texas TX, USA; Tel: 713-792-3962; Fax: 713-794-4922; E-mail: rfcasal@mdanderson.org

Ali I. Musani (Ed.)

and therapeutic techniques are beyond the scope of this chapter and will be addressed elsewhere in this book.

HISTORY

Rigid bronchoscopy, introduced by Gustav Killian in 1897, was the primary invasive tool available to pulmonologists for the diagnosis and treatment of bronchial and pulmonary conditions through most of the 20th century [3]. While the rigid instrument remains the preferred tool for therapeutic bronchoscopy, its general application is limited by its invasiveness, requirement for general anesthesia, and inability to reach distal areas or access the upper lobes. The introduction of flexible bronchoscopy has largely overcome these limitations [4].

Shigeto Ikeda developed the first flexible fiberoptic bronchoscope in the 1960s, revolutionizing pulmonary practice [3, 5]. Machida manufactured the first commercially available flexible bronchoscope and commercialized it in 1968, quickly followed by bronchoscopes made by Olympus which also included a working channel through which suction or instruments could be applied [3, 6, 7]. Over the next few years, rapid improvements in image quality, flexibility, and angulation followed. By the mid-1970s, the flexible fiberoptic bronchoscope was being commonly used worldwide. Technological advances continued, with the introduction of the first video bronchoscope by Pentax in 1987. This progress improved the quality of the bronchoscopic image by using a miniaturized video camera rather than optical fibers. That allowed the image enhancement on a large screen rather than just through an eyepiece [3, 5].

Some additional diagnostic and therapeutic techniques were developed to make use of the newly expanded reach given to the bronchoscopist by the advent of flexible bronchoscopy. Many of these techniques were originally used in rigid bronchoscopy but were not widely adopted because of the limitations of reach and flexibility intrinsic to the utilization of the rigid instrument and the discomfort of many pulmonologists with its use. Reynolds *et al.* published the first report of BAL using the flexible bronchoscope in 1974 [8]. This innovation allowed bronchoscopists to obtain material from the lower respiratory tract for analysis conveniently. Rigid bronchoscopy has been used for transbronchial biopsy at various centers for several years. Its use was limited to diffuse lung diseases due to the inability to reach lesions with precision, particularly in the upper lobes [9, 10]. The development of flexible forceps allowed this technique to be adapted to flexible bronchoscopy, increasing the ease and accuracy of TBLB and placing the technique within reach of most general pulmonologists [11 - 13]. First described by Schiepatti in 1948 using a needle inserted using a rigid bronchoscope [14, 15],

TBNA was revived by Wang and colleagues in 1978 and adapted for use through the flexible bronchoscope [16 - 18].

In addition to the development of these basic diagnostic techniques both therapeutic and advanced diagnostic techniques have been developed or adapted for use with the flexible bronchoscope. Therapeutic techniques adapted for use in flexible bronchoscopy include the laser bronchoscopy, flexible cryotherapy probes, electrosurgery using various instruments, argon plasma coagulation, bronchial thermoplasty, and much more [19 - 22]. The rapid development of advanced diagnostic techniques for flexible bronchoscopy has continued, with the advent of autofluorescence bronchoscopy, narrow band imaging, confocal microscopy, optical coherence tomography, endobronchial ultrasound (EBUS), electromagnetic navigation (EMN), and others [23 - 29]. While these and other advanced bronchoscopic techniques are beyond the scope of this chapter and will be reviewed elsewhere in this book, they must be mentioned as further evidence of the ongoing revolution in pulmonary practice that began with the development of flexible bronchoscopy.

INDICATIONS AND CONTRAINDICATIONS FOR FLEXIBLE BRONCHOSCOPY

Flexible bronchoscopy is performed for either diagnostic or therapeutic reason. Diagnostic indications predominate. A review of over 4000 flexible bronchoscopies carried out at an academic center over a 5-year period revealed that over 86% of procedures had a diagnostic indication, with only about 10% of procedures performed for a therapeutic one. The remaining 3% were conducted in volunteers for research purposes [30]. The indications for flexible diagnostic bronchoscopy include pulmonary signs and symptoms, abnormal imaging or other diagnostic studies, and indications related to known disease processes [5, 31] as summarized in Table **1**. The bronchoscopist must also remember that a diagnostic procedure occasionally becomes a therapeutic one when there are unexpected bronchoscopic findings or a complication of a diagnostic technique occurs [5]. Therapeutic indications for flexible bronchoscopy are summarized in Table **2**.

Table 1. Indications for Diagnostic Flexible Bronchoscopy.

Pulmonary signs and symptoms
• Unexplained chronic cough
• Hemoptysis
• Stridor
• Unilateral wheezing
• Chronic hoarseness

(Table 1) contd.....

Abnormal diagnostic studies
• Lung nodule or mass
• Intrathoracic lymphadenopathy
• Non-resolving pneumonia or undiagnosed infiltrates
• Cavitary lung lesion
• Bronchial occlusion or obstruction (mucus plugging, foreign body aspiration, tumor)
• Diffuse parenchymal lung disease
• Flow-volume loop suggesting airway obstruction
Related to known disease processes
• Mediastinal staging of lung cancer
• Suspected airway involvement by adjacent tumors (esophageal cancer)
• Early detection of central airway tumor
• Evaluation of tracheobronchomalacia
• Pneumonia in an immunocompromised host
• Benign airway stricture
• Lung transplant surveillance
• Bronchopleural fistula
• Aerodigestive fistula
• Chest trauma
• Thermal or chemical injury of airways
• Endotracheal tube position

Table 2. Indications for Therapeutic Flexible Bronchoscopy

Malignant central airway obstruction
• Mechanical or thermal tumor destruction
• Stenting
Benign central airway obstruction
• Mechanical or thermal dilation or cutting
• Stenting
Aerodigestive fistulas
• Stenting
• Thermal treatment
Bronchopleural fistulas
• Intrabronchial/Endobronchial valves
• Airway spigots
• Sealants
Foreign body removal
Tracheobronchial toilet/mucus plugging
Hemoptysis
• Hemostasis of central lesions
• Airway blockers
Other
• Bronchial thermoplasty
• Bronchoscopic lung volume reduction
• Drainage of abscess or cyst

Flexible bronchoscopy is a very safe procedure with low complication rates. Major complications include significant hemorrhage, pneumothorax requiring chest tube placement, respiratory distress, cardiac arrhythmias, seizures, and cardiopulmonary arrest. Minor complications include laryngospasm, bronchospasm, epistaxis, transient hoarseness, fever, nausea, and cough. Large retrospective surveys evaluating over 68,000 procedures estimate a rate of major complications from 0.08-0.3%, although this may be an underestimate due to response bias related to the study design [32 - 35]. Prospective studies and a more recent large retrospective study of consecutive patients suggest a slightly higher major complication rate, somewhere between 0.1% and 5%, with the majority of major complications related to TBLB [30, 35 - 38]. Mortality is rare, less than 0.04% [34, 35, 39].

There are few absolute contraindications to flexible bronchoscopy. They include refractory hypoxemia, hemodynamic instability, life-threatening arrhythmias, lack of informed consent, inappropriate equipment or facility, and an inexperienced operator [5, 31, 40]. Relative contraindications which increase the risk of flexible bronchoscopy are much more common, and in such cases, the risk and benefit of the procedure must be weighed carefully and measures taken to mitigate the risk when possible. Severe hypoxemia is a relative contraindication to flexible bronchoscopy. It may be preferable to perform the procedure under general anesthesia if it cannot be postponed. Patients who are uncooperative or delirious also have an increased risk of complications and may also benefit from general anesthesia to enable a necessary procedure to be safely performed [5]. While bronchoscopy using moderate sedation is considered safe for patients with stable coronary artery disease, hemodynamic changes associated with the procedure may induce ischemia in rare cases [41]. For this reason, most bronchoscopists postpone elective procedures for at least six weeks after acute coronary syndrome or an episode of decompensated heart failure. The presence of large bullae or extensive emphysema in the area near the target lesion is a relative contraindication to TBLB in patients with poor respiratory function because of the increased risk of symptomatic pneumothorax in that setting [5].

Coagulopathy is another relative contraindication to flexible bronchoscopy, but its importance depends on the type of procedure to be performed. A simple bronchoscopic airway exam and BAL can be conducted with minimal bleeding risk, even in patients with mild coagulopathy. If the coagulopathy is severe and not corrected, the oral route of insertion for the bronchoscope may be preferred. If the planned procedure will require tissue sampling with TBNA, biopsies, or brushing then the correcting the coagulopathy becomes much more important. The risk of bleeding is higher with TBLB than with TBNA or other methods of sampling [5, 30, 35, 42]. Good quality data regarding TBLB in the setting of coagulopathy is scanty. One study reviewed the risk of bleeding from TBLB in 24 patients with thrombocytopenia (less than 60,000/mm^3) due to chemotherapy or bone marrow invasion. In 20 of the cases, patients received a transfusion of platelets within 60 minutes before the procedure. The rate of significant bleeding was 21%, and there was one fatal hemorrhage [43]. Two retrospective studies evaluating the predictive value of pre-bronchoscopy coagulation studies did not show increased risk of bleeding from TBLB in patients with high partial thromboplastin time (PTT), prothrombin time (PT), or international normalized ratio (INR). Only 45 patients had abnormal coagulation parameters (out of a total of 731 who underwent a biopsy in the two studies), and it is likely that some patients with abnormal coagulation studies at who were thought to be at high risk of bleeding were not biopsied [44, 45]. When the relative risk of bleeding for patients in the previous studies was subsequently calculated the confidence intervals were very wide, and stronger evidence is needed before forgoing pre-biopsy assessment of coagulation in patients at risk for bleeding [46]. For this reason, guidelines still recommend checking platelets and coagulation studies before bronchoscopy with planned biopsy, and this is our practice as well [35]. Personal experience and expert opinion suggest that platelet counts below 50,000/mm3, elevated PTT, and INR above 1.5 should be considered relative contraindications to biopsy unless corrected [5].

Medications that may increase bleeding risk must also be considered relative contraindications to flexible bronchoscopy. Although little evidence exists regarding management of anticoagulants for bronchoscopy, recommendations extrapolated from the surgical literature have been incorporated into guidelines for bronchoscopy [47]. Warfarin should be stopped approximately five days before bronchoscopy, and low-molecular-weight heparin should be held for at least 12 hours before the procedure. Direct factor Xa inhibitors such as apixaban, edoxaban, and rivaroxaban and direct thrombin inhibitors such as dabigatran should be held for at least 72 hours before bronchoscopy [35, 48]. There is literature evaluating antiplatelet agents in bronchoscopy, and this is particularly relevant in the current age of drug-eluting coronary stents requiring dual antiplatelet therapy. Daily use of aspirin was not associated with increased risk of bleeding after TBLB in a prospective study of over 1200 patients, 285 of whom were taking aspirin [49]. A prospective study of 604 patients undergoing TBLB, 30 of whom were taking clopidogrel, demonstrated a very high rate of significant bleeding in those patients--89% of patients on clopidogrel alone, and 100% of patients on clopidogrel and aspirin [50]. For this reason, clopidogrel should be stopped if possible 5-7 days before bronchoscopy. Aspirin may be continued. For those patients with drug-eluting coronary stents which have been in place for less than 12 months delaying bronchoscopy is recommended [35]. Interventional cardiology should be consulted for urgent procedures.

BASIC DIAGNOSTIC PROCEDURES IN FLEXIBLE BRONCHOSCOPY

The most important part of a flexible diagnostic bronchoscopy is the planning of the procedure. The patient's clinical presentation, radiographic images, suspected etiology of the condition, and the location of the intrathoracic lesions must be evaluated carefully. This information is used to select the most appropriate procedure or combination of procedures. All flexible diagnostic bronchoscopies should include a thorough airway exam, and detailed knowledge of the anatomy of the bronchial tree is essential to the bronchoscopist. In addition to the visual inspection of the airways flexible bronchoscopy can provide several types of samples. These specimens are useful in diagnosing diseases of the chest. For example, cytology (washings, BAL, brushings, and TBNA), histologic (forceps biopsy, core needle biopsy, and cryo biopsy), and microbiologic samples. Using multiple techniques (such as TBLB, cytology brush, and BAL) to obtain samples tends to increase the diagnostic yield of the procedure [51 - 54].

Bronchial Washings, Bronchial Brushing, and Endobronchial Biopsy

Bronchial washings, brushings, and endobronchial biopsies are taken from the large airways under direct visualization, although cytology brushes can be used to take samples from peripheral parts of the lung as well. They are frequently used together to diagnose visible endobronchial malignancy or pulmonary infections [51, 53]. Bronchial washing just involves the instillation of saline through the working channel of the bronchoscope into the airway. The bronchoscopist then suctions the saline (mixed with local secretions and cellular elements) back through the bronchoscope and into a fluid trap. Available evidence does not suggest that waiting until after forceps biopsy to obtain bronchial washings increases yield, although this is a common practice [52, 54].

Bronchial brushing can be used to obtain cytologic or microbiologic samples in the large airways under direct visualization or in the peripheral airways using fluoroscopic guidance. A variety of brushes is available to the bronchoscopist. The brush is kept in its protective sheath until the distal end of the sheath exits the working channel of the bronchoscope. Then the sheath is positioned near the target site, an assistant advance the brush out from the sheath, and vigorous brushing of the lesion is carried out. The brush is then retracted back into the sheath before being removed from the working channel. The overall diagnostic yield of brushing for malignancy in visible endobronchial lesions is around 60-90% [51, 53, 54].

The same flexible forceps used for TBLB are also used for endobronchial biopsies. The forceps are advanced through the working channel of the bronchoscope. Once they emerge from the channel, the forceps are positioned near the target lesion and opened by an assistant. The bronchoscopist then advances the forceps until the lesion is within their jaws. The assistant closes the forceps around the tissue, and they are then retracted through the working channel of the bronchoscope to retrieve the biopsy. Several biopsies of the lesion are recommended. Diagnostic yield of endobronchial biopsy for visible endobronchial tumors ranges from 78%-94% [51 - 54].

Bronchoalveolar Lavage

Bronchoalveolar lavage is used to obtain diagnostic material from the distal airways and alveoli. Although guidelines exist highlighting that the technique is not standardized across centers [55]. In general, after the airway examination the bronchoscope is advanced to the targeted segment (usually the most abnormal appearing portion of the lung by imaging) and wedged into a bronchus in the 4th or 5th generation. Then serial aliquots of 30-60 mL of sterile saline are instilled *via* the working channel of the bronchoscope. A total of 100-300 mL is typical of most institutions, although the optimal total volume is not known. The saline (mixed with contents of the lower respiratory tract) is then aspirated with the syringes used to instill it or using the suction of the bronchoscope [5, 55]. It is believed that smaller amounts of fluid (60 mL or less) sample primarily the small bronchi, while amounts of 120 mL or larger fill the entire segment more evenly, leading to sampling of fluid from the alveoli as well [56]. The proportion of the instilled volume of fluid recovered is typically 40-60%, with optimal sampling yielding at least 30% of the total instilled volume [55, 57]. Return is diminished with loss of elastic recoil of the airways which leads to easy collapse with suctioning. BAL is very safe with extremely low complication rates, most commonly transient hypoxemia and fever [5].

The differential cell count of BAL fluid in a healthy adult nonsmoker should have 80-95% macrophages, 5-15% lymphocytes, less than 3% neutrophils, and less than 1% eosinophils [55, 57, 58]. The normal ratio of CD4:CD8 lymphocytes in BAL fluid is 1.4-1.8 [58].

The most frequent indication for BAL is probably to diagnose or exclude pulmonary infections, especially in immunocompromised patients or those who have nonresolving pneumonias. For bacterial pneumonia the yield of BAL is around 65%. In ventilator-associated pneumonias the yield is slightly higher. It is commonly used to diagnose mycobacterial infections including tuberculosis with yield around 75%, although the sensitivity is lower in than TBLB in cases of military disease [5, 40]. Bronchoscopy is especially useful for diagnosing infections in immunocompromised patients. Indeed, in a study of 95 immunocompromised patients on broad spectrum antibiotics and antifungals,

BAL used to diagnose pneumonia found organisms not targeted by or resistant to current therapy in 40% of cases [59].

In addition to diagnosing pulmonary infections, BAL is also used to evaluate inflammatory processes and malignancies. It is often combined with TBLB to diagnose malignant lung tumors. In diffuse parenchymal lung diseases BAL is most commonly used to help rule out infectious conditions that may mimic non-infectious inflammatory diseases. In a few such inflammatory diseases, such as pulmonary alveolar proteinosis, pulmonary Langerhans cell histiocytosis, and eosinophilic pneumonia, BAL may be diagnostic but these are the exceptions to the general rule [5].

Transbronchial Lung Biopsy

A transbronchial lung biopsy is a technique in which flexible forceps are used to obtain histologic samples of tissue from the lung parenchyma or from localized lesions sufficiently distal that the forceps can no longer be directly visualized. It is used commonly to diagnose infectious and non-infectious diffuse lung diseases as well as lung tumors. It is frequently combined with guidance techniques, such as radial probe-EBUS and electromagnetic navigation, to improve the diagnostic yield for peripheral lung lesions. One of the most common indications for TBLB is diffuse interstitial lung disease (ILD) if clinical, imaging and laboratory evaluation are unable to reach a definite diagnosis. TBLB is typically indicated for diffuse ILD in patients who have atypical patterns of disease on high-resolution CT, have rapidly progressive disease, are younger, are suspected of conditions more likely to respond to therapy, or to rule out infection before a trial of immunosuppressive treatment [5]. The overall yield of TBLB for diffuse ILDs is around 70%. It is higher for those conditions with a centrilobular or bronchogenic distribution, such as sarcoidosis or hypersensitivity pneumonitis [5, 60]. TBLB is also used in conjunction with BAL to diagnose pulmonary infections, especially in patients who are immunocompromised. In such patients, the combination of TBLB and BAL has higher diagnostic yield than either technique alone [61, 62]. The yield of TBLB for focal peripheral lung lesions varies considerably with the location and size of the lesion as well as the other modalities used to guide biopsy. The yield of TBLB for peripheral lung lesions in conjunction with radial probe-EBUS and EMN will be discussed more fully in another part of this book.

Most TBLBs are performed in the bronchoscopy suite using moderate sedation. Contraindications to TBLB under moderate sedation include allergy to the sedatives to be used, excessive cough, and inability to cooperate with the bronchoscopist. Most institutions use fluoroscopy to guide TBLB, especially for localized lesions. Because bleeding encountered after TBLB may prevent other procedures (such as BAL) from being completed successfully, biopsy should be performed after the airway examination and other desired procedures have been completed. The bronchoscope is advanced to the area of interest and wedged gently into the bronchus. The bronchoscope is kept wedged in the airway to isolate potential bleeding and also to allow more rapid completion of the procedure since several biopsies can be taken without moving the scope each time [5]. The closed biopsy forceps are then advanced through the working channel into the airway, and fluoroscopy is activated once the tip of the forceps is outside the working channel of the bronchoscope. The forceps are then advanced to the target area or lesion and opened when they are 0.5-1 cm proximal to the target. The forceps are then advanced to the target or until resistance is encountered and then closed. Care should be taken to avoid taking the biopsy during a coughing episode. The closed forceps is then retracted while carefully watching the visceral pleural line on the fluoroscopy monitor. If the visceral pleura is "tented" in with retraction, then the forceps should be opened and a different less distal site selected to avoid possible pneumothorax [5]. If the visceral pleura is not tented, the forceps are retracted gently into the working channel of the bronchoscope and removed so that the biopsy specimen can be retrieved. Specimens can be used to create touch-preps for rapid on-site cytology assessment and then placed into formalin for final pathology. They can also be placed into saline for microbiologic analysis when indicated. The more biopsies that are taken, the greater the diagnostic yield, which also varies with the underlying disease. A study of 530 consecutive TBLB in 516 immunocompetent patients with chronic diffuse infiltrates, focal peripheral lesions or hilar adenopathy demonstrated a diagnostic yield of 38% when 1-3 specimens were taken compared to a yield of 69% when 6-10 specimens were obtained. The investigators also noted differences in yield for TBLB among different causes of diffuse chronic infiltrates, with better results for hypersensitivity pneumonitis and sarcoidosis than for pulmonary fibrosis or miliary tuberculosis [63]. While taking more biopsies increases diagnostic yield, it also increased the number of complications such as pneumothorax and bleeding. In most cases, 5-7 biopsies should give sufficient yield without unduly increasing the risk to the patient. Larger forceps do not appear to increase the yield over smaller ones [64].

The incidence of pneumothorax with TBLB is influenced by factors including operator experience, type of forceps, number of samples taken, and fluoroscopy guidance [5]. The rate of pneumothorax varies among institutions but is quite small, ranging from 1-5% [30, 36, 39, 65]. Pneumothorax is more common in mechanically ventilated patients, occurring in 7-14% of TBLB procedures, although the information gained changes management in over 40% of cases [66, 67]. Whether or not the use of fluoroscopy to guide TBLB reduces the rate of pneumothorax is controversial. Some investigators have demonstrated a pneumothorax rate of 1% for TBLB without fluoroscopy in 68 patients suspected of having sarcoidosis [65]. However, an extensive mail survey of bronchoscopists in the United Kingdom demonstrated a lower rate of pneumothorax associated with TBLB if fluoroscopy was used, 1.8% with fluoroscopy as opposed to 2.9% without it [39]. Significant bleeding occurs in 2-9% of TBLB procedures [13, 30, 36]. Coagulopathy, uremia, and clopidogrel [43, 47, 50, 68] increase the risk of bleeding with TBLB. Pulmonary hypertension is also thought to increase the risk of bleeding with TBLB although the absolute pressure above which the risk is prohibitive is unknown [47]. Cordasco and colleagues did not identify pulmonary hypertension as a risk factor for bleeding in their retrospective analysis of over 3000 cases in which TBLB or bronchial brushing was used [68]. Another group looked at 37 heart-transplant patients who required TBLB to diagnose pulmonary conditions. No bleeding occurred in the 17 patients with normal mean pulmonary arterial pressures, and moderate bleeding occurred in 3 of 20 patients with mean pulmonary arterial pressures greater than 16 mm Hg. The difference was suggestive of an increased risk, but the number of episodes was too small to reach statistical significance [69]. A subsequent study evaluating TBLB in 24 patients with mild to moderate pulmonary hypertension (compared to 32 controls) did not demonstrate an increased risk of bleeding [70]. Since the evidence is scanty, proceeding with caution seems prudent in patients with pulmonary hypertension. In our practice, we avoid TBLB for patients with systolic pulmonary pressures greater than 50 mm Hg when possible, although we do not consider it an absolute contraindication.

Transbronchial Needle Aspiration

Transbronchial needle aspiration is a very useful technique that uses a small needle advanced through the bronchoscope to sample mediastinal and hilar nodes or masses as well as peripheral lung lesions [17, 18, 71]. Despite its utility, surveys of bronchoscopists have indicated that it is not widely used, primarily because of its perceived low diagnostic yield [1, 2, 72]. The indications for TBNA are summarized in Table **3**. The most common indication for TBNA has historically been for the sampling of hilar or mediastinal lymph nodes and masses. The use of conventional (or blind) TBNA for this purpose has decreased significantly in the last decade since the introduction of convex probe-endobronchial ultrasound (CP-EBUS), which allows real-time ultrasound guidance of TBNA using an integrated ultrasonic bronchoscope [28, 73, 74]. The high diagnostic yield of EBUS-TBNA has led to much of the decline in the use of conventional TBNA for mediastinal and hilar lesions. The use of TBNA for visible endobronchial lesions may also occasionally improve the already-high diagnostic yield of endobronchial forceps biopsy by reaching the core of tumors covered in necrotic material [75]. More recently TBNA has been used more frequently for sampling peripheral lung lesions, often in conjunction with new technologies such as radial probe EBUS, EMN, and virtual bronchoscopy [71, 76]. This section will discuss conventional TBNA, and EBUS-TBNA will be reviewed elsewhere in this book.

Table 3. Indications for Transbronchial Needle Aspiration

Central
• Mediastinal or hilar lymphadenopathy
• Central or endobronchial masses
• Diagnosis/drainage of mediastinal cysts
• Diagnosis/drainage of mediastinal abscesses
• Submucosal injection (glue, cidofovir)
Peripheral
• Diagnosis of peripheral lung lesions
• Insertion of fiducial markers for stereotactic ablative radiation therapy

Needles used for TBNA must be retractable to prevent damage to the bronchoscope. They range in diameter from 19G to 22G, with a typical length of 4-15 mm [77]. Most operators will choose a longer, stiffer needle to sample central structures when the bronchial wall must be penetrated. Shorter and more flexible needles are preferred for sampling peripheral lung lesions [5]. For central lesions the catheter containing the TBNA is passed through the working channel until the metal tip is visible outside the bronchoscope. This technique should be used with the bronchoscope in neutral flexion so as to avoid inadvertent damage to the instrument. The catheter is then withdrawn, exposing the tip of the needle. Once it is visible, the bronchoscope is advanced to the target for puncture and anchored on the wall at an angle as close to 90 degrees as possible. Four techniques are commonly used to penetrate the bronchial wall. In the jabbing method, the bronchoscope is held still, and the needle is quickly advanced through the intercartilaginous space with a quick, firm motion. The piggyback method has the bronchoscopist hold the needle fixed at the entrance to the working channel while the bronchoscope and needle are thrust forward together so that the needle penetrates the wall. In the hub-against-the-wall method, the hub of the needle catheter is placed against the target site while the needle is kept retracted. The needle is then pushed out of the catheter and through the wall into the lesion. Finally, during the cough method, the bronchoscopist employs the jabbing technique while asking the patient to cough to facilitate penetration of the wall with the needle. Once the needle has penetrated the wall suction is applied proximally with a syringe, and the needle is agitated back and forth to collect cellular material. Once the suction is released the needle must be withdrawn entirely into the catheter before it is removed from the bronchoscope. If blood is aspirated into the catheter, it may mean that a large vessel has been punctured, so a new site should be selected [77]. For peripheral TBNA the bronchoscope is advanced to the targeted segment. Then the needle catheter is advanced through the working channel into the airway. Using fluoroscopic guidance (and any other techniques are chosen to aid in navigation) the catheter is advanced to the target lesion, stopping 1-2 cm proximal to the lesion to accommodate the length of the needle. The needle is then pushed out of the catheter into the target lesion, suction is applied, and it is agitated within the target for a few seconds to obtain cellular material. Suction is then released, and the needle is withdrawn into the catheter before the catheter is removed *via* the bronchoscope [5, 71].

The sensitivity of TBNA for identifying malignant involvement of the mediastinum ranges from 40-80%, and despite the lack of randomized controlled trials, it has largely been replaced by EBUS-TBNA for this purpose [18, 78, 79]. Likewise, TBNA has largely been replaced by EBUS-TBNA for sarcoidosis, with a randomized trial showing its inferiority to EBUS-TBNA for diagnosing stage I and II sarcoidosis [80]. The yield of TBNA for mycobacterial or fungal lymphadenitis is variable, but when correlated with cytology showing granulomas may demonstrate added benefit in this setting as well [81, 82]. Using TBNA for peripheral lung nodules has grown in popularity in the last decade in with the availability of new tools for guided bronchoscopy [RP-EBUS, EMN] which are addressed elsewhere in this book. In addition to the availability of guided bronchoscopy, the yield of TBNA for peripheral lesions is influenced by the lesion size, location, and relationship to the bronchus [83]. TBNA has been shown to improve the diagnostic yield for conventional bronchoscopic techniques for peripheral lesions, perhaps because it can penetrate the bronchial wall [71, 84, 85].

Transbronchial needle aspiration is a very safe technique. Damage to the bronchoscope is probably the most common complication of its use [5, 77]. Being careful to keep the needle withdrawn inside the catheter during insertion and removal as well as holding the scope in neutral flexion during insertion minimize this risk. Other complications, such as pneumothorax or bleeding, are exceedingly rare [77, 85, 86].

CONCLUSION

Flexible bronchoscopy has revolutionized pulmonary practice since its inception in the late 1960s. Basic flexible bronchoscopic procedures such as brushings, BAL, TBLB, and TBNA remain essential tools in the armamentarium of the pulmonologist, even in the current era of rapidly advancing technology.

CONFLICT OF INTEREST

The authors declare no conflict of interest, financial or otherwise.

ACKNOWLEDGEMENTS

Declared none.

REFERENCES

[1] Prakash UB, Offord KP, Stubbs SE. Bronchoscopy in North America: the ACCP survey. Chest 1991; 100(6): 1668-75.
[http://dx.doi.org/10.1378/chest.100.6.1668] [PMID: 1959412]

[2] Colt HG, Prakash UB, Offord KP. Bronchoscopy in North America: Survey by the American Association for Bronchology, 1999. Journal of Bronchology 2000; 7(1): 8-25.
[http://dx.doi.org/10.1097/00128594-200007010-00004]

[3] Becker HD. Bronchoscopy: the past, the present, and the future. Clin Chest Med 2010; 31(1): 1-18.
[http://dx.doi.org/10.1016/j.ccm.2009.11.001] [PMID: 20172428]

[4] Dutau H, Vandemoortele T, Breen DP. Rigid bronchoscopy. Clin Chest Med 2013; 34(3): 427-35.
[http://dx.doi.org/10.1016/j.ccm.2013.04.003] [PMID: 23993814]

[5] Casal RF, Ost DE, Eapen GA. Flexible bronchoscopy. Clin Chest Med 2013; 34(3): 341-52.
[http://dx.doi.org/10.1016/j.ccm.2013.03.001] [PMID: 23993807]

[6] Ikeda S, Yanai N, Ishikawa S. Flexible bronchofiberscope. Keio J Med 1968; 17(1): 1-16.
[http://dx.doi.org/10.2302/kjm.17.1] [PMID: 5674435]

[7] Ikeda S, Tsuboi E, Ono R, Ishikawa S. Flexible bronchofiberscope. Jpn J Clin Oncol 1971; 1(1): 55-65.
[PMID: 20736215]

[8] Reynolds HY, Newball HH. Analysis of proteins and respiratory cells obtained from human lungs by bronchial lavage. J Lab Clin Med 1974; 84(4): 559-73.
[PMID: 4412011]

[9] Andersen HA, Fontana RS, Harrison EG Jr. Transbronchoscopic lung biopsy in diffuse pulmonary disease. Dis Chest 1965; 48: 187-92.
[http://dx.doi.org/10.1378/chest.48.2.187] [PMID: 14333652]

[10] Andersen HA, Fontana RS. Transbronchoscopic lung biopsy for diffuse pulmonary diseases: technique and results in 450 cases. Chest 1972; 62(2): 125-8.
[http://dx.doi.org/10.1378/chest.62.2.125] [PMID: 5050217]

[11] Levin DC, Wicks AB, Ellis JH Jr. Transbronchial lung biopsy *via* the fiberoptic bronchoscope. Am Rev Respir Dis 1974; 110(1): 4-12.
[PMID: 4545899]

[12] Scheinhorn DJ, Joyner LR, Whitcomb ME. Transbronchial forceps lung biopsy through the fiberoptic bronchoscope in Pneumocystis carinii pneumonia. Chest 1974; 66(3): 294-5.
[http://dx.doi.org/10.1378/chest.66.3.294] [PMID: 4547596]

[13] Hanson RR, Zavala DC, Rhodes ML, Keim LW, Smith JD. Transbronchial biopsy *via* flexible fiberoptic bronchoscope; results in 164 patients. Am Rev Respir Dis 1976; 114(1): 67-72.
[PMID: 937843]

[14] Schieppati E. La punción mediastinal a través de la carina traqueal. Rev Asoc Med Argent 1949; 63(663-664): 497-9.
[PMID: 15395728]

[15] Schieppati E. Mediastinal lymph node puncture through the tracheal carina. Surg Gynecol Obstet 1958; 107(2): 243-6.
[PMID: 13580767]

[16] Wang KP, Terry P, Marsh B. Bronchoscopic needle aspiration biopsy of paratracheal tumors. Am Rev Respir Dis 1978; 118(1): 17-21.
[PMID: 677557]

[17] Wang KP, Terry PB. Transbronchial needle aspiration in the diagnosis and staging of bronchogenic carcinoma. Am Rev Respir Dis 1983; 127(3): 344-7.
[PMID: 6830056]

[18] Wang KP, Brower R, Haponik EF, Siegelman S. Flexible transbronchial needle aspiration for staging of bronchogenic carcinoma. Chest 1983; 84(5): 571-6.
[http://dx.doi.org/10.1378/chest.84.5.571] [PMID: 6313305]

[19] Dumon JF, Reboud E, Garbe L, Aucomte F, Meric B. Treatment of tracheobronchial lesions by laser photoresection. Chest 1982; 81(3): 278-84.
[http://dx.doi.org/10.1378/chest.81.3.278] [PMID: 7056101]

[20] Mathur PN, Wolf KM, Busk MF, Briete WM, Datzman M. Fiberoptic bronchoscopic cryotherapy in the management of tracheobronchial obstruction. Chest 1996; 110(3): 718-23.
[http://dx.doi.org/10.1378/chest.110.3.718] [PMID: 8797417]

[21] Sheski FD, Mathur PN. Endobronchial electrosurgery: argon plasma coagulation and electrocautery. Semin Respir Crit Care Med 2004; 25(4): 367-74.
[http://dx.doi.org/10.1055/s-2004-832709] [PMID: 16088479]

[22] Cox G, Miller JD, McWilliams A, Fitzgerald JM, Lam S. Bronchial thermoplasty for asthma. Am J Respir Crit Care Med 2006; 173(9): 965-9.
[http://dx.doi.org/10.1164/rccm.200507-1162OC] [PMID: 16456145]

[23] Lam S, Hung JY, Kennedy SM, *et al.* Detection of dysplasia and carcinoma in situ by ratio fluorometry. Am Rev Respir Dis 1992; 146(6): 1458-61.
[http://dx.doi.org/10.1164/ajrccm/146.6.1458] [PMID: 1280929]

[24] Shibuya K, Hoshino H, Chiyo M, *et al.* High magnification bronchovideoscopy combined with narrow band imaging could detect capillary loops of angiogenic squamous dysplasia in heavy smokers at high risk for lung cancer. Thorax 2003; 58(11): 989-95.
[http://dx.doi.org/10.1136/thorax.58.11.989] [PMID: 14586056]

[25] Thiberville L, Moreno-Swirc S, Vercauteren T, Peltier E, Cavé C, Bourg Heckly G. *In vivo* imaging of the bronchial wall microstructure using fibered confocal fluorescence microscopy. Am J Respir Crit Care Med 2007; 175(1): 22-31.
[http://dx.doi.org/10.1164/rccm.200605-684OC] [PMID: 17023733]

[26] Tsuboi M, Hayashi A, Ikeda N, *et al.* Optical coherence tomography in the diagnosis of bronchial lesions. Lung Cancer 2005; 49(3): 387-94.
[http://dx.doi.org/10.1016/j.lungcan.2005.04.007] [PMID: 15922488]

[27] Becker HD. Endobronchial ultrasound--a new perspective in bronchology. Ultraschall Med 1996; 17(3): 106-12.
[http://dx.doi.org/10.1055/s-2007-1003156] [PMID: 8767647]

[28] Yasufuku K, Chiyo M, Sekine Y, *et al.* Real-time endobronchial ultrasound-guided transbronchial needle aspiration of mediastinal and hilar lymph nodes. Chest 2004; 126(1): 122-8.
[http://dx.doi.org/10.1378/chest.126.1.122] [PMID: 15249452]

[29] Schwarz Y, Mehta AC, Ernst A, *et al.* Electromagnetic navigation during flexible bronchoscopy. Respiration 2003; 70(5): 516-22.
[http://dx.doi.org/10.1159/000074210] [PMID: 14665778]

[30] Pue CA, Pacht ER. Complications of fiberoptic bronchoscopy at a university hospital. Chest 1995; 107(2): 430-2.
[http://dx.doi.org/10.1378/chest.107.2.430] [PMID: 7842773]

[31] Waxman AB. Flexible bronchoscopy: indications, contraindications, and consent.Introduction to Bronchoscopy. 1st ed. New York: Cambridge University Press 2009; pp. 78-84.

[32] Credle WF Jr, Smiddy JF, Elliott RC. Complications of fiberoptic bronchoscopy. Am Rev Respir Dis 1974; 109(1): 67-72.
[PMID: 4809166]

[33] Suratt PM, Smiddy JF, Gruber B. Deaths and complications associated with fiberoptic bronchoscopy. Chest 1976; 69(6): 747-51.
[http://dx.doi.org/10.1378/chest.69.6.747] [PMID: 1277893]

[34] Ernst A, Silvestri GA, Johnstone D. American College of Chest Physicians. Interventional pulmonary procedures: Guidelines from the American college of chest physicians. Chest 2003; 123(5): 1693-717.
[http://dx.doi.org/10.1378/chest.123.5.1693] [PMID: 12740291]

[35] Du Rand IA, Blaikley J, Booton R, *et al.* British Thoracic Society Bronchoscopy Guideline Group. British Thoracic Society guideline for diagnostic flexible bronchoscopy in adults: accredited by NICE. Thorax 2013; 68 (Suppl. 1): i1-i44.
[http://dx.doi.org/10.1136/thoraxjnl-2013-203618] [PMID: 23860341]

[36] Pereira W Jr, Kovnat DM, Snider GL. A prospective cooperative study of complications following flexible fiberoptic bronchoscopy. Chest 1978; 73(6): 813-6.
[http://dx.doi.org/10.1378/chest.73.6.813] [PMID: 657853]

[37] Dreisin RB, Albert RK, Talley PA, Kryger MH, Scoggin CH, Zwillich CW. Flexible fiberoptic bronchoscopy in the teaching hospital. Yield and complications. Chest 1978; 74(2): 144-9.
[http://dx.doi.org/10.1378/chest.74.2.144] [PMID: 679742]

[38] Zavala DC. Diagnostic fiberoptic bronchoscopy: Techniques and results of biopsy in 600 patients. Chest 1975; 68(1): 12-9.
[http://dx.doi.org/10.1378/chest.68.1.12] [PMID: 168036]

[39] Simpson FG, Arnold AG, Purvis A, Belfield PW, Muers MF, Cooke NJ. Postal survey of bronchoscopic practice by physicians in the United Kingdom. Thorax 1986; 41(4): 311-7.
[http://dx.doi.org/10.1136/thx.41.4.311] [PMID: 3738850]

[40] Prakash UB. Bronchoscopy.Murray and Nadel's Textbook of Respiratory Medicine. 4th ed. Philadelphia: Elsevier Saunders 2005; pp. 617-50.

[41] Matot I, Kramer MR, Glantz L, Drenger B, Cotev S. Myocardial ischemia in sedated patients undergoing fiberoptic bronchoscopy. Chest 1997; 112(6): 1454-8.
[http://dx.doi.org/10.1378/chest.112.6.1454] [PMID: 9404738]

[42] Shofer S, Wahidi MM. Transbronchial Lung Biopsy.Introduction to Bronchoscopy. 1st ed. New York: Cambridge University Press 2009; pp. 98-106.

[43] Papin TA, Lynch JP III, Weg JG. Transbronchial biopsy in the thrombocytopenic patient. Chest 1985; 88(4): 549-52.
[http://dx.doi.org/10.1378/chest.88.4.549] [PMID: 4042705]

[44] Kozak EA, Brath LK. Do "screening" coagulation tests predict bleeding in patients undergoing fiberoptic bronchoscopy with biopsy? Chest 1994; 106(3): 703-5.
[http://dx.doi.org/10.1378/chest.106.3.703] [PMID: 8082343]

[45] Zahreddine I, Atassi K, Fuhrman C, Febvre M, Maitre B, Housset B. Impact of prior biological assessment of coagulation on the hemorrhagic risk of fiberoptic bronchoscopy. Rev Mal Respir 2003; 20(3 Pt 1): 341-6.
[PMID: 12910108]

[46] Segal JB, Dzik WH. Transfusion Medicine/Hemostasis Clinical Trials Network. Paucity of studies to support that abnormal coagulation test results predict bleeding in the setting of invasive procedures: an evidence-based review. Transfusion 2005; 45(9): 1413-25. [http://dx.doi.org/10.1111/j.1537-2995.2005.00546.x] [PMID: 16131373]

[47] Wahidi MM, Rocha AT, Hollingsworth JW, Govert JA, Feller-Kopman D, Ernst A. Contraindications and safety of transbronchial lung biopsy *via* flexible bronchoscopy. A survey of pulmonologists and review of the literature. Respiration 2005; 72(3): 285-95. [http://dx.doi.org/10.1159/000085370] [PMID: 15942298]

[48] Douketis JD, Spyropoulos AC, Spencer FA, *et al.* Perioperative management of antithrombotic therapy: Antithrombotic Therapy and Prevention of Thrombosis. American College of Chest Physicians Evidence-Based Clinical Practice Guidelines Chest. 9th ed. 2012; 141: pp. (2 Suppl)e326S-50S.

[49] Herth FJ, Becker HD, Ernst A. Aspirin does not increase bleeding complications after transbronchial biopsy. Chest 2002; 122(4): 1461-4. [http://dx.doi.org/10.1378/chest.122.4.1461] [PMID: 12377879]

[50] Ernst A, Eberhardt R, Wahidi M, Becker HD, Herth FJ. Effect of routine clopidogrel use on bleeding complications after transbronchial biopsy in humans. Chest 2006; 129(3): 734-7. [http://dx.doi.org/10.1378/chest.129.3.734] [PMID: 16537875]

[51] Lam B, Wong MP, Ooi C, *et al.* Diagnostic yield of bronchoscopic sampling methods in bronchial carcinoma. Respirology 2000; 5(3): 265-70. [http://dx.doi.org/10.1046/j.1440-1843.2000.00258.x] [PMID: 11022989]

[52] Lee HS, Kwon SY, Kim DK, *et al.* Bronchial washing yield before and after forceps biopsy in patients with endoscopically visible lung cancers. Respirology 2007; 12(2): 277-82. [http://dx.doi.org/10.1111/j.1440-1843.2006.01001.x] [PMID: 17298463]

[53] Karahalli E, Yilmaz A, Türker H, Ozvaran K. Usefulness of various diagnostic techniques during fiberoptic bronchoscopy for endoscopically visible lung cancer: should cytologic examinations be performed routinely? Respiration 2001; 68(6): 611-4. [http://dx.doi.org/10.1159/000050581] [PMID: 11786717]

[54] van der Drift MA, van der Wilt GJ, Thunnissen FB, Janssen JP. A prospective study of the timing and cost-effectiveness of bronchial washing during bronchoscopy for pulmonary malignant tumors. Chest 2005; 128(1): 394-400. [http://dx.doi.org/10.1378/chest.128.1.394] [PMID: 16002962]

[55] Meyer KC, Raghu G, Baughman RP, *et al.* American Thoracic Society Committee on BAL in Interstitial Lung Disease. An official American Thoracic Society clinical practice guideline: the clinical utility of bronchoalveolar lavage cellular analysis in interstitial lung disease. Am J Respir Crit Care Med 2012; 185(9): 1004-14. [http://dx.doi.org/10.1164/rccm.201202-0320ST] [PMID: 22550210]

[56] Kelly CA, Kotre CJ, Ward C, Hendrick DJ, Walters EH. Anatomical distribution of bronchoalveolar lavage fluid as assessed by digital subtraction radiography. Thorax 1987; 42(8): 624-8. [http://dx.doi.org/10.1136/thx.42.8.624] [PMID: 3310313]

[57] Hunninghake GW, Gadek JE, Kawanami O, Ferrans VJ, Crystal RG. Inflammatory and immune processes in the human lung in health and disease: evaluation by bronchoalveolar lavage. Am J Pathol 1979; 97(1): 149-206. [PMID: 495693]

[58] The BAL Cooperative Group Steering Committee. Bronchoalveolar lavage constituents in healthy individuals, idiopathic pulmonary fibrosis, and selected comparison groups. Am Rev Respir Dis 1990; 141(5 Pt 2): S169-202. [PMID: 2186681]

[59] Hohenadel IA, Kiworr M, Genitsariotis R, Zeidler D, Lorenz J. Role of bronchoalveolar lavage in immunocompromised patients with pneumonia treated with a broad spectrum antibiotic and antifungal regimen. Thorax 2001; 56(2): 115-20. [http://dx.doi.org/10.1136/thorax.56.2.115] [PMID: 11209099]

[60] Ensminger SA, Prakash UB. Is bronchoscopic lung biopsy helpful in the management of patients with diffuse lung disease? Eur Respir J 2006; 28(6): 1081-4. [http://dx.doi.org/10.1183/09031936.06.00013106] [PMID: 16899488]

[61] Cazzadori A, Di Perri G, Todeschini G, *et al.* Transbronchial biopsy in the diagnosis of pulmonary infiltrates in immunocompromised patients. Chest 1995; 107(1): 101-6. [http://dx.doi.org/10.1378/chest.107.1.101] [PMID: 7813258]

[62] Jain P, Sandur S, Meli Y, Arroliga AC, Stoller JK, Mehta AC. Role of flexible bronchoscopy in immunocompromised patients with lung infiltrates. Chest 2004; 125(2): 712-22. [http://dx.doi.org/10.1378/chest.125.2.712] [PMID: 14769756]

[63] Descombes E, Gardiol D, Leuenberger P. Transbronchial lung biopsy: an analysis of 530 cases with reference to the number of samples. Monaldi Arch Chest Dis 1997; 52(4): 324-9. [PMID: 9401359]

[64] Smith LS, Seaquist M, Schillaci RF. Comparison of forceps used for transbronchial lung biopsy. Bigger may not be better. Chest 1985; 87(5): 574-6. [http://dx.doi.org/10.1378/chest.87.5.574] [PMID: 3987369]

[65] Puar HS, Young RC Jr, Armstrong EM. Bronchial and transbronchial lung biopsy without fluoroscopy in sarcoidosis. Chest 1985; 87(3): 303-6. [http://dx.doi.org/10.1378/chest.87.3.303] [PMID: 3971752]

[66] Papin TA, Grum CM, Weg JG. Transbronchial biopsy during mechanical ventilation. Chest 1986; 89(2): 168-70. [http://dx.doi.org/10.1378/chest.89.2.168] [PMID: 3943376]

[67] O'Brien JD, Ettinger NA, Shevlin D, Kollef MH. Safety and yield of transbronchial biopsy in mechanically ventilated patients. Crit Care Med 1997; 25(3): 440-6. [http://dx.doi.org/10.1097/00003246-199703000-00012] [PMID: 9118660]

[68] Cordasco EM Jr, Mehta AC, Ahmad M. Bronchoscopically induced bleeding. A summary of nine years' Cleveland clinic experience and review of the literature. Chest 1991; 100(4): 1141-7. [http://dx.doi.org/10.1378/chest.100.4.1141] [PMID: 1914575]

[69] Schulman LL, Smith CR, Drusin R, Rose EA, Enson Y, Reemtsma K. Utility of airway endoscopy in the diagnosis of respiratory complications of cardiac transplantation. Chest 1988; 93(5): 960-7. [http://dx.doi.org/10.1378/chest.93.5.960] [PMID: 3282824]

[70] Diaz-Guzman E, Vadi S, Minai OA, Gildea TR, Mehta AC. Safety of diagnostic bronchoscopy in patients with pulmonary hypertension. Respiration 2009; 77(3): 292-7. [http://dx.doi.org/10.1159/000197465] [PMID: 19174601]

[71] Katis K, Inglesos E, Zachariadis E, *et al.* The role of transbronchial needle aspiration in the diagnosis of peripheral lung masses or nodules. Eur Respir J 1995; 8(6): 963-6. [PMID: 7589384]

[72] Prakash UB, Stubbs SE. The bronchoscopy survey. Some reflections. Chest 1991; 100(6): 1660-7. [http://dx.doi.org/10.1378/chest.100.6.1660] [PMID: 1959411]

[73] Yasufuku K, Pierre A, Darling G, *et al.* A prospective controlled trial of endobronchial ultrasound-guided transbronchial needle aspiration compared with mediastinoscopy for mediastinal lymph node staging of lung cancer. J Thorac Cardiovasc Surg 2011; 142(6): 1393-400 e1.

[74] Herth FJ, Eberhardt R, Vilmann P, Krasnik M, Ernst A. Real-time endobronchial ultrasound guided transbronchial needle aspiration for sampling mediastinal lymph nodes. Thorax 2006; 61(9): 795-8.

[http://dx.doi.org/10.1136/thx.2005.047829] [PMID: 16738038]

[75] Dasgupta A, Jain P, Minai OA, *et al.* Utility of transbronchial needle aspiration in the diagnosis of endobronchial lesions. Chest 1999; 115(5): 1237-41. [http://dx.doi.org/10.1378/chest.115.5.1237] [PMID: 10334133]

[76] Gildea TR, Mazzone PJ, Karnak D, Meziane M, Mehta AC. Electromagnetic navigation diagnostic bronchoscopy: a prospective study. Am J Respir Crit Care Med 2006; 174(9): 982-9. [http://dx.doi.org/10.1164/rccm.200603-344OC] [PMID: 16873767]

[77] Dasgupta A, Mehta AC, Wang KP. Transbronchial needle aspiration. Semin Respir Crit Care Med 1997; 18(6): 571-81. [http://dx.doi.org/10.1055/s-2007-1009373]

[78] Schenk DA, Bower JH, Bryan CL, *et al.* Transbronchial needle aspiration staging of bronchogenic carcinoma. Am Rev Respir Dis 1986; 134(1): 146-8. [PMID: 3014934]

[79] Hsu LH, Liu CC, Ko JS. Education and experience improve the performance of transbronchial needle aspiration: a learning curve at a cancer center. Chest 2004; 125(2): 532-40. [http://dx.doi.org/10.1378/chest.125.2.532] [PMID: 14769735]

[80] Tremblay A, Stather DR, MacEachern P, Khalil M, Field SK. A randomized controlled trial of standard vs endobronchial ultrasonography-guided transbronchial needle aspiration in patients with suspected sarcoidosis. Chest 2009; 136(2): 340-6. [http://dx.doi.org/10.1378/chest.08-2768] [PMID: 19188547]

[81] Harkin TJ, Ciotoli C, Addrizzo-Harris DJ, Naidich DP, Jagirdar J, Rom WN. Transbronchial needle aspiration (TBNA) in patients infected with HIV. Am J Respir Crit Care Med 1998; 157(6 Pt 1): 1913-8. [http://dx.doi.org/10.1164/ajrccm.157.6.9607093] [PMID: 9620927]

[82] Baran R, Tor M, Tahaoğlu K, *et al.* Intrathoracic tuberculous lymphadenopathy: clinical and bronchoscopic features in 17 adults without parenchymal lesions. Thorax 1996; 51(1): 87-9. [http://dx.doi.org/10.1136/thx.51.1.87] [PMID: 8658377]

[83] Baaklini WA, Reinoso MA, Gorin AB, Sharafkaneh A, Manian P. Diagnostic yield of fiberoptic bronchoscopy in evaluating solitary pulmonary nodules. Chest 2000; 117(4): 1049-54. [http://dx.doi.org/10.1378/chest.117.4.1049] [PMID: 10767238]

[84] Chao TY, Chien MT, Lie CH, Chung YH, Wang JL, Lin MC. Endobronchial ultrasonography-guided transbronchial needle aspiration increases the diagnostic yield of peripheral pulmonary lesions: a randomized trial. Chest 2009; 136(1): 229-36. [http://dx.doi.org/10.1378/chest.08-0577] [PMID: 18812446]

[85] Reichenberger F, Weber J, Tamm M, *et al.* The value of transbronchial needle aspiration in the diagnosis of peripheral pulmonary lesions. Chest 1999; 116(3): 704-8. [http://dx.doi.org/10.1378/chest.116.3.704] [PMID: 10492275]

[86] Harrow EM, Oldenburg FA Jr, Lingenfelter MS, Smith AM Jr. Transbronchial needle aspiration in clinical practice. A five-year experience. Chest 1989; 96(6): 1268-72. [http://dx.doi.org/10.1378/chest.96.6.1268] [PMID: 2582832]

CHAPTER 2

Rigid Bronchoscopy

Hervé Dutau*

Department of Thoracic Oncology, Pleural Diseases and Interventional Pulmonology, North University Hospital, Marseille, France

Abstract: Complex airway diseases represent a therapeutic challenge and require multidisciplinary input including the interventional pulmonologist and thoracic surgeon. Surgery, if feasible, remains the definitive modality. However, minimally invasive endobronchial techniques have resulted in symptom control and, in selected patients, long-term improvements in quality of life. These techniques are, in general, safe and well tolerated when performed by experienced operators. Endobronchial laser therapy, cryotherapy, electrocautery or argon plasma coagulation and photodynamic therapy have been used successfully.

Despite the introduction of new technologies, the rigid bronchoscope remains the method of choice for the treatment of both benign and malignant central airway obstruction. It allows rapid and safe dilation, mechanical debulking, foreign body removal and silicone stent placement. However, it has limited use if lesions are located in the upper lobes or lung periphery but significant technological advances allow for effective treatments using the flexible bronchoscope. Rigid and flexible bronchoscopes should be seen as complementary procedures and most cases will require the use of both modalities.

Keywords: Airway compression, Airway stenosis, Airway stenting, Bronchial stenosis, Bronchoscopy, Central airway obstruction, Flexible bronchoscopy, Foreign body, Interventional bronchoscopy, Interventional pulmonology, Laser, Lung cancer, Lung transplantation, Rigid bronchoscopy, Silicone stent, Tracheal stenosis.

HISTORICAL BACKGROUND

Gustav Killian first described rigid bronchoscopy for therapeutic airway indications in Freiburg (Germany) in 1895. The first reported procedure involved the removal of a pork bone from the bronchus of a farmer using a rigid esophagoscope. Killian continued to experiment with rigid tubes in both cadavers

* **Corresponding author Hervé Dutau:** Department of Thoracic Oncology, Pleural Diseases and Interventional Pulmonology, North University Hospital, Chemin des Bourrely, 13015, Marseille, France; TeL: +33 4 91 96 59 87; Fax: +33 4 91 96 59 90; E-mail: herve.dutau@mail.ap-hm.fr

and patients and, in 1898, described the successful removal of foreign bodies in three more cases. The technique was further advanced by the discovery of the anaesthetizing effect of locally applied cocaine. At the same time, on the other side of the Atlantic Ocean, Chevalier Jackson was instrumental in developing the modern rigid bronchoscope. In 1904, he developed an endoscope with a small light at the distal end. He pioneered endobronchial treatment for the complications of tuberculosis, which was the leading cause of airway disease during the first half on the twentieth century. He is also credited with the first reported endoluminal mechanical resections of endobronchial tumours. Other significant historical advances included the optical telescope by Broyles and the solid rod lens optical system by Hopkins [1]. Modern bronchoscopy benefited from the vision of Shigeto Ikeda, a Japanese pulmonologist, who developed the flexible bronchoscope using optic fibers [1], which radically transformed the diagnostic workup for lung cancer and visualization of the bronchial tree. It is less invasive, does not require a general anesthesia and provides superior visualization of smaller peripheral airways. The rigid bronchoscope was regarded as obsolete and was virtually abandoned in favor of the flexible bronchoscope. Few endoscopists were exposed to the technique and adequate training became a rarity.

However, some European physicians continued to use the rigid system for the treatment of airway diseases, including the father of modern therapeutic bronchoscopy, Jean-François Dumon, who is regarded as a pioneer in the field of interventional pulmonary medicine. He was one of the first bronchoscopists [2 - 5] to use laser therapy in the airway and standardized its utilization [6, 7]. Another major advance was the invention of a dedicated silicone stent for the trachea and bronchi [8]. Before the era of the Dumon stents, the only available option for re-establishing patency of the trachea post-operatively was the the Montgomery T-tube which required a tracheotomy for placement [9]. The combination of laser debulking of the endoluminal component and post-resection endotracheal stent placement when there is concurrent extrinsic compression allowed for immediate and lasting palliation of malignant central airway obstruction. This allowed pulmonologists to treat central airway diseases that had formerly been considered either completely untreatable or treatable only *via* extensive and often prohibitively dangerous surgical procedures.

RIGID BRONCHOSCOPY EQUIPMENT [10]

The modern rigid bronchoscope is essentially a straight, hollow stainless steel tube and has not significantly changed from the equipment developed by Chevalier Jackson. It is available in various lengths and diameters ranging from 5 mm to 13.5 mm. The barrel wall is 2–3 mm thick and the internal diameter is uniform throughout. The distal end of most bronchoscopes is beveled, allowing atraumatic passage through the vocal cords. The bevel can also be used to "core out" an endobronchial tumor and to "corkscrew" the bronchoscope through tight stenosis [10, 11]. Slits in the distal wall of the bronchoscope allow contralateral ventilation during intubation of a main bronchus. The tracheoscope is shorter in length compared with the bronchoscope and has no ventilation slits. The proximal end of the bronchoscope consists of a central opening and various side ports for connection of jet ventilation or conventional ventilation devices as well as a source of illumination. The Efer–Dumon rigid bronchoscope (Fig. **1**), manufactured by EFER Endoscopy (La Ciotat, France) and the Dutau-Novatech rigid bronchoscope (Fig. **2**), manufactured by Novatech SA (La Ciotat, France), have a universal proximal head that can be connected to all the bronchoscope barrels. In addition, the various sized barrels are color-coded. Other manufacturers of rigid bronchoscopy equipment include the TEXAS Rigid Integrated Bronchoscope (Fig. **3**) from Richard Wolf (Knittlingen, Germany) and Karl Storz (Tuttlingen, Germany) (Fig. **4**). Illumination in modern rigid bronchoscopes is provided by a xenon light source with a prismatic light deflector that is attached proximally to allow full use of the bronchoscope lumen. A Hopkins rod rigid telescope is passed through the central opening of the bronchoscope barrel. The bronchoscopist can either look down the eyepiece of the telescope, or a charge-coupled chip video camera can be connected to the eyepiece for visualization on a monitor. This also allows the physician to record procedures. Before the development of the flexible bronchoscope, angled telescopes were needed in order to view all bronchial subdivisions but currently most endoscopists would prefer to pass a flexible bronchoscope *via* the barrel of the rigid bronchoscope for this purpose. The Texas rigid bronchoscope is the first fully integrated rigid bronchoscope with a semiflexible endoscope inside. The benefit of the Texas system is the full inner lumen of the rigid bronchoscope. The semiflexible endoscope is attachable to a separate channel inside the tube.

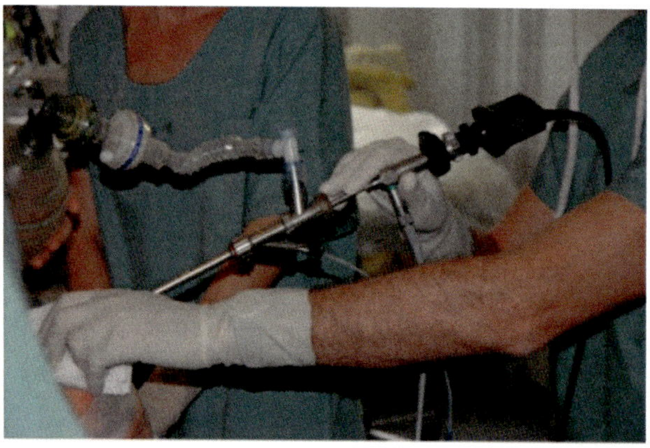

Fig. (1). The EFER-Dumon rigid bronchoscope.

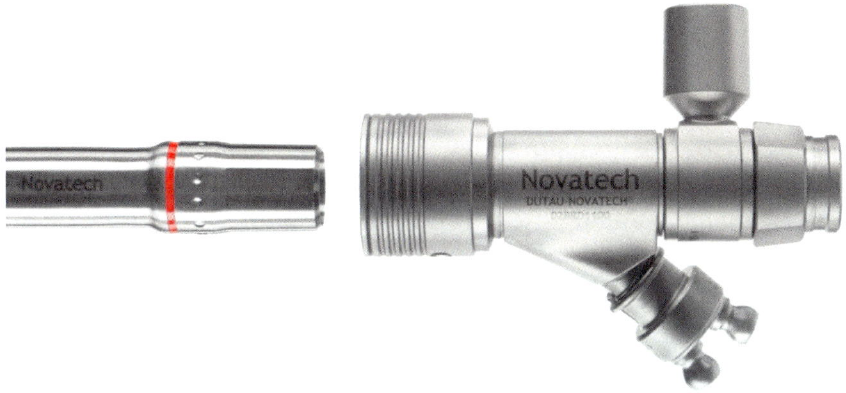

Fig. (2). The Dutau-Novatech rigid bronchoscope.

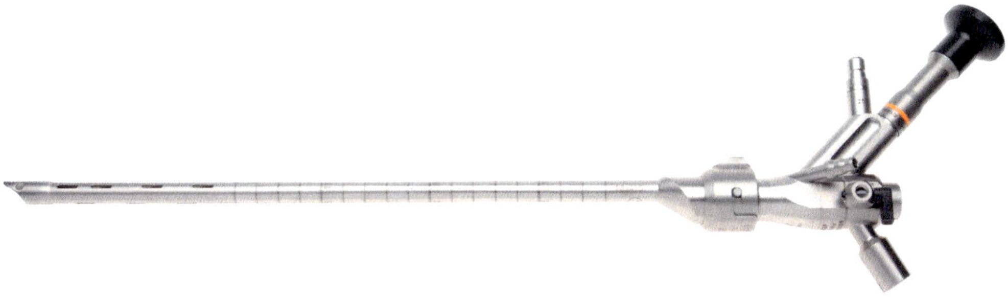

Fig. (3). The STORZ rigid bronchoscope.

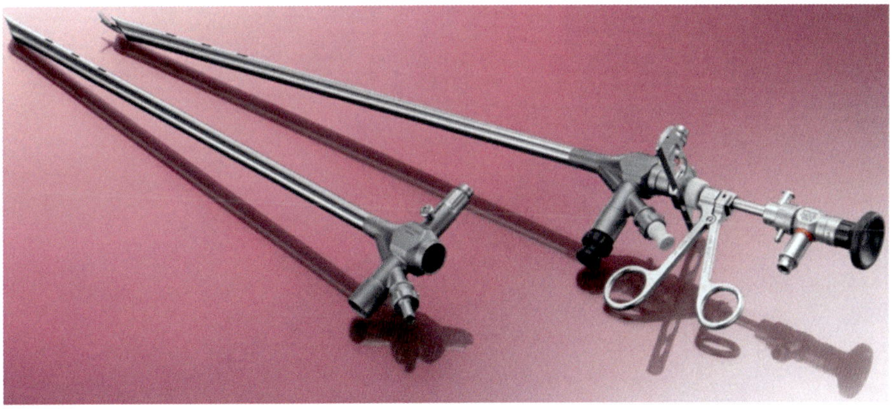

Fig. (4). The Texas rigid bronchoscope.

Various accessory instruments including forceps, suction catheters, laser fibers and stent delivery systems are used during rigid bronchoscopy by passage *via* the proximal opening.

RIGID BRONCHOSCOPY TECHNIQUE [10]

After induction of anesthesia, the patient's head is partially extended and the bronchoscope is introduced in the midline with the bevel anteriorly (Fig. **5**). Care should be taken to avoid trauma to the patient's upper teeth during intubation by protection with the bronchoscopist's finger or the use of a protective guard. The bronchoscope is advanced under the epiglottis and rotated 90° to allow atraumatic passage through the vocal cords. Once the trachea is entered, the bronchoscope is rotated back 90° and advanced to the lower trachea. To enter one side of the bronchial tree, the patient's head is rotated towards the contralateral shoulder. When using the tracheoscope, thinner diameter bronchoscope barrels can be inserted through the lumen of the tracheoscope. There is therefore no need to remove the latter or to reintubate the patient. A flexible bronchoscope can also be passed through the lumen of the rigid bronchoscope to allow inspection of distal airways. In addition, the flexible scope is essential for airway toileting and specimen collection. The use of both bronchoscopes is often used by interventional pulmonologists during therapeutic bronchoscopy. An alternative technique of intubation involves the use of a laryngoscope to lift the epiglottis anteriorly and guide the passage of the bronchoscope to the level of the vocal cords.

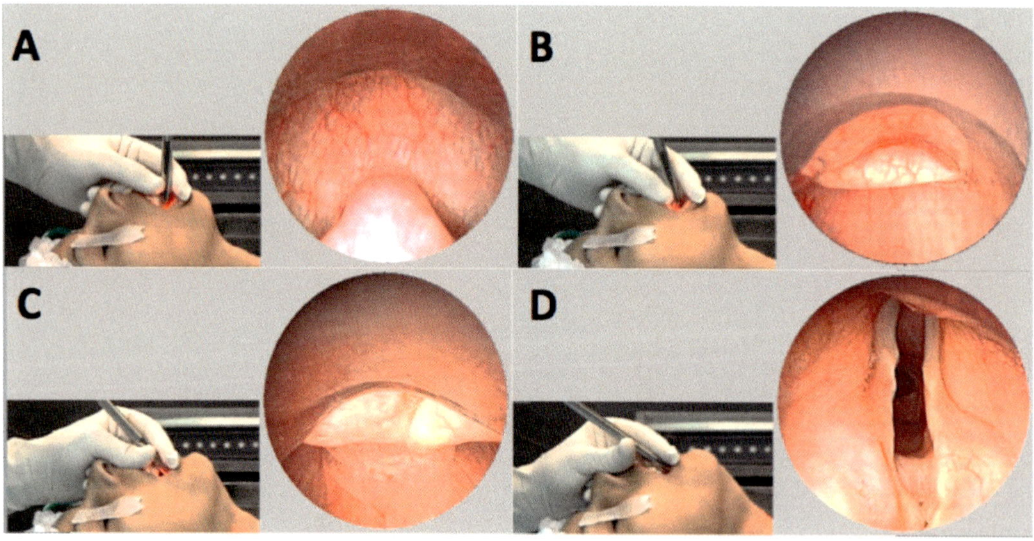

Fig. (5). Rigid bronchoscopy intubation landmarks: **A**: Uvula; **B**: Epiglottis; **C**: Aryhthenoïds; **D**: Vocal cords.

RIGID BRONCHOSCOPY INDICATIONS

The rigid bronchoscope is an invaluable tool in interventional bronchoscopy [12 - 14]. It allows, with maximal safety and under general anesthesia, adequate ventilation of the patient through a side port, efficient suctioning of blood, secretions, pus and smoke *via* large suction catheters, and the use of accessory instruments (laser probes, cryoprobes, rigid forceps, *etc.*) [10].

It also allows therapeutic interventions such as dilation of stenoses or extrinsic compression, and mechanical coring and debulking of endoluminal tumors using the distal sharp bevel to rapidly recanalize the airway [15]. In addition, a foreign body can safely be removed using the rigid forceps. The rigid bronchoscope is the instrument of choice in case of acute respiratory failure secondary to endoluminal obstruction as it allows for a rapid procedure, while maintaining airway patency and adequate ventilation. Due to obvious anatomical limitations, however, its use is not suitable for upper lobe disease. A rigid bronchoscope is required for silicone stent placement using a dedicated rigid loading system.

Treatment of central airway obstruction with a flexible bronchoscope alone is not generally recommended, particularly in the case of tracheal lesions. Its small working channel may not be sufficient to prevent airway flooding in case of massive bleeding. Biopsy forceps have a small diameter and can only sample small tumor fragments, leading to long and fastidious procedures [1]. In an attempt to overcome this, metallic snares or baskets have been developed, in` order to remove larger pieces of tumors or foreign bodies [10]. Rigid and flexible bronchoscopy remain complementary techniques, and most pulmonologists will use both instruments concurrently during interventions. Flexible bronchoscopy is an important tool with easy maneuverability that allows exploration and clearing of the peripheral airways. In addition, flexible bronchoscopy is the only tool available for the treatment of upper lobe obstruction. A variety of tools (laser, thermocoagulation, argon plasma coagulation and cryoprobes) can be introduced in its working channel.

Foreign Bodies (FB) [16]

The use of rigid bronchoscopy *versus* flexible bronchoscopy has been widely debated in the literature [17, 18]. The rigid bronchoscope provides excellent access to the subglottic airways and passage of the rigid grasping forceps. Optical forceps allow direct visualization of the FB and optically guided grasping. Alternatively, a rigid telescope and a forceps can be used coaxially through the bronchoscope (Fig. **6**). During the extraction procedure, it is crucial not to push the FB distally with the bronchoscope, the forceps, or the suction catheter. If blood and secretions are present proximally to the FB, these should be cleared by careful suctioning. The optical forceps is then advanced in the bronchial axis, a few millimeters proximal to the FB. For smooth and rounded FBs, the key is to grip the largest volume of the FB. In this setting, the smooth forceps (foreign body forceps) are preferred to the sharp alligator forceps. The forceps' cups are opened maximally and the forceps is advanced under visual control using great care not to push the FB downwards. The FB is then gently but securely gripped. Both forceps and FB are pulled up, a few millimeters distal to the tip of the bronchoscope, and then the instruments and FB are withdrawn en bloc from the trachea. Alligator forceps are used for grasping sharp or irregular FBs. In case of large, hard FBs, such as pistachio shells, breaking the FB into two or three fragments may help extraction. In contrast, vigorous grasping of friable FBs, such as peanuts, should be avoided, since it may result in maceration and distal wedging of small fragments. Heavy FBs, such as metallic FBs, tend to move distally due to gravity; in this setting, it may be helpful to place the patient in the Trendelenburg position. During the last step of extraction, the FB can be lost accidentally, either because it is blocked in the narrow glottic area, or because there was some inappropriate coaxial movement between the bronchoscope and the forceps, causing the tip of the bronchoscope to push the FB out of the forceps' cups or jaws. If this occurs, the operator should first carefully inspect the oral cavity and the larynx with the laryngoscope and grasp the FB with a Magill forceps, if possible, prior to reintubating the trachea with the bronchoscope. Once the FB is removed, the trachea is reintubated with the rigid bronchoscope and the airways are carefully re-examined, ideally with a fiberoptic bronchoscope passed through the rigid tube, to rule out another FB or residual fragments [19].

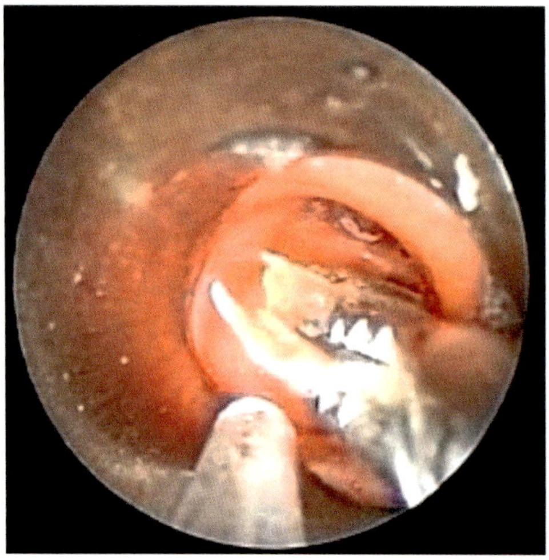

Fig. (6). Foreign body removal using the rigid bronchoscope.

Silicone Stent Placement

The main purpose of stents designed for use in the central airways (trachea, mainstem bronchi and, in select cases, lobar bronchi) is to restore patency of the airway to as close a normal caliber as possible. Any endoluminal pathology responsible for debilitating symptoms such as dyspnea and associated with a significant reduction in airway luminal diameter (greater than 50%) may be an indication for a silicone airway stent [20, 21].

Five major indications have been established [20]:

1. Extrinsic compression from tumours or lymph nodes,
2. Stabilization of airway patency after endoscopic removal of intraluminally growing cancer,
3. Treatment of benign strictures,
4. Stabilization of collapsing airways (malacia and polychondritis),
5. Treatment of fistulas (*e.g.* stump dehiscences or tracheoesophageal fistulas)

Endoluminally growing tumours should be treated initially by laser resection, for example, and then a stent should be placed if it is still necessary. Treating benign lesions requires particular caution, as stents may cause more harm in the long run, even if early benefit is often noted [21]. In general, only removable stents should be used for these indications until a multidisciplinary team has determined inoperability [21].

Airway stents are generally divided in two types: the silicone stents and the metallic stents [21]. The Dumon stent (Tracheobronxane®, Novatech, La Ciotat, France) remains the reference standard as it is the most commonly placed stent worldwide. This airway stent has a simple design consisting of a silicone tube with small studs on the external surface to reduce the risk of migration [8]. They have become, de facto, the gold standard for the treatment of benign and malignant stenoses over the past 10 years [21]. There are 2 specific designs: straight and Y-shaped (for disease involving the carina) [22]. Stents are available in various lengths and diameters to accommodate both pediatric [23] and adult anatomy. For irregularly-shaped stenoses, *i.e.* those with marked reduced central airway caliber as compared to the extremities, specialized hourglass-shaped stents are available [24]. These hourglass-shaped stents are particularly useful in cases of short benign tracheal disease. Ideally, Dumon stents have to be inserted through a dedicated rigid bronchoscope (Fig. **7**). The commercialized introducer set includes a loading tool and a pusher. A Dumon stent can be repositioned, removed and replaced at any time with ease using standard grasping rigid forceps.

Malignant Airway Stenosis

Bronchial obstruction is frequently encountered during the course of bronchial carcinoma: more than 30% of bronchial carcinomas present with central airway obstruction [25].

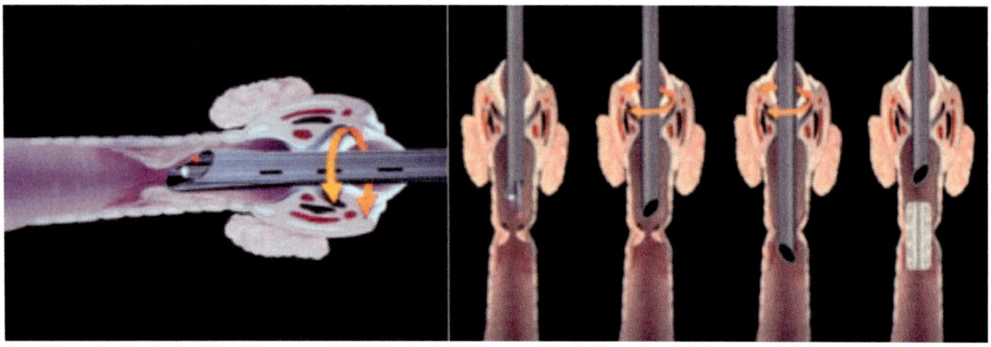

Fig. (7). Silicone stent placement with the rigid bronchoscope.

Such obstructions may lead to specific complications, including reduced survival and decreased quality of life [26]. However, the vast majority of patients still die from general complications caused by their primary intrathoracic disease or extrathoracic extension, and only about 35% from local complications: severe hemoptysis, lung infections or asphyxia [26]. Given that oncologic treatments do not generally result in prompt improvement in patients' symptoms [27, 28], endoscopic treatments are necessary adjuncts to the tailored management of patients at all stages of the disease (neoadjuvant, adjuvant and palliative). In addition, bronchial obstruction-related complications (atelectasis, respiratory insufficiency or distress, repeated infections) are likely to interfere with optimal oncologic treatments, such as chemotherapy or radiotherapy. Malignant airway obstruction is often classified based on the type of airway involvement [29]. Airway involvement can be intrinsic, limited to endoluminal involvement, an extrinsic compression or a mixed condition with both tumor within the airway (*i.e.* intrinsic), and external compression of the airway (*i.e.* extrinsic) [14, 29]. In summary [14, 29], purely intrinsic involvement can often be managed with debulking techniques to remove the endoluminal tumor. The rigid bronchoscope is then the instrument of choice. Three steps can be described. The first one is coagulation and devascularization of the tumor, the second is mechanical coring, and the third is coagulation of the tumoral base (Fig. **8**). This technique is called laser (or electrocautery, or argon plasma) assisted mechanical debulking. On occasions, a stent may be placed as a bridge to chemo-radiotherapy or alternatively may be considered as a permanent solution when the risk of local recurrence is high. Extrinsic compression without intra-luminal disease is readily treated with dilation followed by stenting. Mixed (intrinsic and extrinsic) obstruction is usually managed with both debulking and stent insertion. Usually, benefits noted after successful bronchoscopic treatment of obstruction last for 2 to 3 months [30]. Benefit duration after stent placement is generally reported to be around 4 months before tumoral stent overgrowth [31], but this duration can be increased with the use of effective oncologic treatments (*i.e.* chemo- and/or radiotherapy) [32].

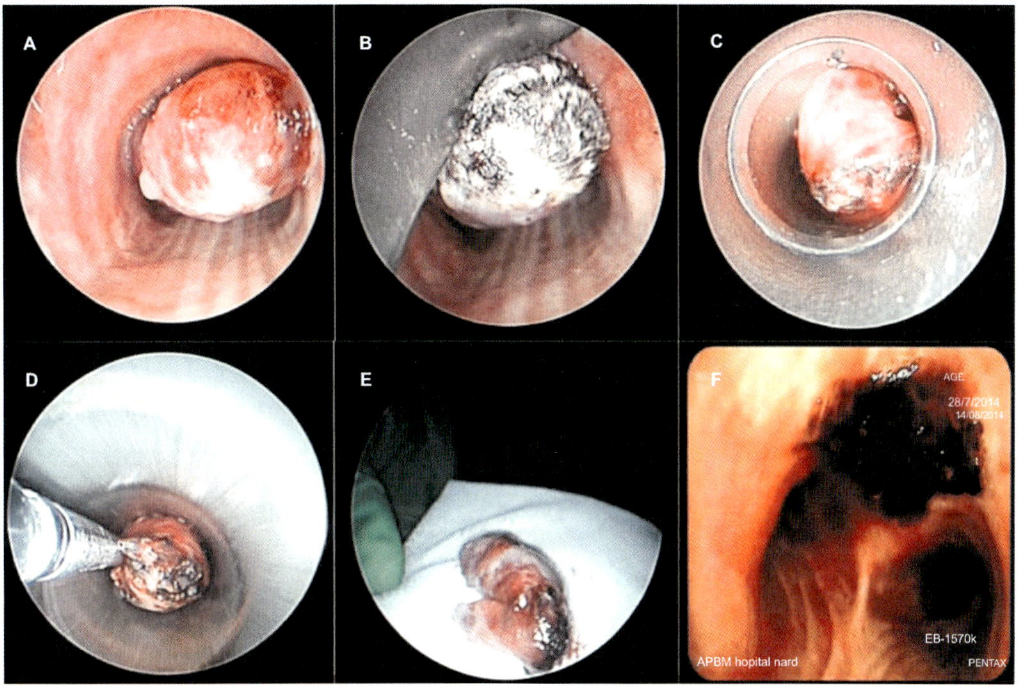

Fig. (8). The various stages of laser assisted mechanical debulking: **A**: A tumor obstructing the trachea ; **B**: Coagulation of the lesion with laser; **C**: Mechanical resection using the bevel of the rigid bronchoscope; **D** and **E**: removal of a large piece of tumor with a rigid forceps, **F**: carbonisation of the tumour base with laser.

Other indications for endobronchial treatment include endobronchial metastases (*e.g.* esophageal, thyroid, renal cell carcinoma, colon and melanoma) or alternatively low grade primary tumors (*e.g.* adenoid cystic carcinomas, typical or atypical carcinoids).

Benign Airway Stenosis

Post Intubation or Post-Tracheostomy Tracheal Stenosis (PITTS)

Despite the decreasing incidence of post-intubation or post-tracheostomy tracheal stenosis (PITTS), management of such conditions remains challenging. Indeed, even if surgical repair (sleeve resection) is the best definitive solution, approximately 50% of patients present with acute respiratory distress prompting emergent less invasive endoscopic treatments as a bridge to surgery or as definitive treatment in cases with contra-indications to surgery [33]. Moreover, tracheal stenosis can recur after tracheal sleeve resection.

One can divide PITTS into two different types: the web-like PITTS (disease of the tracheal mucosa sparing the cartilaginous rings) and the complex PITTS (involving deterioration of the cartilaginous support) [34]. The web-like PITTS is generally successfully treated by radial mucosal incisions followed by mechanical dilation [35]. The success rate is close to 90%, after one to three sessions [36]. For the complex PITTS, mechanical dilation alone is most of the time not sufficient [34]. In case of surgical contra-indication, the next step would be the placement of a stent in order to maintain the long term patency of the tracheal lumen and prevent recurrence [34].

The choice of stent is important. Self-expandable metallic stents (SEMS) have shown to make potentially operable PITTS inoperable because of the severe complications associated with the technique [37]. These prompted the FDA to publish recommendations to limit the use of SEMS in benign tracheal stenosis [38]. Silicone stents are more suitable because of their easy removal and are not likely to jeopardize a future surgery. Long-term results (no recurrence after stent removal at one year) vary from 40% when the stent is placed for 6 months up to 70% when the stent remains in place for 18 months [34, 36, 39, 40]. One should also take into account the fact that silicone stents require surveillance and may present complications like migrations, granulations, and/or mucus obstructions that can affect the quality of life of the patient [41]. Migration is probably the most challenging complication in this indication, with an incidence ranging from 11 to 17.5% [33], especially when the stenosis is close to the vocal cords. This can be reduced by the use of a dedicated hour-glass silicone stent [24] or by external fixation [42, 43]. Endoscopic techniques represent, in about 50% of cases, a very efficient treatment for PITTS, but many questions remain regarding its long term efficacy and its impact on the quality of life when compared to surgery.

Bronchial Stenosis Following Lung Transplantation (LT)

Improvement in surgical techniques, immunosuppressive regimen and post-operative care have resulted in markedly improved clinical outcomes, as airway complication rates have decreased, presently ranging from 5 to 30% with an associated mortality rate of 2-3% [44 - 49].

Several endoscopic interventions may allow effective management of LT-related airway complications. Such procedures include cryotherapy, laser photoresection, balloon bronchoplasty, electrocautery, brachytherapy, airway dilation using rigid bronchoscope and stent placement [50]. Stent placement is usually considered for bronchomalacia, bronchial stenosis, combined stenosis and malacia, or bronchial dehiscence when these conditions are responsible for respiratory symptoms, persistent decline in lung function or post-obstructive complications such as mucus retention and/or infection. Although many studies have previously described management of LT-related airway complications with SEMS, little data are available with regard to the use of silicone stents for this indication. Stent placement can result in mucosal ischemia, and re-stenosis is a common finding. While the overall results (survival and clinical outcome) favour stent placement, a high rate of stent-related problems such as scarring, mucus plugging, bacterial colonisation and migration have to be accepted with currently available stents. It is advisable to select a stent that can be removed if necessary without causing further tissue damage. Recently, our group has published a retrospective study on Dumon stent placement in anastomotic stenosis after lung transplantation [51]. These stents could be removed definitively in 70% of the patients without further recurrence [51].

ANESTHESIA

Rigid bronchoscopy brings together a unique set of conditions that result in a significant challenge for the anesthetist and endoscopist alike. This includes the necessity of both specialties to share the same airway during the procedure. In addition, the airway is often significantly compromised by the underlying disease. Finally, most patients will be of advanced age and have multiple pulmonary and non-pulmonary comorbidities which will complicate the management of the case.

Ideally, all cases should be assessed pre-operatively to address any reversible conditions which may adversely affect the outcome of the procedure. This assessment should address the cardiovascular and pulmonary system. All imaging should be reviewed to document the location of the obstruction and assess how this will interfere with ventilation. Finally, performing routine blood tests including coagulation and arterial gases may be beneficial. Unfortunately, most patients present as emergent cases, and there is therefore no time to perform an in-depth pre-operative assessment.

In the setting of rigid bronchoscopy, general anesthesia is required and various techniques have been employed. This includes spontaneous ventilation with manual assistance, jet ventilation, inhalation ventilation and mechanical ventilation. In the case of an obstructed airway, jet ventilation carries an increased risk for barotrauma if expiration is obstructed. To address this potential complication, the Richard Wolf Company has developed the Hemer rigid bronchoscope with a measuring tube connected to the bronchoscope lumen allowing measurement of inspiratory and expiratory pressures, as well as oxygen and carbon dioxide concentrations. Generally, anesthesia is induced using a combination of a benzodiazepine, such as midazolam, and an opiate, such as remifentanil. Anesthesia is maintained using different techniques, frequently chosen based on the experience of the anesthetist. These include target-controlled infusion devices, simple infusion devices and "top up" according to the desired level of sedation. There is insufficient evidence to recommend one technique over another and the choice of anesthetic agent and mode of ventilation is often made after discussion between the anesthetists and endoscopists at individual centers. Irrespective of the technique employed, it is imperative that members of the team have a good working relationship, as both the anesthetist and endoscopists need to work in unison during the procedure [52, 53].

RIGID BRONCHOSCOPY COMPLICATIONS

Despite the multitude of indications and procedures: Sex, age, and the aim of the procedure are not associated with complications [54].

Unlike flexible bronchoscopy, rigid bronchoscopy is performed in the operating room under general anesthesia. Performing rigid bronchoscopy under general anesthesia adds the potential complication of operator and anesthesiologist sharing the airway but also adds a degree of safety by allowing the operator to focus on airway intervention, while the anesthesiologist prevents and manages mechanical and systemic complications as they arise [54, 55]. Here the anesthesiologists, with the bronchoscope operator, need to navigate the multiple approaches to airway management, such as apneic oxygenation, spontaneous ventilation (assisted or otherwise), controlled mechanical ventilation, high frequency, and manual jet ventilation [56]. The type and rate of complications of rigid bronchoscopy are similar to those of flexible bronchoscopy and can likewise be divided into mechanical and systemic complications. Complications in either category can potentially result in death.

The most common mechanical complications of rigid bronchoscopy are trauma to the teeth, lips, oropharynx, vocal cords or other glottic structures, laryngospasm, mucosal tear, pneumothorax, and hemorrhage, and death [54, 57 - 59]. Systemic complications include vasovagal syncope, hypoxemia, hypercapnia, medication effects of general anesthesia, arrhythmia, post-procedural respiratory failure, and death [54, 56-61].

Relatively few prospective studies provide quantifiable complication rates during and after rigid bronchoscopy, so the true rate of complications resulting from the procedure is difficult to pinpoint and will vary by operator experience and institution. However, advances in equipment, monitoring, and anesthetic drugs have increased the overall margin of safety for rigid bronchoscopy. One retrospective study reviewed 775 cases of rigid bronchoscopy in a university hospital between 1992 and 1999 and found that 86.7% of cases occurred without any of the above listed complications [54]. In this study 103/775 (13.3%) of cases had complications, which included bleeding (6.6%), respiratory failure (5.3%), cough (0.6%), death (0.4%), and arrhythmia (0.3%). A lesion at or near the carina had the highest correlation with procedural complications [54]. Furthermore, rigid bronchoscopy seems to be safe to use in neurosurgery patients with space-occupying lesions [60].

Another notable retrospective study compared the complication rate of flexible bronchoscopy under topical anesthesia with the complication rate of rigid bronchoscopy under general anesthesia [58]. Lukomsky *et al.*, reviewed 3,449 rigid bronchoscopy procedures and complications associated with rigid bronchoscopy occurred in 173 of 3,449 cases (5%); four rigid bronchoscope cases were complicated by pneumothorax and six cases were complicated by death (four due to hypoxia) resulting in a fatality rate of 0.17% [58].

RIGID BRONCHOSCOPY TRAINING AND COMPETENCY

The American College of Chest Physicians (ACCP), American Thoracic Society (ATS) and European Respiratory Society (ERS) have recommended a minimum number of 20 rigid bronchoscopy procedures for initial competency [12, 13]. This number is solely based on expert-opinion, as opposed to discernible scientific evidence. Recent guidelines from ACCP have acknowledged this limitation [62]. Multiple studies have shown that trainees can show significant variation in the rate at which they acquire procedural skills, leading to operators with differing skill levels at these recommended "threshold" numbers, hence concluding that performance-based metrics be incorporated into the process of competency assessment [63, 64].

In order to address the need for competency-based assessment of rigid bronchoscopy, an objective, 23- point, checklist-based instrument, the Rigid-bronchoscopy Tool for Assessment of Skills and Competence (RIGID-TASC) has been developed recently [65]. This instrument assesses the basic competency of an operator in performing rigid bronchoscopic intubation and central airway navigation.

CONCLUSION [66]

The rigid bronchoscope is the instrument of choice in the vast majority of bronchoscopic therapeutic procedures. Indeed, the rigid bronchoscope is not only a tool to visualize the airway but also a therapeutic instrument in itself or in association with other endoscopic techniques. Most of the scientific associations (ERS, ATS, ACCP) agree on this point. Rigid bronchoscopy requires training and a dedicated facility or easy access to an operating room with anesthetic support.

Moreover, rigid bronchoscopy is mandatory in airway stenting when using silicone stents, which still represent the gold standard. Interventional bronchoscopy is a minimally invasive option in a variety of cases, and can occasionally represent a bridge to definitive surgical management. In case of surgical contra-indications, endoscopic techniques are acceptable definitive palliation interventions.

CONFLICT OF INTEREST

Dr Dutau: Consultant for Novatech, La Ciotat, France.

ACKNOWLEDGEMENTS

Declared none.

REFERENCES

[1] Becker HD, Marsh BR. History of the rigid bronchoscope.Interventional Bronchoscopy Basel, Karger, Prog Respir Res. 2000; 30: pp. 2-15.

[2] Toty L, Personne C, Colchen A, Vourc'h G. Bronchoscopic management of tracheal lesions using the YAG laser. Thorax 1981; 36: 175-8. [http://dx.doi.org/10.1136/thx.36.3.175] [PMID: 7197061]

[3] Dumon JF, Reboud E, Garbe L, Aucomte F, Meric B. Treatment of tracheobronchial lesions by laser photoresection. Chest 1982; 81(3): 278-84. [http://dx.doi.org/10.1378/chest.81.3.278] [PMID: 7056101]

[4] Unger M. Bronchoscopic utilization of the Nd:YAG laser for obstructing lesions of the trachea and bronchi. Surg Clin North Am 1984; 64(5): 931-8. [http://dx.doi.org/10.1016/S0039-6109(16)43435-3] [PMID: 6208622]

[5] Kvale PA, Eichenhorn MS, Radke JR, Miks V. YAG laser photoresection of lesions obstructing the central airways. Chest 1985; 87(3): 283-8. [http://dx.doi.org/10.1378/chest.87.3.283] [PMID: 3971751]

[6] Dumon JF, Meric B, Bourcereau J, *et al.* Principles for safety in application of Nd: YAG laser in bronchology. Chest 1984; 86: 278-84. [http://dx.doi.org/10.1378/chest.86.2.163]

[7] Dumon JF, Shapshay S, Bourcereau J, *et al.* Principles for safety in application of neodymium-YAG laser in bronchology. Chest 1984; 86(2): 163-8. [http://dx.doi.org/10.1378/chest.86.2.163] [PMID: 6547662]

[8] Dumon JF. A dedicated tracheobronchial stent. Chest 1990; 97(2): 328-32. [http://dx.doi.org/10.1378/chest.97.2.328] [PMID: 1688757]

[9] Montgomery WW. Silicone tracheal cannula. Ann Otol Rhinol Laryngol 1980; 89(6 Pt 1): 521-8. [http://dx.doi.org/10.1177/000348948008900607] [PMID: 7458139]

[10] Plekker D, Koegelenberg CF, Bolliger CT. Different techniques of bronchoscopy. Eur Respir Mon 2010; 48: 1-17.

[11] Ayers ML, Beamis JF Jr. Rigid bronchoscopy in the twenty-first century. Clin Chest Med 2001; 22(2): 355-64. [http://dx.doi.org/10.1016/S0272-5231(05)70049-6] [PMID: 11444118]

[12] Bolliger CT, Mathur PN, Beamis JF, *et al.* European Respiratory Society/American Thoracic Society. ERS/ATS statement on interventional pulmonology. Eur Respir J 2002; 19(2): 356-73. [http://dx.doi.org/10.1183/09031936.02.00204602] [PMID: 11866017]

[13] Ernst A, Silvestri GA, Johnstone D. American College of Chest Physicians. Interventional pulmonary procedures. Chest 2003; 123(5): 1693-717. [http://dx.doi.org/10.1378/chest.123.5.1693] [PMID: 12740291]

[14] Ernst A, Feller-Kopman D, Becker HD, Mehta AC. Central airway obstruction. Am J Respir Crit Care Med 2004; 169(12): 1278-97. [http://dx.doi.org/10.1164/rccm.200210-1181SO] [PMID: 15187010]

[15] Seijo LM, Sterman DH. Interventional pulmonology. N Engl J Med 2001; 344(10): 740-9. [http://dx.doi.org/10.1056/NEJM200103083441007] [PMID: 11236779]

[16] Delage A, Marquette CH. Airway foreign bodies: clinical presentation, diagnosis and treatment. Eur Respir Mon 2010; 48: 135-48.

[17] Martinot A, Closset M, Marquette CH, *et al.* Indications for flexible *versus* rigid bronchoscopy in children with suspected foreign-body aspiration. Am J Respir Crit Care Med 1997; 155(5): 1676-9. [http://dx.doi.org/10.1164/ajrccm.155.5.9154875] [PMID: 9154875]

[18] Prakash UB, Midthun DE, Edell ES. Indications for flexible *versus* rigid bronchoscopy in children with suspected foreign-body aspiration. Am J Respir Crit Care Med 1997; 156(3 Pt 1): 1017-9. [PMID: 9310030]

[19] Kim IG, Brummitt WM, Humphry A, Siomra SW, Wallace WB. Foreign body in the airway: A review of 202 cases. Laryngoscope 1973; 83(3): 347-54. [http://dx.doi.org/10.1288/00005537-197303000-00004] [PMID: 4690025]

[20] Wood DE, Liu YH, Vallières E, Karmy-Jones R, Mulligan MS. Airway stenting for malignant and benign tracheobronchial stenosis. Ann Thorac Surg 2003; 76(1): 167-72. [http://dx.doi.org/10.1016/S0003-4975(03)00033-X] [PMID: 12842534]

[21] Freitag L. Airway Stents.Interventional Pulmonology Eur Respir Mon. Strausz J, Bolliger CT. 2010; 18: pp. 190-217. [http://dx.doi.org/10.1183/1025448x.00991409]

[22] Dutau H, Toutblanc B, Lamb C, Seijo L. Use of the Dumon Y-stent in the management of malignant disease involving the carina: a retrospective review of 86 patients. Chest 2004; 126(3): 951-8. [http://dx.doi.org/10.1378/chest.126.3.951] [PMID: 15364778]

[23] Fayon M, Donato L, de Blic J, *et al.* French experience of silicone tracheobronchial stenting in children. Pediatr Pulmonol 2005; 39(1): 21-7. [http://dx.doi.org/10.1002/ppul.20136] [PMID: 15532081]

[24] Vergnon JM, Costes F, Polio JC. Efficacy and tolerance of a new silicone stent for the treatment of benign tracheal stenosis: preliminary results. Chest 2000; 118(2): 422-6. [http://dx.doi.org/10.1378/chest.118.2.422] [PMID: 10936135]

[25] Minna JD, Higgins GA, Glatstein EJ. Cancer of the lung.Cancer principles and practice of oncology. 3rd ed. Philadelphia: JB Lippincott Co 1989; pp. 591-705.

[26] Stanley KE. Prognostic factors for survival in patients with inoperable lung cancer. J Natl Cancer Inst 1980; 65(1): 25-32. [PMID: 6930515]

[27] Parrat E, Pujol JL, Gautier V, Michel FB, Godard P. Chest tumor response during lung cancer chemotherapy. Computed tomography vs fiberoptic bronchoscopy. Chest 1993; 103(5): 1495-501. [http://dx.doi.org/10.1378/chest.103.5.1495] [PMID: 8387421]

[28] Chetty KG, Moran EM, Sassoon CS, Viravathana T, Light RW. Effect of radiation therapy on bronchial obstruction due to bronchogenic carcinoma. Chest 1989; 95(3): 582-4.

[http://dx.doi.org/10.1378/chest.95.3.582] [PMID: 2920587]

[29] Vergnon JM. Les traitements endoscopiques du cancer bronchique. Rev Mal Respir 2008; 25: 3S160-6.
[http://dx.doi.org/10.1016/S0761-8425(08)82022-0]

[30] Mohsenifar Z, Jasper AC, Koerner SK. Physiologic assessment of lung function in patients undergoing laser photoresection of tracheobronchial tumors. Chest 1988; 93(1): 65-9.
[http://dx.doi.org/10.1378/chest.93.1.65] [PMID: 3335169]

[31] Vergnon J-M, Costes F, Bayon MC, Emonot A. Efficacy of tracheal and bronchial stent placement on respiratory functional tests. Chest 1995; 107(3): 741-6.
[http://dx.doi.org/10.1378/chest.107.3.741] [PMID: 7533070]

[32] Han CC, Prasetyo D, Wright GM. Endobronchial palliation using Nd:YAG laser is associated with improved survival when combined with multimodal adjuvant treatments. J Thorac Oncol 2007; 2(1): 59-64.
[http://dx.doi.org/10.1097/JTO.0b013e31802bff2d] [PMID: 17410011]

[33] Baugnée PE, Marquette CH, Ramon P, Darras J, Wurtz A. Endoscopic treatment of post-intubation tracheal stenosis. Apropos of 58 cases. Rev Mal Respir 1995; 12(6): 585-92.
[PMID: 8677352]

[34] Brichet A, Verkindre C, Dupont J, *et al.* Multidisciplinary approach to management of postintubation tracheal stenoses. Eur Respir J 1999; 13(4): 888-93.
[http://dx.doi.org/10.1034/j.1399-3003.1999.13d32.x] [PMID: 10362058]

[35] Mehta AC, Lee FY, Cordasco EM, Kirby T, Eliachar I, De Boer G. Concentric tracheal and subglottic stenosis. Management using the Nd-YAG laser for mucosal sparing followed by gentle dilatation. Chest 1993; 104(3): 673-7.
[http://dx.doi.org/10.1378/chest.104.3.673] [PMID: 8365273]

[36] Galluccio G, Lucantoni G, Battistoni P, *et al.* Interventional endoscopy in the management of benign tracheal stenoses: definitive treatment at long-term follow-up. Eur J Cardiothorac Surg 2009; 35(3): 429-33.
[http://dx.doi.org/10.1016/j.ejcts.2008.10.041] [PMID: 19084420]

[37] Gaissert HA, Grillo HC, Wright CD, Donahue DM, Wain JC, Mathisen DJ. Complication of benign tracheobronchial strictures by self-expanding metal stents. J Thorac Cardiovasc Surg 2003; 126(3): 744-7.
[http://dx.doi.org/10.1016/S0022-5223(03)00361-1] [PMID: 14502148]

[38] FDA. U.S. Food and Drug Administration. FDA Public Health Notification: Complications from metallic tracheal stents in patients with benign airway disorders. 2005. Available at: www.fda.gov/MedicalDevices/Safety/AlertsandNotices/PublicHealthNotifications/UCM062115

[39] Martinez-Ballarin JI, Diaz-Jimenez JP, Castro MJ, Moya JA. Silicone stents in the management of benign tracheobronchial stenoses. Tolerance and early results in 63 patients. Chest 1996; 109(3): 626-9.
[http://dx.doi.org/10.1378/chest.109.3.626] [PMID: 8617068]

[40] Cavaliere S, Bezzi M, Toninelli C, Foccoli P. Management of post-intubation tracheal stenoses using the endoscopic approach. Monaldi Arch Chest Dis 2007; 67(2): 73-80.
[PMID: 17695689]

[41] Bolliger CT, Probst R, Tschopp K, Solèr M, Perruchoud AP. Silicone stents in the management of inoperable tracheobronchial stenoses. Indications and limitations. Chest 1993; 104(6): 1653-9.
[http://dx.doi.org/10.1378/chest.104.6.1653] [PMID: 7504608]

[42] Miwa K, Takamori S, Hayashi A, Fukunaga M, Shirouzu K. Fixation of silicone stents in the subglottic trachea: preventing stent migration using a fixation apparatus. Ann Thorac Surg 2004; 78(6): 2188-90.

[http://dx.doi.org/10.1016/j.athoracsur.2003.10.085] [PMID: 15561074]

[43] Colt HG, Harrell J, Neuman TR, Robbins T. External fixation of subglottic tracheal stents. Chest 1994; 105(6): 1653-7. [http://dx.doi.org/10.1378/chest.105.6.1653] [PMID: 8205856]

[44] Mulligan MS. Endoscopic management of airway complications after lung transplantation. Chest Surg Clin N Am 2001; 11(4): 907-15. [PMID: 11780302]

[45] Alvarez A, Algar J, Santos F, *et al.* Airway complications after lung transplantation: A review of 151 anastomoses. Eur J Cardiothorac Surg 2001; 19(4): 381-7. [http://dx.doi.org/10.1016/S1010-7940(01)00619-4] [PMID: 11306300]

[46] Shennib H, Massard G. Airway complications in lung transplantation. Ann Thorac Surg 1994; 57(2): 506-11. [http://dx.doi.org/10.1016/0003-4975(94)91038-3] [PMID: 8311631]

[47] Colt HG, Janssen JP, Dumon JF, Noirclerc MJ. Endoscopic management of bronchial stenosis after double lung transplantation. Chest 1992; 102(1): 10-6. [http://dx.doi.org/10.1378/chest.102.1.10] [PMID: 1623735]

[48] Ruttmann E, Ulmer H, Marchese M, *et al.* Evaluation of factors damaging the bronchial wall in lung transplantation. J Heart Lung Transplant 2005; 24(3): 275-81. [http://dx.doi.org/10.1016/j.healun.2004.01.008] [PMID: 15737753]

[49] de Hoyos AL, Patterson GA, Maurer JR, Ramirez JC, Miller JD, Winton TL. Pulmonary transplantation. Early and late results. J Thorac Cardiovasc Surg 1992; 103(2): 295-306. [PMID: 1735996]

[50] Santacruz JF, Mehta AC. Airway complications and management after lung transplantation: ischemia, dehiscence, and stenosis. Proc Am Thorac Soc 2009; 6(1): 79-93. [http://dx.doi.org/10.1513/pats.200808-094GO] [PMID: 19131533]

[51] Dutau H, Cavailles A, Sakr L, *et al.* Silicone stent placement for the management of anastomotic airway complications in lung transplant recipients: a retrospective study: Short and long terms outcome. J Heart Lung Transplant 2010; 29: 658-64. [http://dx.doi.org/10.1016/j.healun.2009.12.011] [PMID: 20133161]

[52] Lorx A, Valkó L, Pénzes I. Anaesthesia for interventional bronchoscopy.Interventional Pulmonology. Plymouth, UK: European Respiratory Society Monograph 2010; Vol. 48: pp. 18-32. [http://dx.doi.org/10.1183/1025448x.00990209]

[53] Sarkiss M. Anesthesia for bronchoscopy and interventional pulmonology: from moderate sedation to jet ventilation. Curr Opin Pulm Med 2011; 17(4): 274-8. [http://dx.doi.org/10.1097/MCP.0b013e3283471227] [PMID: 21519266]

[54] Drummond M, Magalhaes A, Hespanhol V, Marques A. Rigid bronchoscopy: Complications in a university hospital. J Bronchol 2003; 10: 177-81. [http://dx.doi.org/10.1097/00128594-200307000-00003]

[55] Dincq AS, Gourdin M, Collard E, *et al.* Anesthesia for adult rigid bronchoscopy. Acta Anaesthesiol Belg 2014; 65(3): 95-103. [PMID: 25470890]

[56] Pathak V, Welsby I, Mahmood K, Wahidi M, MacIntyre N, Shofer S. Ventilation and anesthetic approaches for rigid bronchoscopy. Ann Am Thorac Soc 2014; 11(4): 628-34. [http://dx.doi.org/10.1513/AnnalsATS.201309-302FR] [PMID: 24635585]

[57] Petrella F, Borri A, Casiraghi M, Cavaliere S, Donghi S, Galetta D, *et al.* Operative rigid bronchoscopy: Indications, basic techniques and results. Multimed Man Cardiothorac Surg 2014; 2014

[58] Lukomsky GI, Ovchinnikov AA, Bilal A. Complications of bronchoscopy: comparison of rigid

bronchoscopy under general anesthesia and flexible fiberoptic bronchoscopy under topical anesthesia. Chest 1981; 79(3): 316-21.
[http://dx.doi.org/10.1378/chest.79.3.316] [PMID: 7471862]

[59] Facciolongo N, Patelli M, Gasparini S, *et al.* Incidence of complications in bronchoscopy. Multicentre prospective study of 20,986 bronchoscopies. Monaldi Arch Chest Dis 2009; 71(1): 8-14.
[PMID: 19522159]

[60] Grosu HB, Morice RC, Sarkiss M, *et al.* Safety of flexible bronchoscopy, rigid bronchoscopy, and endobronchial ultrasound-guided transbronchial needle aspiration in patients with malignant space-occupying brain lesions. Chest 2015; 147(6): 1621-8.
[http://dx.doi.org/10.1378/chest.14-1704] [PMID: 25393333]

[61] Tomaske M, Gerber AC, Weiss M. Anesthesia and periinterventional morbidity of rigid bronchoscopy for tracheobronchial foreign body diagnosis and removal. Paediatr Anaesth 2006; 16(2): 123-9.
[http://dx.doi.org/10.1111/j.1460-9592.2005.01714.x] [PMID: 16430406]

[62] Ernst A, Wahidi MM, Read CA, *et al.* Adult Bronchoscopy Training: Current State and Suggestions for the Future: CHEST Expert Panel Report. Chest 2015; 148(2): 321-32.
[http://dx.doi.org/10.1378/chest.14-0678] [PMID: 25674901]

[63] Wahidi MM, Silvestri GA, Coakley RD, *et al.* A prospective multicenter study of competency metrics and educational interventions in the learning of bronchoscopy among new pulmonary fellows. Chest 2010; 137(5): 1040-9.
[http://dx.doi.org/10.1378/chest.09-1234] [PMID: 19858234]

[64] Wahidi MM, Hulett C, Pastis N, *et al.* Learning experience of linear endobronchial ultrasound among pulmonary trainees. Chest 2014; 145(3): 574-8.
[http://dx.doi.org/10.1378/chest.13-0701] [PMID: 24114380]

[65] Mahmood K, Wahidi MM, Osann KE, *et al.* Development of a Tool to Assess Basic Competency in the Performance of Rigid Bronchoscopy. Ann Am Thorac Soc 2016; 13(4): 502-11.
[PMID: 26989810]

[66] Dutau H, Vandemoortele T, Breen DP. Rigid bronchoscopy. Clin Chest Med 2013; 34(3): 427-35.
[http://dx.doi.org/10.1016/j.ccm.2013.04.003] [PMID: 23993814]

CHAPTER 3

Bronchoscopy Training: Principles and Practice

Lakshmi Mudambi and **George A. Eapen***

MD Anderson Cancer Center, Houston, Texas, USA

Abstract: Bronchoscopy education and training form a foundation for novice bronchoscopists to acquire skills necessary to provide optimal patient care. This chapter reviews the process of instructional design, the application of teaching and learning principles to bronchoscopy education, the use of the Accreditation Council for Graduate Medical Education's Core Competencies to guide curricula development in bronchoscopy education, the current literature regarding training practices and tools available to develop curricula.

Keywords: Bronchoscopy education, Learning principles, Teaching principles, Training.

INTRODUCTION

Over the last century, medical education in the United States has been increasingly focused on providing evidence-based training. The Flexner report [1] in 1910 provided the initial impetus for the transformation of the medical education system. Residency education is currently governed by the standards laid forth by the Accreditation Council for Graduate Medical Education (ACGME) and these standards evolve as the definitions of adequacy of medical training change over time. While cognitive knowledge acquisition can be readily assessed, determining satisfactory levels of procedural training is particularly challenging since skill acquisition and application are dependent on many variables, which makes assessment somewhat subjective.

Bronchoscopy is an airway visualization platform that is typically combined with an array of diagnostic and therapeutic interventions. It is utilized primarily by pulmonologists and occasionally, by intensivists, surgeons and anesthesiologists. In specialties requiring demonstration of competency in bronchoscopy, the current training model is focused on the teaching and assessment of acquired skills by supervising physicians while trainees attain a designated number of procedures

* **Corresponding author George A. Eapen:** FCT 12.6010, 1400 Pressler St, Unit 1462, Houston, TX 77030, USA; Tel: 713-792-6238; Fax: 713-794-4922; E-mail: geapen@mdanderson.org

Ali I. Musani (Ed.)

assigned arbitrarily by governing bodies. This model has been criticized because it cannot completely ascertain an individual's skill given that clinical scenarios are not uniform; it does, however, serve as an imperfect surrogate of competency during the time of training.

BRONCHOSCOPY EDUCATION

In the United States today, bronchoscopy education is still loosely based on Halsted's philosophy of "see one, do one, teach one". A trainee will observe the procedure and then, perform it under the supervision of a senior physician. As more procedures are performed, the trainee variably gains confidence and competence depending upon the individual's aptitude. The principal drawback of this model is the potential adverse outcomes (including discomfort) that a patient may experience. From a trainee's perspective, the variability of instructors' methodology and the lack of consistency in the training environment or evaluation form barriers to skill acquisition.

Both learning and teaching allow humans to enhance their understanding of the world by synthesizing knowledge with the senses. Educational psychologists have identified over seventy theories of learning styles based on learning paradigms [2]. These paradigms are different ways to view a concept and often mutually exclusive, making comparison of learning theories fundamentally impossible. Still, these paradigms help learners and teachers organize methods to optimize learning. Instructional design, which is the process of analyzing and correcting instructional problems based on learning needs, is a crucial, yet, incompletely explored aspect of bronchoscopy education. Optimal learning is a shared responsibility between teachers and students.

Based on the current theories of learning, a learner-centered approach to teaching has been implemented by many centers of education. We can create a more systematic training process by applying the same principles to bronchoscopy education.

PRINCIPLES OF TEACHING [3]

Understand the Student

Training programs in the United States comply with ACGME standards but student characteristics influence the ability to learn. Specifically for bronchoscopy training, it is important to recognize these variables and adapt instructional methods. Assumptions made about a student before training begins must be justified with evidence. For example, a trainee may have had significant exposure to hi-fidelity bronchoscopy simulation before beginning a pulmonology fellowship but this does not guarantee performance in live patients. Similarly, student's prior knowledge can be accurate or inaccurate and it is the responsibility of a teacher to recognize the baseline and adjust their instructional methods.

Define Learning Objectives

Bloom's taxonomy classifies educational objectives into the domains of cognition, affect and psychomotor. This can be applied to bronchoscopy education.

- The cognitive aspect of bronchoscopy training includes knowledge of indications, complications and alternatives to bronchoscopy, knowledge of technical specifications, ability to interpret radiographic imaging and a broad knowledge of pulmonology. This objective is best achieved through a combination of didactics and multiple clinical scenario immersion with an emphasis on developing sound judgment and critical thinking.
- Developing affective objectives assists in self-realization and is the most fluid domain. The aim is to foster self-awareness about ones abilities, pinpoint areas of excellence and deficit, explore characteristics that have led to these endpoints and promote behaviors that engender lifelong learning.
- For bronchoscopy training, the psychomotor domain can only be developed by "doing". A student must perform bronchoscopies and every opportunity to do so must be offered.

State Expectations

The overarching goal of bronchoscopy training (and all procedural training) is to safely and effectively apply the most appropriate technology and technique to provide clinical benefit to a patient with a particular disease condition. This composite goal requires a broad understanding of the disease pathophysiology, the available techniques and the psychomotor skills to successfully implement them. This may be overwhelming for a novice trainee and a series of intermediate training goals should be implemented to facilitate learning. The crawl, walk, run training methodology [4] enables learners to gain confidence and competence in graduated tasks as experience and judgment is accumulated (Table **1**).

Table 1. Stages in training.

Phase	Description	Scenario
Crawl (Explain and demonstrate)	Trainer describes the task step-by-step and demonstrates proper form, technique and sequence of task performance	Didactic sessions, bedside discussions, low fidelity simulations

(Table 1) contd.....

Phase	Description	Scenario
Walk (Practice)	Trainee performs the assigned tasks in a low stakes, low stress environment with emphasis on proper form, technique and sequence.	Animal models, high fidelity simulations, available training modules.
Run (Perform)	Trainee performs the assigned task under supervision with coaching, as needed, in a live stakes environment at a realistic pace.	Direct patient care

These phases are implemented in sequence, but if the trainee has difficulty with any phase, educators should flexibly revert back to the last successful training phase. Expectations and goals must be repeatedly reinforced by instructors with the understanding that trainees evolve during the course of training. For instance, the initial focus may be learning airway anatomy, visualizing the airways and learning scope manipulation while complementary techniques and tools are introduced periodically throughout training as clinical context and scenarios require.

Prioritize What is Taught

As new technology is introduced and bronchoscopy applications expand, it is necessary to recognize the core learning requirements for the training period. Teach the "essentials" first and build based on what the student accomplishes. Although all students will not become experts in all aspects of bronchoscopy, the scope of training should seek to impart these "building block" skills that enable the trainee to continue to learn and adapt even after completion of the formal training period.

Experts have "Blind Spots"

Experts have access to a broad knowledge base and experiences and in bronchoscopy, years of practice result in fine hand-eye coordination and development of muscle memory, a situation that has been described as "unconscious competence" [5]. This can lead to blurred descriptions of the steps involved in a procedure and diligent instructors must be aware of this to mitigate the training deficiency.

Redefine Your Role

The instructors' role changes as the training process progresses. Based on the student's background, aptitude and proficiency, the teacher's role may transition from a guide, to a collaborator, to a critic and so on. These changes progressively challenge a student to take on greater responsibilities in their decision-making and develop confidence in their abilities.

Refine Your Syllabus and Teaching Style

Most teachers develop a personal teaching plan and unique teaching style through the years. To be a truly effective teacher, flexibility of the syllabus and style based upon 360-degree feedback should be standard practice. Some inferences on effectiveness can also be made by analyzing the performances of previous students. Generally, growth as a teacher depends upon adaptability to the student's needs.

PRINCIPLES OF LEARNING

In a learner-centered model of education, the responsibility of training is shared with the student.

- A learner's fund of knowledge can be variable. Learners should seek to recognize deficiencies and implement corrective measures.
- In procedural training, systematic organization of information and graduated task performance allows for smoother comprehension, retrieval and application.
- Cultivating situational awareness while practicing component skills of bronchoscopy allows integration of these skills.
- Advanced learners are able to identify their strengths and weaknesses, judiciously recognize their own learning styles and self-direct efforts to buttress areas needing improvement.

Both learning and teaching pursue each other constantly in the cycle of education and at any given point, neither is far behind the other. The teacher projects instruction from the foundation of what he was taught. The strength of this foundation depends on the teacher's insight, ability (innate and acquired), interest and clinical experiences. As he imparts his knowledge to the learner, the same characteristics determine how the learner will absorb this information. Much of this process is effort-dependent and as advanced learners, introspection to identify areas of improvement is as important as the teacher correcting obvious errors. However, the significance of clinical experiences under the mentorship of an exemplary teacher is incomparable since this directly impacts the process of learning and ultimately, the outcome for the patient.

Over time, the trainee progresses from a novice through rising levels of proficiency to becoming an educator. Fellowship training would benefit if senior fellows are formally incorporated into the process of procedural education. In the process, the senior fellow learns to become an independent instructor and a malleable mentor to students with different aptitudes while honing their own skills through the exercise of self-examination that teaching entails.

BRONCHOSCOPY AND CORE COMPETENCIES

In 2000, ACGME's Outcome Project established six core competencies with the aim of reliably assessing a trainee's overall performance. The American Board of Medical Specialties has also adopted this model for certification of practicing physicians. Although there are no guidelines or standardized curricula for bronchoscopy education, these six competencies form the structural framework for trainee assessment and are very relevant to bronchoscopy education. The ACGME also mandates the performance of 100 bronchoscopies during a 2 or 3-year fellowship track to graduate [6].

- ***Patient Care***: By incorporating the patient's history, physical examination, laboratory and radiological data and current scientific evidence, a learner must demonstrate the ability to identify an appropriate indication for the bronchoscopy and associated interventions, assess and prepare for potential complications, provide clear counseling to patients and families and finally, safely execute the procedure. Cumulatively, this competency focuses on optimal patient care outcomes.
- ***Medical Knowledge**:* In bronchoscopy training, medical knowledge can be broadly divided into three components: (1) Knowledge of pulmonary disease processes and how bronchoscopy may assist in diagnostics and therapeutics, (2) Knowledge of available instrument characteristics and (3) Knowledge of bronchoscopic techniques. Of the three, the greatest gaps in procedural training are found in knowledge of instrument characteristics and bronchoscopic techniques and warrants constant attention. Bronchoscopic techniques evolve as new technologies are discovered and awareness of these technologies is essential to provide optimal care.
- ***Practice Based Learning and Improvement**:* During the course of training, the student is expected to not only to learn how to perform bronchoscopy but also, to analyze their practice experiences and assimilate observed standards. Self-analysis is encouraged and is a critical life skill for a successful proceduralist.
- ***Systems Based Practice**:* A fundamental facet of an accomplished bronchoscopist is a deep understanding of the healthcare delivery system, which allows them to utilize available resources to maximally benefit the patient.
- ***Professionalism**:* This implies a commitment to continued professional development, self-evaluation and demonstration of the emotional and intellectual characteristics required of an effective physician.
- ***Interpersonal Skills and Communication**:* Bronchoscopy is always a team based task, usually consisting of a proceduralist, a nurse to administer drugs and monitor vital parameters and a bronchoscopy technician who maintains the scopes, processors and assists with the procedure. Additional staff may be necessary based on the complexity and requirements of the procedure. Optimal

team performance involves clear communication and mutually supportive team dynamics. This competency addresses the process of learning to work seamlessly in a team by clarifying team roles, developing healthy working relationships with involved staff and providing detailed and informative instructions effectively. Moving beyond the immediate health care team, the student is also responsible for developing interpersonal and communication skills that fosters rapport with the patient and their families.

CURRENT STATE OF BRONCHOSCOPY EDUCATION

In the last few decades, there have been questions raised about the training practices of fellowship programs and its effects on practicing pulmonologists. One study of fifty-nine pulmonary fellows from multiple regions across the United States found that fellowship programs have markedly diverse approaches to bronchoscopy education [7]. As bronchoscopy experiences differed significantly amongst programs, the perception of proficiency by a fellow was also different [7]. Fellowship program directors also report large variations in the training offered to fellows, particularly in advanced therapeutic procedures [8] with fewer than 30% of programs meeting the competency requirements for Interventional Pulmonary procedures outlined by the ACCP guidelines [9]. Whether reaching the current competency recommendations correlates with good clinical outcomes is not known and critics of the current guidelines emphasize the recommendations are based on expert opinion rather than evidence. However, from studies evaluating competency in other procedural fields [10], it appears that guidelines based on expert opinion tend to underestimate the procedural numbers required to achieve competence. From the viewpoint of a fellow, this unpredictability of the training experience may create a personal lack of confidence in their abilities to handle the challenges posed by clinical practice. Even worse, potential patients cannot be assured that their board certified pulmonologist is actually competent in the procedure he or she is proposing to perform. As such, concerted efforts to identify and implement clear competency based criteria in bronchoscopy training is urgently needed.

Gastroenterologists and cardiologists appear to be ahead of pulmonologists in defining competency metrics for their procedures. With the scope of endoscopy procedures traversing diagnostics to therapeutics in gastroenterology, pivotal studies have challenged the accepted normal standards of competency [10, 11]. They have successfully used hierarchical task analysis to analyze various components of specific procedures and estimate numbers that support a high probability of attaining competency [11]. A recently published systematic review of trainees and competency in endoscopic retrograde cholangiopancreatography also revealed that minimum procedural thresholds had risen much higher than the recommended by current guidelines [12]. In bronchoscopy, there is presently no evidence substantiating the ACCP training recommendations for attaining and maintaining proficiency [9] (Table **2**).

Table 2. Suggested minimal procedural counts for competency.

Procedure	Number for Initial Proficiency	Number to Maintain Competency/year
Flexible Bronchoscopy	100	25
Rigid Bronchoscopy	20	10
TBNA	25	10
Autofluorescence	20	10
EBUS	50	20
Laser	15	10
Electrocautery/APC	15	10
Cryotherapy	10	5
Brachytherapy	5	5
Photodynamic therapy	10	5
Stents	20	10
Thoracic percutaneous needle aspiration/Core Biopsy	10/10	10
Tube Thoracotomy	10	5
Pleuroscopy	20	10
Percutaneous Tracheostomy	20	10

Therefore, the time is right to generate scientific data to describe successfully completed diagnostic and therapeutic bronchoscopic procedures and to develop measurable and meaningful metrics that predict trainee competence with a high degree of confidence. This would redefine the "numbers" recommended to achieve competency and allow a foundation to restructure clinical training programs to meet these requirements.

BRONCHOSCOPY EDUCATION TOOLS

Although flexible bronchoscopy was first introduced by Dr. Shigeto Ikeda in 1966 [13], the metrics of defining competency in the procedure has not been defined. Aside from the program specific curriculum set by individual program directors, there are various resources a student of bronchoscopy can use to broaden their knowledge and sharpen their skills.

Bronchoscopy Simulation

Low and High Fidelity Simulation

Low fidelity bronchoscopy simulation involves the use of real bronchoscopes in physical airway models. Anatomical and non-anatomical low fidelity models are widely available. Made of many different materials, they have diverse applications from practicing difficult airway management to flexible and rigid bronchoscopy. The drawbacks of the low fidelity models are that they lack anatomic realism and can only be used for basic instruction. An underexplored concept is the use three-dimensional (3D) printing to create low cost airway models for practicing bronchoscopy. Recently, a 3D printed bronchial model was used to modify a Y-shaped silicone stent prior to insertion in a post lung transplant patient [14] and to plan an airway intervention in a patient with severe relapsing polychondritis [15]. This provides proof in principle that similar efforts in educational applications may be feasible.

High fidelity simulation consists of a form of virtual bronchoscopy, initially described over a decade ago. Several bronchoscopy simulators are currently available with various distinct features and some incorporate both gastrointestinal and bronchoscopy modules. There are no studies directly comparing these simulators, making it impossible to rank their performance. It has been shown that bronchoscopy simulators can distinguish different levels of training and act as suitable platforms for skill level assessment that correlate to actual practice [16]. Interestingly, a study comparing a low fidelity simulation model (a rubber trachea attached to a laryngotracheal airway) and a high fidelity simulation model (AccuTouch System) to learn the techniques of transbronchial needle aspiration found that the learners preferred the low fidelity model [17]. Other studies evaluating the effectiveness of high fidelity simulation showed that the use of a bronchoscopy simulator improved procedure time, anatomic airway identification and endobronchial ultrasound-transbronchial needle aspiration (EBUS-TBNA) [18 - 21]. The main barrier to widespread adoption of high fidelity simulators is the high acquisition cost.

In general, any simulation model provides an opportunity to practice bronchoscopic techniques without adversely affecting a patient and it does appear that learning basic bronchoscopy and new techniques can be successful in these models. Training programs should make efforts to incorporate simulation training into their curricula.

Bronchoscopy Education Project

Another resource for aspiring bronchoscopists and educators is the Bronchoscopy

Education Project. Developed by Bronchoscopy International, this online project has developed a competency-based curriculum consisting of eBooks, training manuals, patient-centered exercises and assessment tools (Bronchoscopy Self-Assessment Tool and Bronchoscopy Skills and Task Assessment Tools) for instructors and students alike. Some of the assessment tools have been validated in peer reviewed manuscripts [22]. While this site mostly contains the personal opinions, preferences and practices of the content developers, it forms a useful framework for systematized bronchoscopy training and self-study.

Workshops and Hands-on Courses

Other available bronchoscopy education resources include simulation courses and workshops regularly offered by major societies (like the American College of Chest Physicians, the World Association for Bronchology and Interventional Pulmonology and the American Thoracic Society). Generally, these incorporate mixed fidelity hands-on instructional sessions and lectures from prominent experts in the field. Many centers with expertise in bronchoscopy and interventional pulmonology also provide additional periodic workshops and offer internship opportunities as well.

CONCLUSION

In bronchoscopy education, a thoughtful instructional design process is required to construct a curriculum that enhances the probability of learning and attaining competence. Educators have a responsibility to identify deficits in the current process, perform research to determine the factors that influence proficiency in bronchoscopy (including numbers) and make all necessary changes to the training curricula based on the best available evidence. Our solemn duty is to do our best to train and provide training to care for the patients who entrust their lives in our hands.

CONFLICT OF INTEREST

The authors declare no conflict of interest, financial or otherwise.

ACKNOWLEDGEMENTS

Declared none.

REFERENCES

[1] Flexner A. Medical Education in the United States and Canada Bulletin Number Four (The Flexner Report). Carnegie Bulletin 1910; p. 364.

[2] Coffield F, Moseley D, Hall E, Ecclestone K. Learning styles and pedagogy in post 16 learning: a systematic and critical review. Learn Ski Res Cent 2004; p. 84.

[3] ©Copyright 2008, 2015. Eberly center for teaching excellence & educational innovation Carnegie Mellon University 2015.

[4] Department of the Army. Field Manual 7-0: Training for full Spectrum 2008.

[5] Gordon Training International. The four stages of learning any new skill Available at: http://www.gordontraining.com/free-workplace-articles/learning-a-new-skill-is-easier-said-than-done/

[6] Accreditation Council for Graduate Medical Education. Available at: https://www.acgme.org/acgmeweb/tabid/134/ProgramandInstitutionalAccreditation/MedicalSpecialties/InternalMedicine.aspx

[7] Haponik EF, Russell GB, Beamis JF Jr, *et al.* Bronchoscopy training: current fellows' experiences and some concerns for the future. Chest 2000; 118(3): 625-30. [http://dx.doi.org/10.1378/chest.118.3.625] [PMID: 10988182]

[8] Pastis NJ, Nietert PJ, Silvestri GA. American College of Chest Physicians Interventional Chest/Diagnostic Procedures Network Steering Committee. Variation in training for interventional pulmonary procedures among US pulmonary/critical care fellowships: a survey of fellowship directors. Chest 2005; 127(5): 1614-21. [http://dx.doi.org/10.1378/chest.127.5.1614] [PMID: 15888836]

[9] Ernst A, Silvestri GA, Johnstone D. American College of Chest Physicians. Interventional pulmonary procedures. Chest 2003; 123(5): 1693-717. [http://dx.doi.org/10.1378/chest.123.5.1693] [PMID: 12740291]

[10] Watkins JL, Etzkorn KP, Wiley TE, DeGuzman L, Harig JM. Assessment of technical competence during ERCP training. Gastrointest Endosc 1996; 44(4): 411-5. [http://dx.doi.org/10.1016/S0016-5107(96)70090-1] [PMID: 8905359]

[11] Jowell PS, Baillie J, Branch MS, Affronti J, Browning CL, Bute BP. Quantitative assessment of procedural competence. A prospective study of training in endoscopic retrograde cholangiopancreatography. Ann Intern Med 1996; 125(12): 983-9. [http://dx.doi.org/10.7326/0003-4819-125-12-199612150-00009] [PMID: 8967710]

[12] Shahidi N, Ou G, Telford J, Enns R. When trainees reach competency in performing ERCP: a systematic review. Gastrointest Endosc 2015; 81(6): 1337-42. [http://dx.doi.org/10.1016/j.gie.2014.12.054] [PMID: 25841579]

[13] Ikeda S, Yanai N, Ishikawa S. Flexible bronchofiberscope. Keio J Med 1968; 17(1): 1-16. [http://dx.doi.org/10.2302/kjm.17.1] [PMID: 5674435]

[14] Miyazaki T, Yamasaki N, Tsuchiya T, Matsumoto K, Takagi K, Nagayasu T. Airway Stent Insertion Simulated With a Three-Dimensional Printed Airway Model. Ann Thorac Surg Elsevier 2015; 99(1): e21-3. [http://dx.doi.org/10.1016/j.athoracsur.2014.10.021]

[15] Tam MD, Laycock SD, Jayne D, Babar J, Noble B. 3-D printouts of the tracheobronchial tree generated from CT images as an aid to management in a case of tracheobronchial chondromalacia caused by relapsing polychondritis. J Radiol Case Rep 2013; 7(8): 34-43. [http://dx.doi.org/10.3941/jrcr.v7i8.1390] [PMID: 24421951]

[16] Ost D, DeRosiers A, Britt EJ, Fein AM, Lesser ML, Mehta AC. Assessment of a bronchoscopy simulator. Am J Respir Crit Care Med 2001; 164(12): 2248-55. [http://dx.doi.org/10.1164/ajrccm.164.12.2102087] [PMID: 11751195]

[17] Davoudi M, Wahidi MM, Zamanian Rohani N, Colt HG. Comparative effectiveness of low- and high-fidelity bronchoscopy simulation for training in conventional transbronchial needle aspiration and user preferences. Respiration 2010; 80(4): 327-34. [http://dx.doi.org/10.1159/000318674] [PMID: 20616534]

[18] Colt HG, Crawford SW, Galbraith O III. Virtual reality bronchoscopy simulation: a revolution in procedural training. Chest 2001; 120(4): 1333-9.

[http://dx.doi.org/10.1378/chest.120.4.1333] [PMID: 11591579]

[19] Blum MG, Powers TW, Sundaresan S. Bronchoscopy simulator effectively prepares junior residents to competently perform basic clinical bronchoscopy. Ann Thorac Surg 2004; 78(1): 287-91. [http://dx.doi.org/10.1016/j.athoracsur.2003.11.058] [PMID: 15223446]

[20] Stather DR, Maceachern P, Rimmer K, Hergott CA, Tremblay A. Assessment and learning curve evaluation of endobronchial ultrasound skills following simulation and clinical training. Respirology 2011; 16(4): 698-704. [http://dx.doi.org/10.1111/j.1440-1843.2011.01961.x] [PMID: 21355965]

[21] Stather DR, MacEachern P, Chee A, Dumoulin E, Tremblay A. Evaluation of clinical endobronchial ultrasound skills following clinical *versus* simulation training. Respirology 2012; 17(2): 291-9. [http://dx.doi.org/10.1111/j.1440-1843.2011.02068.x] [PMID: 21943051]

[22] Davoudi M, Osann K, Colt HG. Validation of two instruments to assess technical bronchoscopic skill using virtual reality simulation. Respiration 2008; 76(1): 92-101. [http://dx.doi.org/10.1159/000126493] [PMID: 18408359]

CHAPTER 4

Lung Cancer Screening: Past, Present and Future

Nathaniel R. Little[1], **Jeffrey A. Kern**[1,2,3] and **James H. Finigan**[1,2,3,*]

[1] *Division of Pulmonary Sciences and Critical Care Medicine, Department of Medicine, University of Colorado, 127000 East 19th Avenue, Aurora, CO 80045, USA*

[2] *Division of Oncology, Department of Medicine, National Jewish Health, 1400 Jackson Street, Denver CO 80206, USA*

[3] *Division of Pulmonary and Critical Care Medicine, Department of Medicine, National Jewish Health, 1400 Jackson Street, Denver CO 80206, USA*

Abstract: Lung cancer is the leading cause of cancer-related deaths worldwide. While smoking cessation efforts are imperative, development of effective lung cancer screening approaches are essential given current lung cancer prevalence. Historical attempts to screen lung cancer through chest radiography and sputum cytology resulted in earlier diagnosis of lung cancers, without improvement in cancer-related mortality or stage shift. The National Lung Screening Trial (NLST) demonstrated that low-dose computed tomography (LDCT) screening for lung cancer decreases cancer-related and all-cause mortality. Current consensus guidelines recommend annual LDCT screening for individuals at high-risk for the development of lung cancer. Prospective trials are needed to refine selection of optimal screening populations, duration and intervals. Successful implementation of lung cancer screening programs will depend upon creation of a multi-disciplinary team allowing for nodule surveillance with expertise in lung cancer diagnosis and treatment.

Keywords: Chest radiograph, Cost-effectiveness, Guidelines, Low-dose computed tomography, Lung cancer, Lung cancer screening, Lung nodule, National Lung Screening Trial, Overdiagnosis, Smoking cessation.

BURDEN OF DISEASE

Lung cancer remains the leading cause of cancer-related death for both men and women [1] with estimates of mortality in 2015 exceeding 158,000 deaths in the US, and 1.6 million deaths worldwide [2]. Lung cancer is the 3rd leading cause of all-cause mortality in the US [1]. This high mortality rate reflects lung cancer incidence with more than 221,000 estimated new cases in the US and 1.8 million new cases worldwide this year. While evidence suggests that lung cancer

* **Corresponding author James H. Finigan:** Department of Medicine, National Jewish Health, 1400 Jackson Street, K736A, Denver, CO 80206, USA; Tel: 877.225.5654; E-mail: FiniganJ@NJHealth.org

Ali I. Musani (Ed.)

incidence is declining for both sexes, rates of cigarette smoking remain stubbornly high and likely will continue to influence the development of lung cancer for years to come. Moreover, despite significant advances in understanding the molecular underpinnings of lung cancer and subsequent design of new therapies, the overall 5-year survival for lung cancer remains abysmally low (18%) [3], having only minimally changed over the last quarter of a century. Lung cancer's high mortality rate is heavily influenced by the fact that most cases continue to be diagnosed in advanced stages of disease, often precluding cure. Over 70% of all lung cancers are found to be stage 3 or 4 at the time of diagnosis [4]. These characteristics make lung cancer a prime target for intensified efforts focused upon prevention and early diagnosis to identify it at an early stage when cure is an option.

LUNG CANCER SCREENING

Efforts aimed at lung cancer prevention through tobacco cessation are paramount, as an estimated 80-90% of lung cancers are attributed to smoking [5]. However, due to ongoing smoking behavior, efforts to develop effective lung cancer screening approaches are also essential. Lung cancer, similar to other malignancies for which successful screening programs have been implemented, has certain key characteristics that allow for early diagnosis (Table **1**) [6]. With the advent, accuracy, and increasing availability of low-dose CT (LDCT) imaging, an increasing number of lung cancers are now being diagnosed at earlier stages. The 2011 publication of the National Lung Screening Trial (NLST) demonstrated for the first time that lung cancer screening improves cancer-related mortality.

Table 1. Core Principles for Population Cancer Screening

a) High burden of disease
b) Recognition of early or latent asymptomatic disease
c) Understanding of the natural history of disease
d) Beneficial treatment options in patients with recognized disease
e) Screening test with high level of accuracy
f) Screening test offering favorable benefit to risk ratio
g) Delineated plan for determination of which patients are appropriate for treatment
h) Accessibility to facilities able to offer diagnosis and treatment
i) Cost of screening should be balanced in regard to total expenditure on medical care as a whole
j) Screening as an ongoing, dynamic process

Adapted from: Wilson JMG, Junger G. Principles and practices of screening for disease. Geneva, Switzerland: World Health Organization; 1968. Report No.: Public Health Papers No. 34.

HISTORY OF LUNG CANCER SCREENING

Lung Cancer Screening Through Chest Radiography

Over the past 4 decades, numerous lung cancer screening trials have been performed assessing chest radiography with or without sputum cytology as a screening tool for lung cancer. One of the first randomized controlled trials to examine lung cancer screening was the Mayo Lung Project (MLP). This study randomized 9211 men, aged 45 years or older with at least 1 pack-per-day smoking history in the past 1 year to chest x-ray and sputum cytology screening *versus* standard care over a 6 year study period. Following a universal prevalence screen for all participants *via* chest radiograph and pooled sputum cytology analysis, subjects were randomized to either the screening group *versus* the standard of care group, who were recommended to undergo an annual chest x-ray. Results demonstrated that screening with chest x-ray and sputum cytology every 4 months increased the overall lung cancer detection rate, increased detection at earlier stages of disease, and increased resectability. However, no differences in lung cancer-related mortality or all-cause mortality among the screened *versus* unscreened arms were identified [7, 8]. Similar results were seen in screening studies performed at the Johns Hopkins and Memorial Sloan Kettering medical centers, along with an investigation performed in Czechoslovakia. While all of these studies, which utilized some form of chest radiography and sputum cytology at variable intervals, noted increased diagnosis of lung cancer at earlier stages of disease (stage I or II), no difference in mortality was detected between patients in the screening *versus* control groups [9 - 11].

This early lung cancer screening experience demonstrates the chasm that can exist between improved cancer detection and translatable impact upon cancer-related and all-cause mortality. Such discrepancies are likely explained by the presence of lead-time and over-diagnosis bias [8]. Lead-time bias occurs when screening detects cancers earlier than non screen-detected cancers, which are diagnosed because of symptoms, yet there is no difference in mortality. It represents an overestimation of the duration of survival among cases detected through screening, giving the appearance of a useful test. In contrast, over-diagnosis refers to the diagnosis of a slowly growing, indolent cancer that would be unlikely to progress to advanced disease or result in mortality of a particular patient. In an adequately powered, randomized controlled trial, the incidence of cancer should be equal in both the screening and control arms. However, if cancer is found to occur more frequently in the screening arm, it suggests that the difference in cancer diagnoses represents malignancies that would not advance to the point of causing death. Over-diagnosis can result in the performance of unneeded invasive diagnostic testing that can be associated with complications, as well as equally unneeded cancer treatment with adverse effects. While both lead-time and over-diagnosis biases can be present in the background of a particular study, careful examination of the early lung cancer screening studies reveals over-diagnosis at work.

The Mayo Lung Project is an example of over-diagnosis [8]. Longitudinal follow-up of screening and control groups in this study identified that after 8.5 years 206 cancers were diagnosed in the screening arm, compared with only 160 cancers in the control arm. Subsequent analysis at 12 years of surveillance demonstrates a persistent discrepancy of lung cancer prevalence between the screening and control arms (585 cancers vs 500 cancers). It has been speculated, however, that over time, such curves of cancer detection rates might eventually merge to reveal a similar collection of both slowly progressing, non-morbid cancers along with aggressive, potentially lethal disease.

The most recent trial examining lung cancer screening through chest radiography is the Prostate, Lung, Colorectal, and Ovarian (PLCO) trial published in 2011 [12]. Patients, between the ages of 55 and 74 years, were enrolled from 1993 to 2001 at one of 10 study centers. The study group underwent annual screening *via* chest radiograph for 4 years, while the control group received usual care as determined by their treating physician. Overall adherence rates in the screening group across the 4 year period was quite high at 83.5%, while contamination rates in the usual care group (defined as receiving a chest radiograph during the screening interval) remained relatively low at 11%. During the 13 year observation period, no differences in lung cancer detection, clinical stage, histologic grade, or lung cancer mortality were identified. Furthermore, a predefined sub-analysis examining outcomes in a high-risk patient cohort, (patients with at least a 30 pack-year smoking history and either current smokers or quit within the past 15 years), was performed and no statistical differences between the two groups for lung cancer incidence or cancer-related mortality were identified.

It should be noted that while no differences in either lung cancer detection rates or changes in cancer-related mortality were found, a significant number of cancers were ultimately diagnosed after the predetermined screening period. This raises that possibility that extension of screening beyond the 4 years may have yielded a more effective screening intervention. However, based on the predetermined screening interval, the PLCO study corroborates prior study findings that suggest lung cancer screening through chest radiography does not influence cancer diagnosis, or cancer-related mortality in comparison with performance of usual care.

The PLCO trial differed from other chest radiograph screening trials in several ways. First, it was the largest chest radiograph screening study with 154,901 participants randomized into screening *versus* control groups. Second, while the intervention arm received baseline and subsequent radiographs on an annual basis, the control arm did not receive either baseline or subsequent imaging unless determined necessary by a treating physician. Third, sputum cytology was not included as part of the intervention protocol. Finally, given the overall study breadth of the PLCO to investigate other malignancies aside from lung (prostate, colorectal, ovarian); smoking history was not required as a mandatory criterion for participant enrollment. Thus the PLCO trial serves as a more representative evaluation of lung cancer screening within the general population and not specifically aimed at assessing high-risk groups.

Lung Cancer Screening By CT Imaging

Despite some evidence that lung cancer screening by chest radiography could diagnose more lung cancers at early stages of disease, it did not translate into observable benefit in terms of overall survival, or a reduction in the ultimate number of advanced stage lung cancers identified. Thus, more effective screening interventions were needed. The advent of computed tomography (CT) screening, with its initial application in 1971 [13], followed by subsequent improvements in technique and safety over the next 3 decades brought forth a new modality to be investigated for the purposes of lung cancer screening.

Initial trials of lung cancer screening through use of CT imaging consisted of small, single-arm, observational studies that investigated the application of low-dose CT (LDCT) to diagnose early stage disease. LDCT, or helical CT, allows for continuous data acquisition, which results in shorter scan times and significantly reduced radiation exposure [14]. Use of LDCT for thoracic imaging results in radiation exposures of 1-2 mSV, compared with 7 mSV encountered in conventional CT imaging [15]. Kaneko *et al*, comparing the role of LDCT to chest radiography for detection of lung cancer in 1369 high-risk individuals, found that in patients screened annually by both methods over a 2 year period, more peripheral lung cancers were identified by CT than chest radiography [16]. Another early Japanese study by Sone *et al.* found that CT imaging resulted in a higher lung cancer detection rate (0.48%), even in the background of a low-risk cancer population. Furthermore, in this observational study of 5483 patients, CT detected lung cancers of smaller size, as well as more benign lung nodules in comparison to chest radiography [17].

A prospective cohort study, assessing LDCT for early diagnosis of lung cancer performed at the Mayo Clinic, enrolled 1520 high-risk subjects, defined as patients with at least a 20 pack-year smoking history and having actively smoked within the prior 10 years [18]. Patients were monitored with 5 annual LDCT scans (1 prevalence scan at enrollment followed by 4 years of annual incidence scans). After 4 years, 1118 patients had non-calcified lung nodules (74%) of at least 4 mm in size. Within this group, 66 individuals were ultimately diagnosed with lung cancer. The majority of lung cancers identified (61%) were stage I, with an overall lung cancer-related mortality estimated at 2.8%. Despite results that suggested improved identification of early stage lung cancers by LDCT, comparison with prior chest radiograph screening data as part of the Mayo Lung Project showed no statistically significant difference in late stage disease, or cancer-related mortality. Thus it was concluded that true stage shift, *i.e.* detection of increased early stage cancers and fewer late stage cancers, did not occur.

Thus, while LDCT screening was able to detect lung cancers at earlier stages of development in comparison to no screening, the failure to impact mortality demonstrated no effect upon survivorship. Such findings again raised the likelihood of lead-time bias. This study also raised important questions in terms of acceptable limits for false negative rates in a screening test given that 26% of patients were found to have lung nodules in subsequent scans that were missed by the initial baseline scan. Furthermore, only 66 nodules identified by LDCT imaging were lung cancer, while the vast majority of nodules identified were benign. While LDCT may offer a higher degree of resolution and diagnosis of parenchymal abnormalities, this high rate of newly identified abnormalities (whether malignant or benign) resulted in increased utilization of diagnostic testing and definitive intervention to exclude malignancy.

The Early Lung Cancer Action Program (ELCAP) study was a much larger, single arm study that screened patients at high-risk for development of lung cancer. Defined as subjects 60 years or older with at least 10 pack-year smoking history, baseline screening was performed on 31,567 participants. Pulmonary nodules on baseline screening were identified in 4186 (13%) study participants. Of these nodules, 9.7% were found to be lung cancers. Subsequent annual incidence scans (27,456 total annual screens) demonstrated new nodules in 1460 (5%) participants. Within the incidence screens, and in particular newly diagnosed nodules, 5.1% were found to represent lung cancers. The majority of lung cancers diagnosed, either at the baseline or annual screening, were found to be stage I disease (85%). Furthermore, 10-year survival rate for patients diagnosed with stage I disease reached 88%, with those undergoing surgical resection fairing even better at 92%. Lung biopsies were obtained in 535 patients, with 92% demonstrating cancer. These study results are intriguing, given the proportion of early (stage I) lung cancer diagnoses, and the presumption of improved mortality. Equally striking is the respectively low proportion of biopsies performed for ultimately diagnosed benign *versus* malignant disease. This study remains limited by the absence of a control group, which precludes important comparisons of cancer-related mortality.

The Detection and Screening of Early Lung Cancer by Novel Imaging Technology and Molecular Essays (DANTE) trial was a randomized, controlled lung cancer screening trial that compared 5 annual LDCTs to no screening within a high-risk population (60-75 years-old, $\geq$ 20 pack-years smoking history) [19]. Following a baseline assessment of chest radiography and sputum cytology analysis, a total of 2811 men were randomized to either the screening arm, which consisted of annual LDCT for 4 years, or the control arm, which received yearly clinical exams only. Participants were followed for a median duration of 33.7 months. Similar to prior CT screening studies, there was a significant increase in lung cancer diagnoses with screening performed by LDCT (60 vs 34). However, while the number of patients diagnosed with stage I lung cancers was higher in the LDCT group (54 vs 34), both study arms had an equal proportion of advanced lung cancers. Thus, no stage shift was appreciated as a result of LDCT screening. More importantly, no effect was identified in terms of lung cancer-related or all-cause mortality. It should be noted that the rate of invasive procedures (*e.g.*, video-assisted thoracoscopic surgery, CT-guided core biopsy, or bronchoscopy) was significantly higher in the screening arm compared with the control arm (134 vs 54) [19, 20]. Similar to single arm LDCT trials, DANTE suggested that lung cancer screening with LDCT might result in over-diagnosis, with an elevated false-positive rate, and lead to an increased number of unnecessary invasive procedures that would not affect overall mortality. While DANTE advanced the arena of LDCT lung cancer screening trials through its inclusion of a control arm, interpretation of its results and possibly outcome were limited by its small trial size.

NLST—Improved Survival with LDCT

The National Lung Screening Trial (NLST) was the first large-scale, randomized controlled trial using LDCT screening in patients at high risk for lung cancer and this study was also the first to demonstrate that lung cancer screening with LDCTs resulted in a decrease in lung cancer-related mortality. The NLST enrolled 53,454 participants (59% male) across 33 U.S. medical centers at high risk for lung cancer being between 55 and 75 years of age, having at least a 30 pack-year smoking history, and either currently smoking or quit within the prior 15 years [21]. Patients were recruited between August 2002 and April 2004, during which the screening group (26,723 subjects) underwent an initial prevalence LDCT, followed by 2 annual incidence scans. The control group (26,733 subjects) underwent yearly chest radiographs. The median follow-up of patients in both arms was 6.5 years, and the maximum follow-up was 7.4 years. Adherence rates to the screening protocols were high, exceeding 95% in the LDCT group and 93% in the chest radiography group.

Over 2 years of LDCT screening, the rate of positive (or abnormal) imaging was 24.2% in the LDCT group, compared with 6.9% in the chest radiograph group. Among these positive screening tests, the vast majority of radiologic abnormalities were found to represent benign disease (96.4% in the LDCT group and 94.5% in the chest radiograph group). Within this same period of observation, 649 lung cancers were diagnosed in the LDCT group, compared with 279 lung cancers in the chest radiograph group. At the completion of study follow-up however, 1060 and 941 lung cancers had been diagnosed in the LDCT and chest radiograph groups, respectively. Among patients diagnosed with lung cancer, LDCT subjects were more likely to be diagnosed with stage I or II disease, compared with subjects screened by chest radiography (57.1% vs 39.9%). Differing from other studies evaluating LDCT as a screening modality for lung cancer, cancer-related mortality was decreased in the LDCT group compared with the chest radiograph group (247 deaths per 100,000 person-years vs 309 deaths per 100,000 person years). Overall mortality was also significantly reduced in the LDCT screening group. The relative risk reduction by LDCT screening was estimated to be 20.3% (95% confidence interval [CI] 6.8% - 26.7%, p = 0.004), and the number needed to treat to prevent 1 lung cancer death with LDCT was 320.

BEYOND NLST

As a result of the findings from the NLST study, with reductions in both cancer-related and all-cause mortality in patients screened with LDCT, multiple international oncologic, pulmonary, and surgical organizations adopted recommendations to include annual LDCT as the screening modality of choice for individuals at high risk for the development of lung cancer (Table 2). Furthermore, in the U.S., the Centers for Medicare & Medicaid Services (CMS) have recently issued a national coverage determination (NCD) for Medicare coverage of screening for lung cancer with LDCT, moving this screening method from an investigational practice to a new standard of care of lung cancer detection [22].

Despite acceptance and cautious adoption of LDCT screening for lung cancer, numerous questions still exist regarding appropriate implementation and potential downstream effects of lung cancer screening by LDCT. One issue relates to which patients should receive lung cancer screening to maximize survival benefit and minimize any associated risks. While the majority of LDCT screening guidelines

Table 2. Current Consensus Guidelines for Use of LDCT In Lung Cancer Screening.

Organization	Recommendations	Year Published
US Preventative Services Task Force (USPSTF)[a]	Annual LDCT screening in adults aged 55-80, who have at least a 30 pack-year smoking history who currently smoke or have quit within the past 15 years. Screening should be discontinued once a patient has not smoked for more than 15 years, developed a life expectancy limiting illness, or refuses curative thoracic surgery if indicated.	December 2013
American College of Chest Physicians (ACCP)/American Society for Clinical Oncology (ASCO)[b]	Annual LDCT screening in adults aged 55-74, who have at least a 30 pack-year smoking history who currently smoke or have quit within the past 15 years. Screening should only be performed in settings capable of offering comprehensive care similar to that provided in the NLST trial.	May 2013
American Association of Thoracic Surgery (AATS)[c]	Annual LDCT screening in adults aged 55-79, who have at least a 30 pack-year smoking history who currently smoke or have quit within the past 15 years. Long-term cancer survivors should be offered second primary lung cancer screening through age 79. Annual LDCT screening should also be offered to adults age 50, with at least a 20 pack-year smoking history if cumulative devlopment of lung cancer exceeds 5% or greater over the proceeding 5 years.	May 2012
American Cancer Society (ACS)[d]	Annual LDCT screening in adults aged 55-74, who have at least a 30 pack-year smoking history who currently smoke or have quit within the past 15 years. Thorough informed consent and shared decision-making should be offered to patient prior to screening, along with smoking cessation counseling.	March 2013
European Respiratory Society (ERS), European Society of Radiology (ESR)[e]	Annual LDCT screening in adults aged 55-80, who have at least a 30 pack-year smoking history who currently smoke or have quit within the past 15 years. Multidisciplinary medical resources, shared decision-making, and smoking cessation interventions should be offered.	April 2015

Data from:

[a]Final Update Summary: Lung Cancer Screening. U.S. Preventive Services Task Force. July 2015.

[b]Detterbeck FC, Mazzone PJ, Naidich DP, *et al.* Screening for lung cancer: diagnosis and management of lung cancer, 3rd ed: American College of Chest Physicians evidence-based clinical practical guidelines. Chest 2013;143(5 Suppl):e78S-92S.

[c]Jaklitsch MT, Jacobson FL, Austin JH, *et al.* The American Association for Thoracic Surgery guidelines for lung cancer screening using low-dose computed tomography scans for lung cancer survivors and other high-risk groups. J Thorac Cardiovasc Surg 2012;144:33-38.

[d]Wender R, Fontham ETH, Barrera E, *et al.* American Cancer Society lung cancer screening guidelines. CA: A Cancer Journal for Clinicians 2013;63(2):106-117.

[e]Kauczor H, Bonomo L, Gaga M, *et al.* ESR/ERS white paper on lung cancer screening. European Respiratory Journal, E-published April 30, 2015.

currently draw from the NLST inclusion criteria, multiple European studies are ongoing to refine an ideal screening population and how patients are followed. Differing slightly from NLST in terms of patient recruitment, screening interval, as well as screening duration, the NELSON trial, a Dutch-Belgian randomized controlled trial is being performed to assess differences in lung cancer mortality between patients receiving LDCT screening vs control populations [23]. Eligibility for this trial extends into a slightly younger population of high-risk smokers (50 to 75 years of age), a slightly lower pack year smoking history (at least 15 cigarettes for more than 25 years or at least 10 cigarettes for more than 30 years), and a more recent period of tobacco exposure (patients currently smoking or quit within 10 years). The screening strategy assessed in the NELSON trial relies upon volumetric change of a nodule over time to determine benign from malignant nodules. This strategy is based on the principle that cancers increase in size at a greater rate than benign processes. Thus, the investigators postulated that a long volume doubling time (>400 days) predicted benign disease and might be used to reduce follow-up imaging and invasive diagnostic testing. Evaluation of nodules (classified as negative, positive, or indeterminate) uses a two-step approach. Screening tests with indeterminate nodules lead to follow-up imaging to determine the nodule's volume doubling time and classify the screening test as negative or positive. The study is ongoing, though preliminary results show that among 15,822 participants randomized to either LDCT screening or control groups, with a median follow-up exceeding 8 years, 187 patients were diagnosed with 196 screen-detected lung cancers. An additional 34 patients were diagnosed with 35 interval cancers, identified in the subsequent screening interval. For the 3 screening rounds combined and a 2-year follow-up; sensitivity, specificity, positive predictive value, and negative predictive value were 84.6%, 98.6%, 40.4%, and 99.8% respectively. Most notably, retrospectively identified interval cancers compared with screen-detected cancers were diagnosed at later stages of disease, and had a higher likelihood of squamous cell carcinoma, with a lower likelihood of adenocarcinoma. The Danish Randomized Lung Cancer CT Screening Trial (DLCST), a much smaller study temporally coordinated with the NELSON trial has demonstrated an increase in diagnosis of lower stage non-small cell lung cancer as well [24]. However, no mortality advantage has been detected, possibly as a result of the study's small sample size. Additional ongoing randomized studies examining appropriate LDCT screening populations and screening intervals include the Multi-centric Italian Lung Detection Trial (MILD) [25], the German Lung Cancer Screening Intervention Study (LUSI) [26], the Italian Lung Cancer Computed Tomography Screening Trial (ITALUNG) [27], and the United Kingdom Lung Cancer Screening Trial (UKLS) [28].

The issue of appropriate patient selection for LDCT lung cancer screening is also being addressed through the application of lung cancer risk prediction models. Kovalchik *et al.* developed an absolute-risk prediction model for lung cancer mortality using demographic and clinical characteristics drawn from retrospective analysis of the NLST radiograph (control) group [29]. Following external validation of the prediction model through NLST-eligible and NLST-ineligible patients who had been enrolled within the PLCO cohort; participants within the NLST LDCT group were stratified into quintiles based upon their 5-year risk of death from lung cancer (Quintile 1 with the lowest risk, Quintile 5 with the highest risk). The number of lung cancer-related deaths per 100,000 person-years prevented in the LDCT group increased according to the risk quintile stratification (0.2 in Quintile 1 vs 12.0 in Quintile 5). Furthermore, the number of false positive results declined across the risk quintiles (1648 in Quintile 1 vs 65 in Quintile 5). Strikingly, an estimated 60% of patients (comprising Quintiles 3-5) were noted to account for more than 88% of screen-prevented lung cancer deaths, whereas the lowest-risk quintile accounted for only 1% of prevented-lung cancer deaths. Such findings may suggest that risk-based approaches to screening may not only improve accuracy and detection of lethal lung cancers, but also aid in minimizing harm from downstream procedures and untoward psychological burden prompted by false positive results. The PLCO(m2012) [30] and Liverpool Lung Project (LLP) [31] also serve as lung cancer mortality risk prediction models based upon patient characteristics such as smoking duration, age, education, BMI, family history, presence of chronic lung disease such as chronic obstructive pulmonary disease, asbestos exposure, and pneumonia history. Risk-based prediction models will, nevertheless, require prospective validation before implementation into future LDCT lung cancer screening guidelines.

Additional issues to be considered in implementation of lung cancer screening with LDCT includes the phenomenon of over-diagnosis. Over-diagnosis is estimated to be an increasingly frequent issue with widespread adoption of LDCT lung cancer screening and expected improvements in radiologic technique. It is notable that most of the increase in lung cancers diagnosed by LDCT in the NLST consisted of bronchioalveolar carcinomas (BAC's). LDCT diagnosed 119 more cancers than chest radiographs, with 75 of these being BAC's. In contrast, other histologic forms of lung cancer were diagnosed at similar rates in both the LDCT and the chest radiograph arms. True BAC, now re-classified as adenocarcinoma in situ (AIS), is thought to be a slowly growing process with little impact on mortality [32, 33]. The evaluation and treatment of cancers unlikely to affect mortality expose patients to unneeded risks, costs, and psychological burden. The evaluation of nodules eventually found to be benign further raises concerns for excess morbidity and expense. To this end, judicious monitoring of observed pulmonary nodules will be required. Based upon the Fleischner Society criteria, the American College of Radiology has implemented the Lung Imaging Reporting and Data System (Lung-RADS™), a protocol for follow-up of screen detected nodules to serve as a quality assurance tool to better standardize reporting of LDCT lung cancer screening and provide management recommendations (TABLE 3) [34]. Lung-RADS assumes that patients in a screening program will receive yearly CTs and therefore recommends fewer short term (3 and 6 month) follow-up CT scans compared to standard Fleischner criteria, which is typically used for nodules detected incidentally outside of the context of a lung cancer screening CT.

Table 3. Lung-RADS Version 1.0 Assessment Categories for the evaluation of non-calcified pulmonary nodules detected by LDCT screening.

Category	Nodule Description	Category	Radiologic Findings	Plan for Follow-up CT Imaging	% Malignancy
Incomplete		0	Prior CT required for comparision Part or all of lungs cannot be examined	Additional lung cancer screening CT or comparison CT is needed	Not applicable
Negative	No nodule	1	No lung nodule		
	Definite benign nodule		Nodule with specfic benign calcifications or fat containing nodule		
Benign Appearance/Behavior		2	Solid nodule: either < 6 mm or new < 4 mm	Continue annual LDCT screening in 12 months	< 1%
	Nodule with very low likelihood of representing active cancer due to size of lack of growth		Part solid nodule: < 6 mm on baseline imaging		
			Non-solid nodule: < 20 mm or ≥ 20 mm unchanged/slow growing		
			Category 3 or 4 nodule unchanged for at least 3 months		
Probably Benign		3	Solid nodule: ≥ 6 to < 8 mm on baseline CT OR new 4 mm to < 6 mm		
	Probable benign finding with short term follow-up recommended Includes nodules with low likelihood of active cancer		Part solid nodule: ≥ 6 mm diameter with solid component <6 mm OR new < 6mm diameter	6 month LDCT screening	1-2%
			Non-solid nodule: ≥ 20 mm on baseline CT or new		
Suspicious		4A	Solid nodule: ≥ 8 mm to < 15 mm on baseline CT OR growing <8 mm OR new 6 to <8 mm		
			Part solid nodule: ≥ 6 mm with solid component ≥ 6 mm to < 8 mm OR with new/growing <4 mm solid component	3 month LDCT; consideration of PET/CT if ≥ 8 mm solid component	5-15%
	Findings for which additional diagnostic testing or tissue sampling is indicated		Endobronchial nodule		
		4B	Solid nodule: ≥ 15 mm OR new/growing and ≥ 8 mm		
			Part solid nodule: with a solid component > 8 mm OR new/growing >4 mm solid component	Chest CT with or without contrast, PET/CT and tissue sampling depending on malignancy probability/comorbdities	> 15%
		4X	Category 3 or 4 nodule with additional features or imaging that increases likelihood of malignancy		
Other	Clinically significant or potentially significant findings, non-lung cancer	S	Modifier-may add category 0-4 coding	As appropriate	Not applicable
History of Lung Cancer	Modifier for patients with prior lung cancer diagnosis who return to screening	C	Modifier-may add category 0-4 coding		

Adapted from: American College of Radiology. Lung CT Screening Reporting and Data System (Lung-RADS). Available at: http://www.acr.org/Quality-Safety/Resources/LungRADS. Accessed August 11, 2015.

Despite findings by the NLST that suggest that LDCT screening can improve survival in patients at risk for lung cancer, screening also opens patients to the risk of radiation exposure as well as increased cost and physical and emotional morbidity associated with follow-up of identified nodules. Increased radiation exposure secondary to LDCT screening is a concern given the heightened risk of cancer secondary to radiation. As previously stated, the dose of radiation with a LDCT is 1-2 mSv compared to 7 mSv from a conventional chest CT [15].

However, a positive scan usually results in subsequent imaging, including diagnostic CT or positron emission tomography (PET) scanning, raising the cumulative radiation exposure. Despite this, it has been estimated that in high-risk patients, the benefits of LDCT screening outweigh risks of radiation-induced malignancy [35]. However, in individuals at low risk of lung cancer, for example non-smokers or younger individuals, the favorable benefit to risk ratio is unlikely to persist [36].

One major issue requiring investigation as LDCT lung cancer screening approaches wide-spread implementation is consideration of cost-effectiveness and potential economic influences of lung cancer screening programs. Many analyses of cost-effectiveness have been performed, with rather broad-ranging estimates, with a spectrum of favorable to unfavorable cost outcomes [37 - 40]. As many of these cost-effective analyses were proposed prior to the publishing of the NLST study, they were not based upon the observed mortality reduction seen in the NLST, nor specifics regarding the LDCT screening protocol in terms of characteristics of patients screened, screening intervals, or duration. One study, performed by McMahon *et al.* simulated an existing patient-level lung cancer model. Costs per quality-adjusted life-year (QALY) gained were estimated for LDCT screening, smoking-cessation alone, or combined programs [41]. Annual screening of current and former smokers aged 50-74 years were estimated to cost between $126,000 and $169,000 per QALY based on 20 pack-year smoking history and between $110,000 and $166,000 per QALY with a 40 pack-year smoking history). If screening was postulated to halve smoking rates, the cost of annual screening was projected to decrease to less than $75,000 per QALY. However, if such impact of LDCT screening upon smoking cessation did occur, screening with LDCT would be no more cost effective than smoking cessation interventions alone. This study suggests that cost-effectiveness may be intimately linked to achievable smoking cessation rates associated with lung cancer screening. Black *et al.,* applying cost-effectiveness analysis to the NLST results, examined mean-life years, QALYs, costs per person, and incremental cost-effectiveness ratios (ICERs) for 3 study groups (LDCT screening, chest radiograph screening, and no screening) [42]. Compared with no screening, LDCT was estimated to cost an additional $1631 per person, provide an additional 0.0316 life-years per person, and 0.0201 QALY's per person. Such estimations translated into an estimated cost of $81,000 per QALY gained, and $52,000 per life-year gained. Both figures appear to fall within range of similar cost-effectiveness seen in screening interventions for other malignancies. Interestingly, subgroup analysis suggests that LDCT screening may be more cost-effective in individuals at highest risk of lung cancer and in women. Regardless, cost-effectiveness estimations are likely to change dramatically following implementation and refinement of lung cancer screening.

A final area of ongoing interest surrounding LDCT screening revolves around the potential for patient distress that is postulated to accompany LDCT screening, identification of abnormalities, and any invasive diagnostic testing that may be required. Only a few studies have evaluated patient distress in the arena of LDCT screening, although there is suggestion that limited short-term psychological discomfort may result from the process of LDCT screening [43]. It should be noted, however, that no studies have demonstrated long-term psychological impediment or reduction in overall quality of life due to lung cancer screening. Regardless, such theoretical concerns should inform clinicians of the necessity to obtain appropriate informed consent and invite patients into the process of shared decision-making when considering LDCT screening in the high-risk patient population.

FUTURE DIRECTIONS

Even in the wake of widespread implementation of LDCT screening for lung cancer, other approaches beyond thoracic imaging are also under study including independent assays or used in combination with imaging for lung cancer screening and diagnosis. The use of biologic markers, such as those based upon differential gene expression between patients with malignant and non-malignant disease, is in development. A recent study examined a bronchial-airway gene-expression classifier for the purposes of improving the diagnostic performance of bronchoscopy in the diagnosis of lung cancer [44]. In indeterminate-risk patients, a negative gene-expression classifier in conjunction with a non-diagnostic bronchoscopic evaluation, provided support to allow for a more conservative approach to subsequent diagnostic testing. Application of similar differential genomic approaches through analysis of airway epithelium or blood-based tissues could someday be utilized for primary or secondary lung cancer screening. Additional methods including exhaled breath analysis for volatile compounds [45], serum measurement of tumor specific proteins [46], differential quantitation of tumor-specific antibodies [47], and micro-RNA's are currently under development. While not currently influencing the standard of care, these techniques may prove essential diagnostic tools for the early detection of lung cancer in high-risk populations moving forward.

CONCLUSION

We believe that lung cancer screening is important, considering disease prevalence and the impact screening could have worldwide. Screening will undoubtedly evolve over time and may move toward other modalities, either in addition to, or beyond our current use of LDCT imaging. But for today, imaging has to be the screening methodology. While LDCT remains central to effective screening, it should be viewed only as a single pillar in the framework of a high-quality, multi-disciplinary lung cancer screening program. As LDCT screening extends into wide-spread availability and adoption, the overall impact of lung cancer screening programs will depend upon adherence and implementation of core components necessary for success. These components, including clear communication with patients about the risks and benefits of lung cancer screening, a commitment to smoking cessation counseling, tracking of LDCT results to ensure proper follow-up of positive scans, and appropriate referral for non-nodule findings detected on LDCT such as airways disease and emphysema, lie at the root of lung cancer screening.

Lung cancer programs will, first and foremost, need to determine which individuals in their local region are most likely to receive benefit from LDCT screening. While current consensus guidelines rely upon inclusion criteria of screened participants in the NLST, extrapolation to other high-risk populations likely to receive benefit will need to be assessed. For example, the USPFTF has extended the upper age limit of screening to 80 year-olds based upon modeling performed by the Cancer Intervention and Surveillance Modeling Network through the Agency for Healthcare Research and Quality [48]. The National Comprehensive Cancer Network (NCCN) defines "high risk" as age greater than 50 with a 20 pack year smoking history and a risk factor for lung cancer such as having other chronic lung diseases like chronic obstructive pulmonary disease [49]. Individual screening programs will need to rely upon prospective trials and internal programmatic review to assess whether expansion of inclusion criteria is generalizable to their own population. Additional determinations regarding duration of LDCT screening and imaging intervals will need to be reviewed on a local level as well. Ongoing studies are likely to inform these screening dimensions in the future.

Another important component necessary for lung cancer screening relates to the parameters that trigger nodule surveillance and downstream diagnostic intervention. Nodule characteristics such as size, composition, and rate of interval progression will need to be determined to inform screening policy. The importance of programmatic reporting, data capture, and adherence to pre-determined diagnostic algorithms for identified nodules cannot be understated. While manual triage of reported findings is possible, utilization of automated systems through the electronic medical record to trigger appropriate provider alerts as well as to allow for an automated patient contact for follow-up imaging is attractive. Regardless of the reporting system employed, a critical component of lung cancer screening effectiveness will depend upon the creation of a multidisciplinary team capable of providing necessary diagnostic and therapeutic intervention for nodule evaluation and lung cancer treatment. Subspecialty care provided by pulmonologists, thoracic surgeons, radiologists, radiation oncologists, medical oncologists, and smoking cessation specialists will be necessary to obtain similar survival outcomes and the low complication rates appreciated in the NLST.

Finally, the cornerstone to any effective lung cancer screening program relies upon unwavering dedication to efforts of smoking cessation. Whether through offerings of formal smoking cessation programs or simply informed discussions between providers and individuals at the initiation of lung cancer screening and its continuation, the opportunities to intervene are significant. Future successes in modifying smoking behavior will affect not only lung cancer screening moving forward, but more importantly, hopefully reduce the profound impact of this deadly disease in the future.

SUMMARY

Lung cancer is the leading cause of cancer-related deaths worldwide, with the majority of diagnoses associated with tobacco smoke exposure. While smoking prevention and cessation efforts are central to reducing lung cancer incidence and cancer-related mortality, development of effective lung cancer screening approaches are essential given current lung cancer prevalence. Historical attempts to screen lung cancer through chest radiography and sputum cytology resulted in earlier diagnosis of lung cancers, without improvement in cancer-related mortality or stage shift. The National Lung Screening Trial (NLST) was the first trial to successfully demonstrate that low-dose computed tomography (LDCT) screening for lung cancer decreases cancer-related and all-cause mortality. Current consensus guidelines recommend annual LDCT screening for individuals at high-risk for the development of lung cancer. Prospective trials are needed to refine selection of optimal screening populations, duration and intervals. Successful implementation of lung cancer screening programs will require a multi-disciplinary approach to care allowing for nodule surveillance with expertise in lung cancer diagnosis and treatment.

CONFLICT OF INTEREST

The authors declare no conflict of interest, financial or otherwise.

ACKNOWLEDGEMENTS

Declared none.

REFERENCES

[1] Centers for Disease Control and Prevention National Center for Health Statistics.. CDC WONDER On-line Database, compiled from Compressed Mortality File 1999-2012 Series 20 No 2R. 2014.

[2] American Cancer Society. Cancer Facts and Figures 2015. Atlanta: American Cancer Society 2015.

[3] Siegel R, Ma J, Zou Z, Jemal A. Cancer statistics, 2014. CA Cancer J Clin 2014; 64(1): 9-29. [http://dx.doi.org/10.3322/caac.21208] [PMID: 24399786]

[4] Siegel R, Naishadham D, Jemal A. Cancer statistics, 2012. CA Cancer J Clin 2012; 62(1): 10-29. [http://dx.doi.org/10.3322/caac.20138] [PMID: 22237781]

[5] U.S. Department of Health and Human Services. The Health Consequences of Smoking: A Report of the US Surgeon General. 2004.

[6] Wilson JM, Junger G. Principles and practices of screening for disease. Geneva, Switzerland: World Health Organization; 1968 Report No: Public Health Papers No 34 1968.

[7] Fontana RS, Sanderson DR, Woolner LB, Taylor WF, Miller WE, Muhm JR. Lung cancer screening: the Mayo program. J Occup Med 1986; 28(8): 746-50. [http://dx.doi.org/10.1097/00043764-198608000-00038] [PMID: 3528436]

[8] Marcus PM, Bergstralh EJ, Zweig MH, Harris A, Offord KP, Fontana RS. Extended lung cancer incidence follow-up in the Mayo Lung Project and overdiagnosis. J Natl Cancer Inst 2006; 98(11): 748-56. [http://dx.doi.org/10.1093/jnci/djj207] [PMID: 16757699]

[9] Frost JK, Ball WC Jr, Levin ML, *et al.* Early lung cancer detection: results of the initial (prevalence) radiologic and cytologic screening in the Johns Hopkins study. Am Rev Respir Dis 1984; 130(4): 549-54. [PMID: 6091505]

[10] Flehinger BJ, Melamed MR, Zaman MB, Heelan RT, Perchick WB, Martini N. Early lung cancer detection: results of the initial (prevalence) radiologic and cytologic screening in the Memorial Sloan-Kettering study. Am Rev Respir Dis 1984; 130(4): 555-60. [PMID: 6091506]

[11] Kubík A, Polák J. Lung cancer detection. Results of a randomized prospective study in Czechoslovakia. Cancer 1986; 57(12): 2427-37. [http://dx.doi.org/10.1002/1097-0142(19860615)57:12<2427::AID-CNCR2820571230>3.0.CO;2-M] [PMID: 3697941]

[12] Oken MM, Hocking WG, Kvale PA, *et al.* PLCO Project Team. Screening by chest radiograph and lung cancer mortality: the Prostate, Lung, Colorectal, and Ovarian (PLCO) randomized trial. JAMA 2011; 306(17): 1865-73. [http://dx.doi.org/10.1001/jama.2011.1591] [PMID: 22031728]

[13] Beckmann EC. CT scanning the early days. Br J Radiol 2006; 79(937): 5-8. [http://dx.doi.org/10.1259/bjr/29444122] [PMID: 16421398]

[14] Itoh S, Ikeda M, Isomura T, *et al.* Screening helical CT for mass screening of lung cancer: application of low-dose and single-breath-hold scanning. Radiat Med 1998; 16(2): 75-83. [PMID: 9650893]

[15] Mettler FA Jr, Huda W, Yoshizumi TT, Mahesh M. Effective doses in radiology and diagnostic nuclear medicine: a catalog. Radiology 2008; 248(1): 254-63. [http://dx.doi.org/10.1148/radiol.2481071451] [PMID: 18566177]

[16] Kaneko M, Eguchi K, Ohmatsu H, *et al.* Peripheral lung cancer: screening and detection with low-dose spiral CT *versus* radiography. Radiology 1996; 201(3): 798-802. [http://dx.doi.org/10.1148/radiology.201.3.8939234] [PMID: 8939234]

[17] Sone S, Takashima S, Li F, *et al.* Mass screening for lung cancer with mobile spiral computed tomography scanner. Lancet 1998; 351(9111): 1242-5. [http://dx.doi.org/10.1016/S0140-6736(97)08229-9] [PMID: 9643744]

[18] Swensen SJ, Jett JR, Hartman TE, *et al.* CT screening for lung cancer: five-year prospective

experience. Radiology 2005; 235(1): 259-65.
[http://dx.doi.org/10.1148/radiol.2351041662] [PMID: 15695622]

[19] Infante M, Cavuto S, Lutman FR, *et al.* DANTE Study Group. A randomized study of lung cancer screening with spiral computed tomography: three-year results from the DANTE trial. Am J Respir Crit Care Med 2009; 180(5): 445-53.
[http://dx.doi.org/10.1164/rccm.200901-0076OC] [PMID: 19520905]

[20] Infante M, Chiesa G, Solomon D, *et al.* DANTE Study Group. Surgical procedures in the DANTE trial, a randomized study of lung cancer early detection with spiral computed tomography: comparative analysis in the screening and control arm. J Thorac Oncol 2011; 6(2): 327-35.
[http://dx.doi.org/10.1097/JTO.0b013e318200f523] [PMID: 21178639]

[21] Aberle DR, Adams AM, Berg CD, *et al.* National Lung Screening Trial Research Team. Reduced lung-cancer mortality with low-dose computed tomographic screening. N Engl J Med 2011; 365(5): 395-409.
[http://dx.doi.org/10.1056/NEJMoa1102873] [PMID: 21714641]

[22] Centers for Medicare & Medicaid Services (CMS). Decision Memo for Screening for Lung Cancer with Low Dose Computed Tomography (LDCT) (CAG-00439N). 2015.

[23] Horeweg N, Scholten ET, de Jong PA, *et al.* Detection of lung cancer through low-dose CT screening (NELSON): a prespecified analysis of screening test performance and interval cancers. Lancet Oncol 2014; 15(12): 1342-50.
[http://dx.doi.org/10.1016/S1470-2045(14)70387-0] [PMID: 25282284]

[24] Saghir Z, Dirksen A, Ashraf H, *et al.* CT screening for lung cancer brings forward early disease. The randomised Danish Lung Cancer Screening Trial: status after five annual screening rounds with low-dose CT. Thorax 2012; 67(4): 296-301.
[http://dx.doi.org/10.1136/thoraxjnl-2011-200736] [PMID: 22286927]

[25] Pastorino U, Rossi M, Rosato V, *et al.* Annual or biennial CT screening *versus* observation in heavy smokers: 5-year results of the MILD trial. Eur J Cancer Prev 2012; 21(3): 308-15.
[http://dx.doi.org/10.1097/CEJ.0b013e328351e1b6] [PMID: 22465911]

[26] Becker N, Motsch E, Gross ML, *et al.* Randomized study on early detection of lung cancer with MSCT in Germany: results of the first 3 years of follow-up after randomization. J Thorac Oncol 2015; 10(6): 890-6.
[http://dx.doi.org/10.1097/JTO.0000000000000530] [PMID: 25783198]

[27] Lopes Pegna A, Picozzi G, Mascalchi M, *et al.* ITALUNG Study Research Group. Design, recruitment and baseline results of the ITALUNG trial for lung cancer screening with low-dose CT. Lung Cancer 2009; 64(1): 34-40.
[http://dx.doi.org/10.1016/j.lungcan.2008.07.003] [PMID: 18723240]

[28] McRonald FE, Yadegarfar G, Baldwin DR, *et al.* The UK Lung Screen (UKLS): demographic profile of first 88,897 approaches provides recommendations for population screening. Cancer Prev Res (Phila) 2014; 7(3): 362-71.
[http://dx.doi.org/10.1158/1940-6207.CAPR-13-0206] [PMID: 24441672]

[29] Kovalchik SA, Tammemagi M, Berg CD, *et al.* Targeting of low-dose CT screening according to the risk of lung-cancer death. N Engl J Med 2013; 369(3): 245-54.
[http://dx.doi.org/10.1056/NEJMoa1301851] [PMID: 23863051]

[30] Tammemägi MC, Katki HA, Hocking WG, *et al.* Selection criteria for lung-cancer screening. N Engl J Med 2013; 368(8): 728-36.
[http://dx.doi.org/10.1056/NEJMoa1211776] [PMID: 23425165]

[31] Raji OY, Duffy SW, Agbaje OF, *et al.* Predictive accuracy of the Liverpool Lung Project risk model for stratifying patients for computed tomography screening for lung cancer: a case-control and cohort validation study. Ann Intern Med 2012; 157(4): 242-50.
[http://dx.doi.org/10.7326/0003-4819-157-4-201208210-00004] [PMID: 22910935]

[32] Travis WD, Brambilla E, Noguchi M, *et al.* International association for the study of lung cancer/american thoracic society/european respiratory society international multidisciplinary classification of lung adenocarcinoma. J Thorac Oncol 2011; 6(2): 244-85. [http://dx.doi.org/10.1097/JTO.0b013e318206a221] [PMID: 21252716]

[33] Russell PA, Wainer Z, Wright GM, Daniels M, Conron M, Williams RA. Does lung adenocarcinoma subtype predict patient survival?: A clinicopathologic study based on the new International Association for the Study of Lung Cancer/American Thoracic Society/European Respiratory Society international multidisciplinary lung adenocarcinoma classification. J Thorac Oncol 2011; 6(9): 1496-504. [http://dx.doi.org/10.1097/JTO.0b013e318221f701] [PMID: 21642859]

[34] Pinsky PF, Gierada DS, Black W, *et al.* Performance of Lung-RADS in the National Lung Screening Trial: a retrospective assessment. Ann Intern Med 2015; 162(7): 485-91. [http://dx.doi.org/10.7326/M14-2086] [PMID: 25664444]

[35] Bach PB, Mirkin JN, Oliver TK, *et al.* Benefits and harms of CT screening for lung cancer: a systematic review. JAMA 2012; 307(22): 2418-29. [http://dx.doi.org/10.1001/jama.2012.5521] [PMID: 22610500]

[36] Berrington de González A, Kim KP, Berg CD. Low-dose lung computed tomography screening before age 55: estimates of the mortality reduction required to outweigh the radiation-induced cancer risk. J Med Screen 2008; 15(3): 153-8. [http://dx.doi.org/10.1258/jms.2008.008052] [PMID: 18927099]

[37] Marshall D, Simpson KN, Earle CC, Chu C. Potential cost-effectiveness of one-time screening for lung cancer (LC) in a high risk cohort. Lung Cancer 2001; 32(3): 227-36. [http://dx.doi.org/10.1016/S0169-5002(00)00239-7] [PMID: 11390004]

[38] Wisnivesky JP, Mushlin AI, Sicherman N, Henschke C. The cost-effectiveness of low-dose CT screening for lung cancer: preliminary results of baseline screening. Chest 2003; 124(2): 614-21. [http://dx.doi.org/10.1378/chest.124.2.614] [PMID: 12907551]

[39] Mahadevia PJ, Fleisher LA, Frick KD, Eng J, Goodman SN, Powe NR. Lung cancer screening with helical computed tomography in older adult smokers: a decision and cost-effectiveness analysis. JAMA 2003; 289(3): 313-22. [http://dx.doi.org/10.1001/jama.289.3.313] [PMID: 12525232]

[40] Manser R, Dalton A, Carter R, Byrnes G, Elwood M, Campbell DA. Cost-effectiveness analysis of screening for lung cancer with low dose spiral CT (computed tomography) in the Australian setting. Lung Cancer 2005; 48(2): 171-85. [http://dx.doi.org/10.1016/j.lungcan.2004.11.001] [PMID: 15829317]

[41] McMahon PM, Kong CY, Bouzan C, *et al.* Cost-effectiveness of computed tomography screening for lung cancer in the United States. J Thorac Oncol 2011; 6(11): 1841-8. [http://dx.doi.org/10.1097/JTO.0b013e31822e59b3] [PMID: 21892105]

[42] Black WC, Gareen IF, Soneji SS, *et al.* National Lung Screening Trial Research Team. Cost-effectiveness of CT screening in the National Lung Screening Trial. N Engl J Med 2014; 371(19): 1793-802. [http://dx.doi.org/10.1056/NEJMoa1312547] [PMID: 25372087]

[43] Slatore CG, Sullivan DR, Pappas M, Humphrey LL. Patient-centered outcomes among lung cancer screening recipients with computed tomography: a systematic review. J Thorac Oncol 2014; 9(7): 927-34. [http://dx.doi.org/10.1097/JTO.0000000000000210] [PMID: 24922011]

[44] Silvestri GA, Vachani A, Whitney D, *et al.* AEGIS Study Team. A bronchial genomic classifier for the diagnostic evaluation of lung cancer. N Engl J Med 2015; 373(3): 243-51. [http://dx.doi.org/10.1056/NEJMoa1504601] [PMID: 25981554]

[45] Mazzone PJ. Analysis of volatile organic compounds in the exhaled breath for the diagnosis of lung cancer. J Thorac Oncol 2008; 3(7): 774-80.
[http://dx.doi.org/10.1097/JTO.0b013e31817c7439] [PMID: 18594325]

[46] Ostroff RM, Bigbee WL, Franklin W, *et al.* Unlocking biomarker discovery: large scale application of aptamer proteomic technology for early detection of lung cancer. PLoS One 2010; 5(12): e15003.
[http://dx.doi.org/10.1371/journal.pone.0015003] [PMID: 21170350]

[47] Boyle P, Chapman CJ, Holdenrieder S, *et al.* Clinical validation of an autoantibody test for lung cancer. Ann Oncol 2011; 22(2): 383-9.
[http://dx.doi.org/10.1093/annonc/mdq361] [PMID: 20675559]

[48] Agency for Healthcare Research and Quality. Benefits and harms of computed tomography lung cancer screening programs for high-risk populations. Agency for Healthcare Research and Quality. Rockville MD, Ed. 2013. AHRQ Publication No. 13-05196-EF-2

[49] Wood DE, Kazerooni E, Baum SL, *et al.* National comprehension cancer network. Lung cancer screening, version 1.2015: featured updates to the NCCN guidelines. J Natl Compr Canc Netw 2015; 13(1): 23-34.
[http://dx.doi.org/10.6004/jnccn.2015.0006] [PMID: 25583767]

CHAPTER 5

Electromagnetic Navigational Bronchoscopy

Akrum Al Zubaidi[*, 1], **Srinivas R Mummadi**[2] and **Peter Y. Hahn**[2]

[1] *Division of Pulmonary, Critical Care and Sleep Medicine, Department of Medicine, National Jewish Health, Denver, Colorado CO, USA*

[2] *Metro Health-University of Michigan Health, Wyoming MI, USA*

Abstract: Electromagnetic navigation bronchoscopy (EMN) is a platform that has been used to diagnose peripheral pulmonary nodules for over 10 years. The basic components of EMN consist of planning software, a location board that emit low frequency electromagnetic waves, computed tomography scan used to reconstruct a three dimensional map, a sensor and computer integration. There is a disparity between reports of diagnostic accuracy of the navigational platforms. This chapter discusses technical aspects of the procedure in addition to review the literature on diagnostic accuracy of ENB, inherent limitations to diagnostic accuracy and methods to increase yield. Also discussed are other applications of ENB in addition to future directions of ENB.

Keywords: Bronchoscopy, Electromagnetic navigation bronchoscopy, Solitary pulmonary nodule.

INTRODUCTION

Pulmonary nodules are being seen in increasing numbers yearly along with the number of chest CT scans. Up to 1.5 million nodules are identified each year without an increase in the number of lung cancers identified each year [1]. Given the enormous and growing burden that pulmonary nodules place on healthcare systems, the ACCP has updated their guidelines in 2013 to be aligned with Fleischner Society guidelines. Per these guidelines, patients with pulmonary nodules are to be risk stratified by evaluating the patients pretest probability of malignancy, assessment of ability to undergo invasive procedure, and applying shared decision-making [2, 3].

* **Corresponding author Akrum Al Zubaidi:** Division of Pulmonary, Critical Care and Sleep Medicine, Department of Medicine, National Jewish Health, Denver, Colorado CO, USA; Tel: 877.225.5654; aknelle@hotmail.com; al-zubaidia@njhealth.org

Ali I. Musani (Ed.)

Generally speaking, patients fall into one of three management pathways; radiological monitoring, tissue biopsy or surgical resection. In a patient with an indeterminate pulmonary nodule with a pretest probability of 5-65% or higher and who wishes to undergo a minimally invasive procedure it is recommended that the patient undergo tissue sampling *via* bronchoscopy or trans-thoracic needle aspiration (TTNA). The most appropriate biopsy technique can be a challenging clinical decision based on risk benefit analysis and variables such as tumor size, bronchus sign, and location among others (Table **1**).

Table 1. Factors associated with higher diagnostic yield in navigational bronchoscopy.

Patient characteristics
Greater nodule size [21]
Air-bronchus sign [22, 23]
Non-lower lobe location [22]
Operator/center characteristics
Number of procedures performed [16]
Application of TBNA [5, 22]
Usage of radial EBUS to aid in localization [24]
Reduced registration error [13]
Availability of ROSE [13]
Preponderance of lung cancer patients [5]
Catheter suction technique [25]

The diagnostic sensitivity of TTNA is high, especially for the larger peripheral-based lung lesion, and TTNA is a relatively rapid procedure. TTNA's sensitivity falls for smaller or more central lesions, where the false negative rate can approach 25% to 30%. The risk of pneumothorax (9-54%) and bleeding increases with central biopsies. Furthermore, TTNA usually does not provide information about nodal staging [4].

The yield of traditional fluoroscopic guided bronchoscopy has been disappointingly low especially with small and peripheral lesions. Techniques like EMN guided biopsy offer the possibility of improved yield for such lesions. Advantages of using a bronchoscopic technique rather than TTNA are its superior safety profile, ability to stage in one procedure and improved diagnostic rates of more central lesions. The ability to perform bronchoscopic biopsy of peripheral pulmonary nodules using an electromagnetic navigation system allows the bronchoscopist to steer the scope and catheter through the bronchial tree to the target lesion.

DESCRIPTION OF PROCEDURE

Various commercial vendors produce electro-magnetic navigational (EMN) systems [5]. Electromagnetic Navigational Bronchoscopy consists of: planning software, a location board which emit low frequency electromagnetic waves, extended working channel (EWC), locatable guide (LG) which contains sensors that allow tracking of position and orientation throughout the electromagnetic field.

PLANNING

CT images in Digital Imaging and Communications In Medicine (DICOM) format must be obtain in a pre-determined protocol with specific slice thickness, convolution and overlap that is loaded onto the planning station and software. The planning software reconstructs the images into a multiplanar format as well as a three dimensional virtual bronchoscopic view (Fig. **1**).

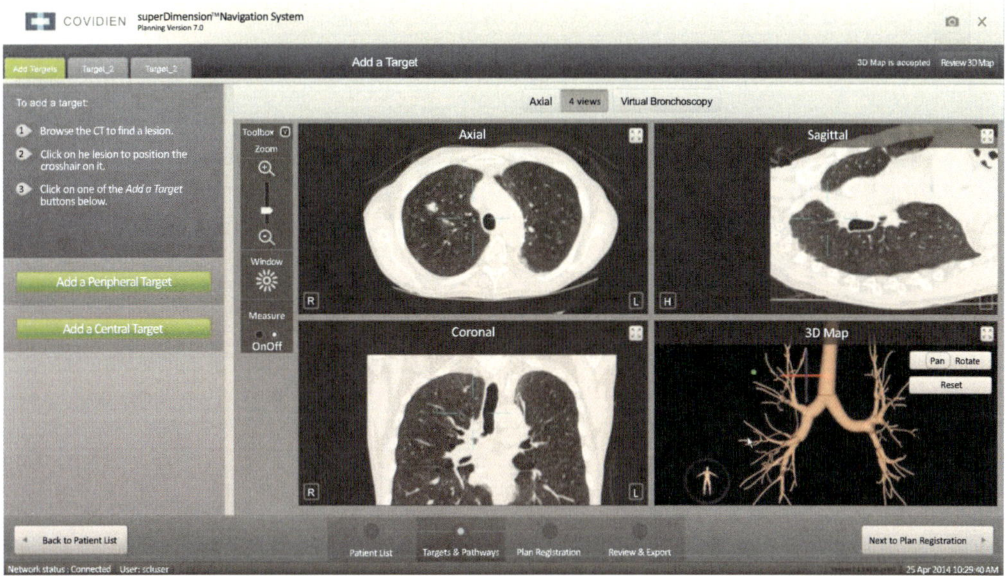

Fig. (1). Planning screen showing multiplanar format and 3D reconstructed tracheobronchial tree.

The target lesion(s) is outlined and a pathway is mapped by tracing points to the nearest bronchus to the trachea. Multiple pathways can be planned leading to the targeted lesion(s). Once planning is complete a virtual bronchoscopy (Show figure) can be visualized that replicates the route that the bronchoscopist will actually perform during the procedure. Registration of six anatomical points will also be captured and marked for the purpose of manual registration if needed during the actual procedure. Data will be saved to a USB drive for use on the system located in the procedure room.

PRE-PROCEDURE SET UP

Metal objects, equipment and mobile devices that may interfere with the electromagnetic field are to be moved further than one meter from the patient's bed. The location board is placed underneath the patient's mattress in a location that captures the patients region of interest. Three location pads are placed on the patient's chest to enable tracking of the locatable guide.

DESCRIPTION OF PROCEDURE

A surveillance bronchoscopy is done to examine the airways to at least the first sub segmental regions in order to exclude endobronchial lesions in addition to clear any secretions. The locatable guide and the extended working channel are then inserted through the working channel of the bronchoscope until 8mm of the locatable guide is visible. Registration is then completed by touching registration points that correspond to anatomical landmarks that provide data for location and orientation of the locatable guide in regards to the patient's actual anatomy. Registration is measured as Average Fiducial Target Registration Error and divergence should be less than 5mm. If divergence is greater than 5mm reduced navigational accuracy can occur and registration should be repeated to decrease the amount of divergence.

The procedure screen can be customized to the operators' preference to include axial, sagittal, coronal, 3D dynamic map, 3D static map, video bronchoscope, virtual bronchoscope, maximum intensity projection and other views to display the planned pathway in addition to location of LG along this pathway (Fig. **2**). The target is also shown in addition to the distance to target among other data points which aid in navigation of the LG/EWC to the lesion. Once the bronchoscopist follows the pathway to a sub segment which leads to the target the bronchoscope is wedged into that sub segment. The EWC and LG are slowly advanced keeping either waypoints or target in aim. The LG can be aimed in multiple directions to make turns into branches along the path by turning the handle in which the EWC has a set flex angle.

Once the LG tip is aligned with and in close proximity to the target lesion the EWC is locked into position on the bronchoscope. At this point the LG can be removed and a radial probe EBUS and/or fluoroscopy can be used to confirm EWC position and saved for use when tools are inserted into the EWC. The biopsy tools are then inserted through the EWC in a similar fashion to the LG and samples are obtained (Fig. **3**).

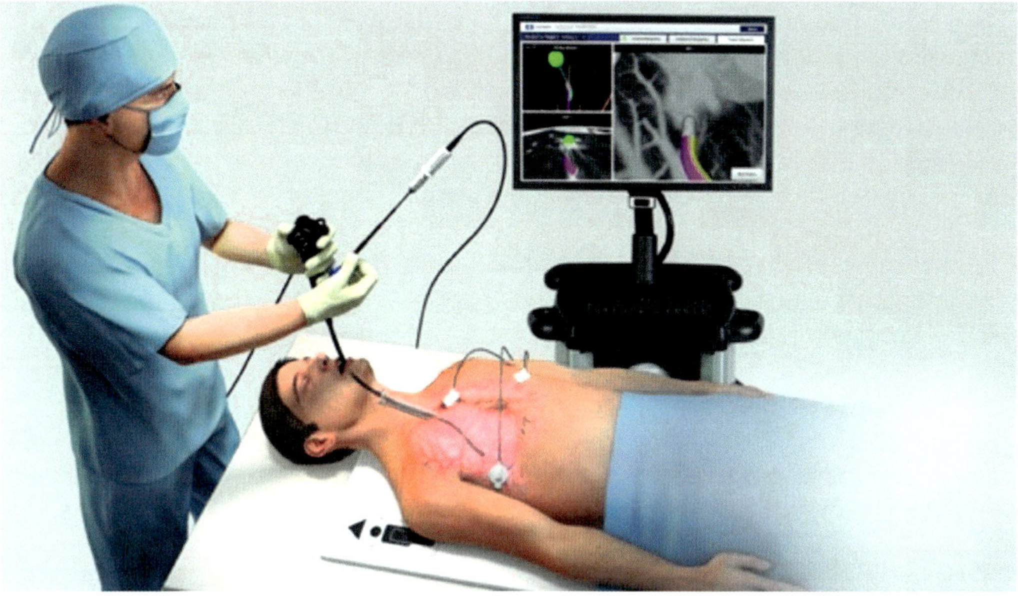

Fig. (2). Procedure Screen displaying custom operator views.

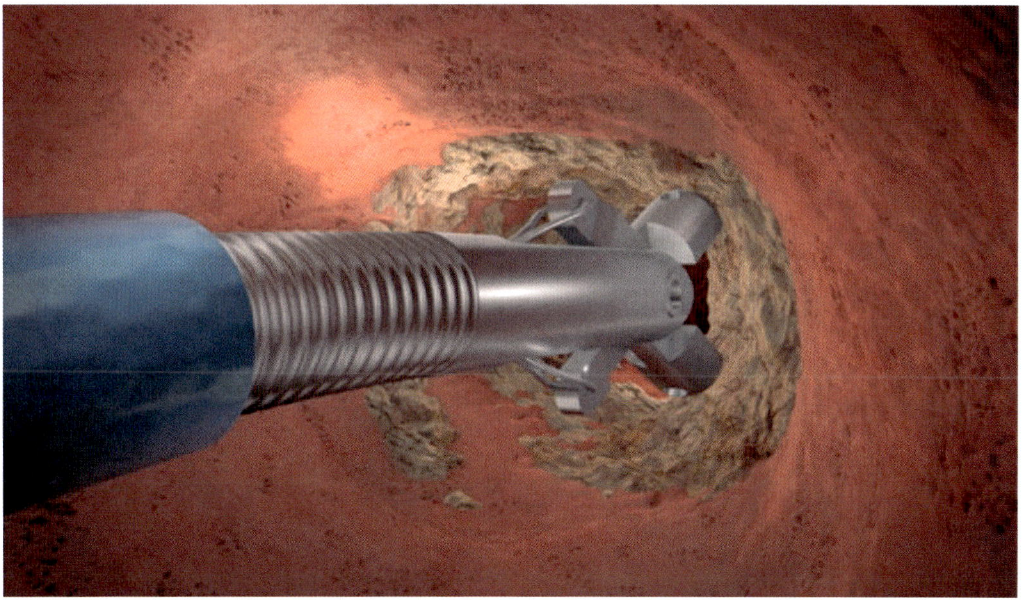

Fig. (3). Biopsy forceps sampling lesion through extended working channel.

DIAGNOSTIC ACCURACY

There is a disparity between reports of diagnostic accuracy of the navigational platforms. This is attributed to studying differing cohorts of patients as well as varying definitions of diagnostic yield [6]. Earlier studies were done at clinical centers of excellence and had high rates of lung cancer prevalence (high pre-test probability for lung cancer in patient cohorts). This could have theoretically led to an overestimation of positive results and thus aid in publication bias [5]. A more recent meta-analysis of initial studies from centers well versed in navigational bronchoscopy (n=1,106 patients) reported a pooled sensitivity and specificity of 82% (95% CI, 78-85%) and 100% (95% CI, 98-100%), respectively [7]. More useful measures of clinical utility (likelihood ratios) reveal an important facet of navigational bronchoscopy's utility in day to day clinical situations [8]. The pooled negative likelihood ratio (LR- of 0.2) reported in the study reflects a moderate decrease in the post test probability (30%) of the suspected disease after a negative bronchoscopy result [7]. On the same token, the reported high positive likelihood ratio (LR + of 18.75) reflects the importance of positive navigational bronchoscopy results in increasing the posttest probability of the suspected disease by an impressive large magnitude.

More recently, data from a longitudinal registry spanning over 4 years revealed a rather surprising result [5]. Conventional bronchoscopy outperformed navigational bronchoscopy in terms of diagnostic performance [n=581 patients]. The registry was comprised of community and academic medical centers. More importantly, the registry did not have a preponderance of lung cancer patients as seen in earlier navigational bronchoscopy studies. The registry analysis revealed a tendency to use it for smaller lesions (<= 2cm). This subgroup likely represents a diagnostically challenging cohort. Such a selection bias could explain the observed lower diagnostic yield in the navigational bronchoscopy cohort of AQuIRE registry [9]. Other factors such as the presence of strong ancillary services (CT surgery, Interventional radiology) can affect the selection of candidates for navigational bronchoscopy and thus the yield in a plausible manner.

WHAT CAN BE DONE TO INCREASE YIELD?

Peripheral application of TBNA is strongly associated with improved yield in all types of bronchoscopy including navigational bronchoscopy [5]. TBNA sampling was found to be relatively underutilized in day to day clinical practice as gleaned from the results of the AQuIRE registry. Various authors have reported a consistent increase in diagnostic yield after combining additional modalities (Radial-EBUS, Rapid Onsite Evaluation) with the EMN platform [5, 10]. In fact, the application of radial-EBUS leads to a synergistic effect which has been shown in multiple studies [5, 11]. Usage of rapid on site cytology evaluation (ROSE) improves yield in diagnostic navigational bronchoscopy [12, 13].

Type of anesthesia does not seem to affect the diagnostic yield of navigation bronchoscopy in controlled clinical trials as well as registry studies [5, 11].

In this era of precision and personalized medicine, a diagnosis of the sub-type of lung cancer is no longer the end point in clinical decision-making. The obtained samples should be adequate to allow for molecular testing. In a study comprising 65 procedures, 17 patients were eligible for further molecular testing [14]. Navigational bronchoscopy specimens were adequate in 16/17 patients, thus establishing its effectiveness for this purpose [14].

The steep learning curve inherent in a complex multi-stage activity such as navigation bronchoscopy impacts diagnostic yield and results in increased utilization of resource [15, 16]. Efforts should be made to reduce the steepness of such a learning curve. A thorough knowledge of correlating chest imaging with endoscopic appearance of airways is recommended to overcome the barrier of increased time spent in navigation. That means the location of interest should be defined at the segmental level with reasonable clarity after examination of chest CT images and before planning is commenced *(e.g., Left upper Lobe, Anterior sub segment)*. Various resources exist in aiding the trainee bronchoscopist in developing the skillset of correlating CT images with endoscopic landmarks [17]. Cadaveric models to simulate navigation to peripheral pulmonary lesions have been described [18].

INHERENT LIMITATIONS THAT CAN AFFECT DIAGNOSTIC YIELD

The extended working channel allows the navigational bronchoscopist to reach areas previously considered unreachable in an accurate manner. This vaunted ability also introduces a theoretical limitation that could affect diagnostic yield. Biopsies performed *via* the EWC tend to be limited to a specified location leading to an “all or none” phenomenon in terms of diagnostic performance [9].

Respiratory variation can also affect the diagnostic yield especially considering the fact that navigational sampling is relatively confined to a narrow focus. It has been shown that lesions move on an average by 17.6 mm between end-inspiration and expiration [19]. Such respiratory variation occurred in a larger magnitude in the lower lobes [19]. This could explain the association between lower lobe nodules and decreased navigation bronchoscopy yields [11, 20].

OTHER APPLICATIONS OF THE NAVIGATION PLATFORM

The primary application of navigational bronchoscopy is to aid the bronchoscopist in diagnostic sampling of peripheral lung lesions. Peripheral lung lesions are defined as beyond the segmental bronchus thus ruling out endobronchial biopsy.

Other applications have also been described.

Navigational bronchoscopy has been used to aid in localization of small non-visible, non-palpable peripheral lung lesions and subsequent insertion of fiducials/methylene blue dye [26 - 29]. This helps in image guided radiotherapy sessions as well as aiding the surgeon in quick localization of the target area to be subjected to wedge resection [30].

Navigational bronchoscopy has been described to aid in trans-bronchial needle aspiration (TBNA) of mediastinal and hilar lymph nodes [31]. In a prospective randomized controlled trial, diagnostic yield in the navigational arm was superior to conventional bronchoscopy (72.8% vs 42.3%, $p<0.005$) [31]. However, other dedicated bronchoscopy platforms (convex-EBUS) exist for sampling mediastinal and hilar lymph nodes and it is the authors' experience to use convex EBUS platform for this purpose.

Insertion of brachytherapy catheters with therapeutic intent has also been described [32]. Animal studies have demonstrated the feasibility of bronchoscopy guided radio frequency ablation of early stage cancerous lesions; however significant technological limitations are existing in this application [33].

COMPLICATIONS

Due to the likely area of sampling being closer to the visceral pleura, there is a theoretical concern for iatrogenic pneumothoraces. However, a systematic review of collective navigational experience revealed a low incidence of pneumothoraces (0.5%) requiring chest tube insertion [7]. Electromagnetic navigation platform's magnetic field can interfere with implanted cardioverter-defibrillators (ICD). In a study comprising 13 patients using ICD's, real time testing revealed a pattern of faithful working and rescue of patients in whom ventricular fibrillation was induced [34, 35]. Overall, electromagnetic navigation appears to be safe in patients with implanted pacemakers and ICD's. However, careful monitoring of these patients during navigational bronchoscopy is recommended.

FUTURE DIRECTIONS

Nonsurgical approaches to peripheral lung nodules are clearly not standardized. Randomized controlled trials are needed to compare navigational platforms with non-navigational platforms. Inconclusive diagnostic results from navigational bronchoscopy resulting in additional procedures are a concern. Multiplatform approaches to peripheral lung lesions in a single procedural setting are evolving (using bronchial genomic classifiers [36], radial EBUS, navigational bronchoscopy and navigational trans thoracic needle aspiration during a single procedural setting) [37]. It remains to see if such a combined approach will increase the diagnostic accuracy of sampling peripheral lesions as well as avoid unnecessary continued testing. Given the initial cost of acquiring navigational platforms and additional repetitive costs incurred by pre-procedural imaging, time spent and using proprietary tools, further cost effectiveness studies are needed [38]. The potential for applying curative treatments (*e.g. radiofrequency ablation in a "heat and destroy" session*) [39] for stage 1 lung cancer patients during a diagnostic navigation session is very promising. Further refinement of technology and clinical trials are needed to confirm the role of navigational bronchoscopy in the management of peripheral lung lesions.

CONFLICT OF INTEREST

Dr. Hahn is a Consultant, Medtronic SuperDimension and Auris Surgical Robotics.

ACKNOWLEDGEMENTS

Declared none.

REFERENCES

[1] Gould MK, Tang T, Liu IL, *et al.* Recent Trends in the Identification of Incidental Pulmonary Nodules. Am J Respir Crit Care Med 2015; 192(10): 1208-14. [http://dx.doi.org/10.1164/rccm.201505-0990OC] [PMID: 26214244]

[2] Gould MK, Donington J, Lynch WR, *et al.* Evaluation of individuals with pulmonary nodules: when is it lung cancer? Diagnosis and management of lung cancer American College of Chest Physicians evidence-based clinical practice guidelines Chest. 3rd ed. 2013; 143: pp. (5 Suppl)e93S-e120S.

[3] MacMahon H, Austin JH, Gamsu G, *et al.* Fleischner Society. Guidelines for management of small pulmonary nodules detected on CT scans: a statement from the Fleischner Society. Radiology 2005; 237(2): 395-400. [http://dx.doi.org/10.1148/radiol.2372041887] [PMID: 16244247]

[4] Yung RC. Tissue diagnosis of suspected lung cancer: selecting between bronchoscopy, transthoracic needle aspiration, and resectional biopsy. Respir Care Clin N Am 2003; 9(1): 51-76. [http://dx.doi.org/10.1016/S1078-5337(02)00083-7] [PMID: 12820712]

[5] Ost DE, Ernst A, Lei X, *et al.* AQuIRE Bronchoscopy Registry. Diagnostic Yield and Complications of Bronchoscopy for Peripheral Lung Lesions. Results of the AQuIRE Registry. Am J Respir Crit Care Med 2016; 193(1): 68-77. [http://dx.doi.org/10.1164/rccm.201507-1332OC] [PMID: 26367186]

[6] Gex G, Pralong JA, Combescure C, Seijo L, Rochat T, Soccal PM. Diagnostic yield and safety of electromagnetic navigation bronchoscopy for lung nodules: a systematic review and meta-analysis. Respiration 2014; 87(2): 165-76. [http://dx.doi.org/10.1159/000355710] [PMID: 24401166]

[7] Zhang W, Chen S, Dong X, Lei P. Meta-analysis of the diagnostic yield and safety of electromagnetic navigation bronchoscopy for lung nodules. J Thorac Dis 2015; 7(5): 799-809. [PMID: 26101635]

[8] Deeks JJ, Altman DG. Diagnostic tests 4: likelihood ratios. BMJ 2004; 329(7458): 168-9.

[http://dx.doi.org/10.1136/bmj.329.7458.168] [PMID: 15258077]

[9] Ferguson JS, Sonetti DA. Surprised but Not Shaken: AQuIRE Sheds New Light on Innovations in Bronchoscopy. Am J Respir Crit Care Med 2016; 193(1): 9-10. [http://dx.doi.org/10.1164/rccm.201509-1907ED] [PMID: 26720786]

[10] Steinfort DP, Bonney A, See K, Irving LB. Sequential multimodality bronchoscopic investigation of peripheral pulmonary lesions. Eur Respir J 2016; 47(2): 607-14. [http://dx.doi.org/10.1183/13993003.00786-2015] [PMID: 26541529]

[11] Bowling MR, Kohan MW, Walker P, Efird J, Ben Or S. The effect of general anesthesia *versus* intravenous sedation on diagnostic yield and success in electromagnetic navigation bronchoscopy. J Bronchology Interv Pulmonol 2015; 22(1): 5-13. [http://dx.doi.org/10.1097/LBR.0000000000000120] [PMID: 25590477]

[12] Loo FL, Halligan AM, Port JL, Hoda RS. The emerging technique of electromagnetic navigation bronchoscopy-guided fine-needle aspiration of peripheral lung lesions: promising results in 50 lesions. Cancer Cytopathol 2014; 122(3): 191-9. [http://dx.doi.org/10.1002/cncy.21373] [PMID: 24323803]

[13] Karnak D, Ciledağ A, Ceyhan K, Atasoy C, Akyar S, Kayacan O. Rapid on-site evaluation and low registration error enhance the success of electromagnetic navigation bronchoscopy. Ann Thorac Med 2013; 8(1): 28-32. [http://dx.doi.org/10.4103/1817-1737.105716] [PMID: 23440066]

[14] Ha D, Choi H, Almeida FA, *et al.* Histologic and molecular characterization of lung cancer with tissue obtained by electromagnetic navigation bronchoscopy. J Bronchology Interv Pulmonol 2013; 20(1): 10-5. [http://dx.doi.org/10.1097/LBR.0b013e31828197e9] [PMID: 23328135]

[15] Stather DR, Maceachern P, Chee A, Dumoulin E, Tremblay A. Trainee impact on advanced diagnostic bronchoscopy: an analysis of 607 consecutive procedures in an interventional pulmonary practice. Respirology 2013; 18(1): 179-84. [http://dx.doi.org/10.1111/j.1440-1843.2012.02270.x] [PMID: 23016797]

[16] Lamprecht B, Porsch P, Wegleitner B, Strasser G, Kaiser B, Studnicka M. Electromagnetic navigation bronchoscopy (ENB): Increasing diagnostic yield. Respir Med 2012; 106(5): 710-5. [http://dx.doi.org/10.1016/j.rmed.2012.02.002] [PMID: 22391437]

[17] Shah P. Atlas of Flexible Bronchoscopy. CRC Press 2011. [http://dx.doi.org/10.1201/b13458]

[18] Chen A, Machuzak M, Edell E, Silvestri GA. Peripheral bronchoscopy training using a human cadaveric model and simulated tumor targets. J Bronchology Interv Pulmonol 2016; 23(1): 83-6. [http://dx.doi.org/10.1097/LBR.0000000000000200] [PMID: 26348696]

[19] Chen A, Pastis N, Furukawa B, Silvestri GA. The effect of respiratory motion on pulmonary nodule location during electromagnetic navigation bronchoscopy. Chest 2015; 147(5): 1275-81. [http://dx.doi.org/10.1378/chest.14-1425] [PMID: 25357229]

[20] Eberhardt R, Anantham D, Ernst A, Feller-Kopman D, Herth F. Multimodality bronchoscopic diagnosis of peripheral lung lesions: a randomized controlled trial. Am J Respir Crit Care Med 2007; 176(1): 36-41. [http://dx.doi.org/10.1164/rccm.200612-1866OC] [PMID: 17379850]

[21] Jensen KW, Hsia DW, Seijo LM, *et al.* Multicenter experience with electromagnetic navigation bronchoscopy for the diagnosis of pulmonary nodules. J Bronchology Interv Pulmonol 2012; 19(3): 195-9. [http://dx.doi.org/10.1097/LBR.0b013e3182616ece] [PMID: 23207460]

[22] Balbo PE, Bodini BD, Patrucco F, *et al.* Electromagnetic navigation bronchoscopy and rapid on site evaluation added to fluoroscopy-guided assisted bronchoscopy and rapid on site evaluation: improved

yield in pulmonary nodules. Minerva Chir 2013; 68(6): 579-85.
[PMID: 24193290]

[23] Gaeta M, Pandolfo I, Volta S, *et al.* Bronchus sign on CT in peripheral carcinoma of the lung: value in predicting results of transbronchial biopsy. AJR Am J Roentgenol 1991; 157(6): 1181-5.
[http://dx.doi.org/10.2214/ajr.157.6.1950861] [PMID: 1950861]

[24] Chee A, Stather DR, Maceachern P, *et al.* Diagnostic utility of peripheral endobronchial ultrasound with electromagnetic navigation bronchoscopy in peripheral lung nodules. Respirology 2013; 18(5): 784-9.
[http://dx.doi.org/10.1111/resp.12085] [PMID: 23521707]

[25] Eberhardt R, Morgan RK, Ernst A, Beyer T, Herth FJ. Comparison of suction catheter *versus* forceps biopsy for sampling of solitary pulmonary nodules guided by electromagnetic navigational bronchoscopy. Respiration 2010; 79(1): 54-60.
[http://dx.doi.org/10.1159/000232394] [PMID: 19648733]

[26] Tay JH, Wallbridge PD, Larobina M, Russell PA, Irving LB, Steinfort DP. Electromagnetic Navigation Bronchoscopy-directed Pleural Tattoo to Aid Surgical Resection of Peripheral Pulmonary Lesions. J Bronchology Interv Pulmonol 2015.
[PMID: 26496089]

[27] Sun J, Mao X, Xie F, Han B, Chen H. Electromagnetic navigation bronchoscopy guided injection of methylene blue combined with hookwire for preoperative localization of small pulmonary lesions in thoracoscopic surgery. J Thorac Dis 2015; 7(12): E652-6.
[PMID: 26793384]

[28] Anayama T, Qiu J, Chan H, *et al.* Localization of pulmonary nodules using navigation bronchoscope and a near-infrared fluorescence thoracoscope. Ann Thorac Surg 2015; 99(1): 224-30.
[http://dx.doi.org/10.1016/j.athoracsur.2014.07.050] [PMID: 25442988]

[29] Krimsky WS, Minnich DJ, Cattaneo SM, *et al.* Thoracoscopic detection of occult indeterminate pulmonary nodules using bronchoscopic pleural dye marking. J Community Hosp Intern Med Perspect 2014; 4: 4.
[http://dx.doi.org/10.3402/jchimp.v4.23084] [PMID: 24596652]

[30] Steinfort DP, Siva S, Kron T, *et al.* Multimodality guidance for accurate bronchoscopic insertion of fiducial markers. J Thorac Oncol 2015; 10(2): 324-30.
[http://dx.doi.org/10.1097/JTO.0000000000000389] [PMID: 25616177]

[31] Diken ÖE, Karnak D, Çiledağ A, *et al.* Electromagnetic navigation-guided TBNA vs conventional TBNA in the diagnosis of mediastinal lymphadenopathy. Clin Respir J 2015; 9(2): 214-20.
[http://dx.doi.org/10.1111/crj.12126] [PMID: 25849298]

[32] Harms W, Krempien R, Grehn C, Hensley F, Debus J, Becker HD. Electromagnetically navigated brachytherapy as a new treatment option for peripheral pulmonary tumors. Strahlenther Onkol 2006; 182(2): 108-11.
[http://dx.doi.org/10.1007/s00066-006-1503-2] [PMID: 16447018]

[33] Tsushima K, Koizumi T, Tanabe T, *et al.* Bronchoscopy-guided radiofrequency ablation as a potential novel therapeutic tool. Eur Respir J 2007; 29(6): 1193-200.
[http://dx.doi.org/10.1183/09031936.00111306] [PMID: 17360727]

[34] Magnani A, Balbo P, Facchini E, Occhetta E, Marino P. Lack of interference of electromagnetic navigation bronchoscopy to implanted cardioverter-defibrillator: in-vivo study. Europace 2014; 16(12): 1767-71.
[http://dx.doi.org/10.1093/europace/euu156] [PMID: 25082949]

[35] Magnani A, Matheoud R, Brambilla M, *et al.* In vitro tests of electromagnetic interference of electromagnetic navigational bronchoscopy to implantable cardioverter defibrillators. Europace 2012; 14(7): 1054-9.
[http://dx.doi.org/10.1093/europace/eur417] [PMID: 22277644]

[36] Silvestri GA, Vachani A, Whitney D, *et al.* AEGIS Study Team. A bronchial genomic classifier for the diagnostic evaluation of lung cancer. N Engl J Med 2015; 373(3): 243-51. [http://dx.doi.org/10.1056/NEJMoa1504601] [PMID: 25981554]

[37] Arias S, Lee H, Semaan R, *et al.* Use of Electromagnetic Navigational Transthoracic Needle Aspiration (E-TTNA) for Sampling of Lung Nodules. J Vis Exp 2015; (99): e52723. [PMID: 26067650]

[38] Reynisson PJ, Leira HO, Hernes TN, *et al.* Navigated bronchoscopy: a technical review. J Bronchology Interv Pulmonol 2014; 21(3): 242-64. [http://dx.doi.org/10.1097/LBR.0000000000000064] [PMID: 24992135]

[39] Eberhardt R, Kahn N, Herth FJ. 'Heat and destroy': bronchoscopic-guided therapy of peripheral lung lesions. Respiration 2010; 79(4): 265-73. [http://dx.doi.org/10.1159/000284015] [PMID: 20203535]

CHAPTER 6

Radial Probe Endobronchial Ultrasound Guided Bronchoscopy

David Hsia*

Division of Respiratory and Critical Care Physiology and Medicine, Harbor-UCLA Medical Center, 1000 W. Carson Street, Box 402, Torrance, CA 90509, USA

Abstract: Radial probe endobronchial ultrasonography (EBUS) provides real-time imaging which allows guided exploration of the airways beyond the visual reach of traditional flexible bronchoscopy. Using this technology, bronchoscopists are able to improve successful navigation of biopsy instruments to peripheral lung lesions and substantially improve diagnostic yields. Radial EBUS can also be used to evaluate anatomic structures underlying the mucosal surface, such as for guidance of transbronchial needle aspiration (TBNA), as well as to aid other therapeutic modalities such as the placement of fiducial markers for radiation therapy. Because of this expanded capability to identify precise targets within the lung, guided bronchoscopic navigation technologies now play a significant role in the clinical evaluation of peripheral pulmonary lesions.

Keywords: Bronchoscopic navigation, Diagnostic yields, Flexible bronchoscopy, Radial probe endobronchial ultrasonography (EBUS), Transbronchial needle aspiration (TBNA).

INTRODUCTION

Obtaining tissue samples from peripheral lung lesions is a common diagnostic challenge for physicians. While traditional flexible bronchoscopy provides direct visualization of the large airways as far as fourth or fifth generation airways, unguided transbronchial biopsy of small parenchymal lesions is suboptimal. Traditional flexible bronchoscopy is able to diagnose only about a third of lung cancers <2 cm in diameter, even with the assistance of fluoroscopy [1]. However, outcomes from numerous studies are decidedly even less favorable.

Radial probe endobronchial ultrasound (EBUS) uses an ultrasound transducer affixed to the tip of a flexible catheter which can be introduced through the

* **Corresponding author David Hsia:** Division of Respiratory and Critical Care Physiology and Medicine, Harbor-UCLA Medical Center, 1000 W. Carson Street, Box 402, Torrance, CA 90509, USA; Tel: 310-222-3801; Fax: 310-328-9849; E-mail: dhsia@labiomed.org

Ali I. Musani (Ed.)

working channel of a bronchoscope. The transducer rotates to provide a 360° image around the catheter tip. In 1992, initial investigations by Hürter and Hanrath used a 20-MHz transducer generating a limited resolution image to evaluate both central airway and peripheral lesions [2]. They described their experience evaluating malignant tissue in 74 patients with central airway disease and 26 patients with peripheral lesions. Heinrich Becker was instrumental in the further development of the techniques using radial probe EBUS to sample mediastinal lymph nodes and parenchymal lesions [3].

Since the subsequent development of dedicated linear or convex probe EBUS bronchoscopes for TBNA of mediastinal targets, radial probe EBUS is primarily used to provide real-time confirmation of successful localization of peripheral lung lesions. It can be used as an independent navigation method or in conjunction with other technologies as complementary techniques. The following discussion will include the procedural technique of performing radial probe EBUS, the impact on diagnostic yield, and a comparison to other navigational bronchoscopy methods.

PROCEDURE TECHNIQUE

The radial EBUS probe uses a 20-MHz transducer that spins in a 360° fashion at the end of a flexible catheter. This probe generates a two-dimensional image of the tissue surrounding the transducer. (Fig. **1**) The transducer is connected to a flexible catheter and can be introduced through the working channel of the flexible bronchoscope and into airways distal to the extent of normal visualization. Several probe sizes are commercially available ranging from 1.4 to 1.7 mm in diameter. A separate ultrasound processor is required for the radial EBUS probe and the EBUS image can either be displayed on the same video monitor as the white-light image or on a separate screen.

Since the radial EBUS probe is located within the airways, the ultrasound image represents a circular view around the airway with the probe situated at the center of the image. The probe can be advanced through the airway to systematically explore the lung to the distal extent that the probe can be advanced. The airways are serially explored until the airway with the target lesion is identified based on the ultrasound image. The probe is removed and bronchoscopy biopsy instruments can be introduced into the identified airway. Fluoroscopy can be used to assist in the sampling of the target lesion by biopsy forceps, aspiration needle, and cytology brush.

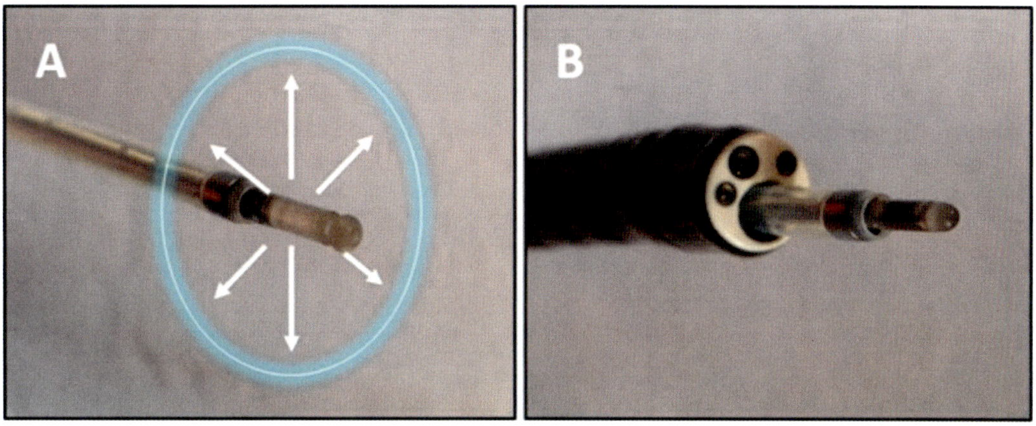

Fig. (1). Radial EBUS probe. (A) The EBUS transducer located in the tip of the probe rotates 360° to generate a two-dimensional circular image around the probe. (B) The radial EBUS probe and guide sheath extended from the working channel of a flexible bronchoscope.

Since the radial EBUS probe must be removed before bronchoscopy biopsy instruments can be inserted, real-time ultrasound visualization of lesion sampling is not possible. An obvious limitation is that biopsy instruments may be inadvertently inserted into the incorrect bronchi, especially if there is branching of the distal airways. In addition, measuring the exact distance that instruments need to be inserted to reach the target lesion is a source of potential error. Fluoroscopy can be used to assure that the path taken during insertion of biopsy instruments mimics the same path traveled during the removal of the radial EBUS probe. And in the event that the target lesion is identifiable on fluoroscopy, the two-dimensional fluoroscopy image can help guide biopsy instruments the proper distance to the target.

The development of the guide sheath technique was able to further minimize this potential problem [4, 5]. For this technique, the radial EBUS probe is introduced through the bronchoscope within a hollow guide sheath catheter. The probe and guide sheath catheter are advanced together as a single unit to explore the distal airways (Fig. **2**). Once the target lesion is identified, the guide sheath is positioned at the proximal edge of the target lesion. The radial EBUS probe is then removed, leaving the guide sheath catheter in place. The guide sheath catheter is then used as an extension of the bronchoscope working channel to introduce biopsy instruments, thereby ensuring that biopsy instruments can be consistently introduced along the same bronchial path. The length of the biopsy instruments can also be pre-marked at the proximal end relative to the guide sheath catheter to indicate when the distal end will emerge from the guide sheath catheter and into the adjacent target lesion. The guide sheath catheter has a radiopaque marker at the distal tip which can be used to assist fluoroscopic visualization and confirmation that the guide sheath catheter has not been displaced during the sampling process. In addition, the radial EBUS probe can be reinserted through the guide sheath catheter after biopsies have been performed to confirm maintenance of proper catheter location throughout the procedure.

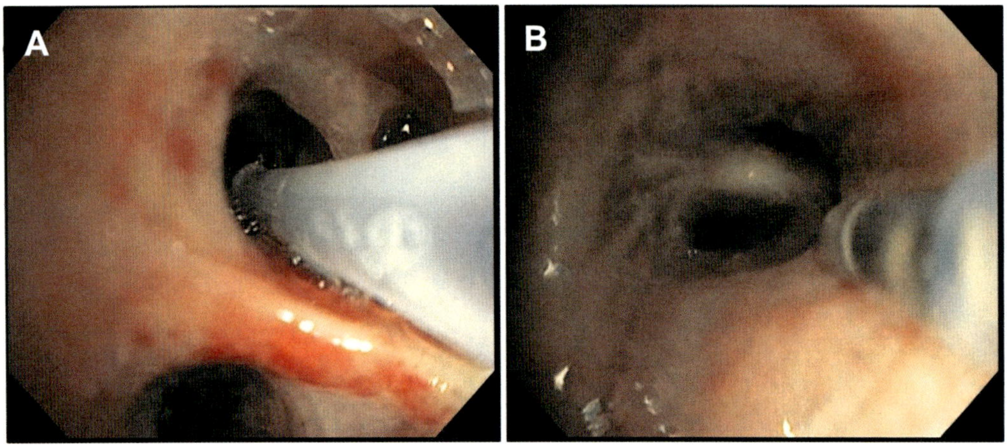

Fig. (2). Use of radial probe EBUS. (A) Introduction of the probe and guide sheath catheter into distal airways to identify peripheral lesions. (B) Evaluation of a proximal airway wall to identify the location of underlying mediastinal lymph nodes and blood vessels.

Localization of the target lesion requires careful pre-procedural evaluation of radiographic images by the bronchoscopist to identify the likely airways leading to the lesion. This requires the bronchoscopist to have refined knowledge of the bronchial tree anatomy. High quality computerized tomography (CT) images will usually permit identification of fourth or fifth generation airways which lead to the lesion. Careful evaluation of coronal and sagittal images in addition to axial plane images is often required to identify the best bronchial pathways to explore during the procedure. A double-hinged directional curette can also be used to assist in the navigation around branching of distal airways. The curette is inserted into the guide sheath to redirect the catheter into a different airway branch. Fluoroscopy is often used to assist in the manipulation of the curette. Lastly, radial EBUS probes can be used in conjunction with other guidance technologies to aid in directing the probe to the appropriate airway. The steerable guide of electromagnetic navigation (EMN) bronchoscopy can be used to direct the guide sheath catheter to the appropriate target location based on pre-planning CT scans, at which point the radial EBUS probe can be inserted to provide real-time confirmation that the target has been accurately localized. Ultrathin bronchoscopes are also useful to permit visual guidance of the guide sheath catheter insertion further into the bronchial tree, provided that the radial EBUS probe or catheter can fit within the working channel.

While radial probe EBUS is primarily used to confirm successful navigation to peripheral lung lesions, it may also be used to identify lymph nodes or masses adjacent to proximal airways that may not be amenable to biopsy *via* convex probe EBUS bronchoscopes. For example, lobar and sub-lobar lymph nodes are sometimes difficult to biopsy with convex probe EBUS bronchoscopes due to the small size of the airways relative to the bronchoscope. Target lesions in an upper lobe bronchi require significant flexion of the bronchoscope which may also pose difficulties for convex probe EBUS bronchoscopes. In contrast, a more flexible diagnostic bronchoscope can be used with a radial EBUS probe to locate the lesion and nearby blood vessels or other underlying structures. Conventional TBNA can then be performed to sample submucosal targets (Fig. **2**).

The radial EBUS probe can be cleaned and reused with a lifespan of approximately 50 cases. The durability of the radial EBUS probe is likely quite variable. One case series reported a considerably greater longevity of 150-200 cases per probe [6], though this may not be consistently reproduced in other institutions.

RADIAL EBUS IMAGING

Use of radial probe EBUS is dependent upon the bronchoscopist's ability to interpret the ultrasound images and determine when the target lesion has been reached. As demonstrated in Fig. (**3**), lung lesions can have different ultrasonographic appearances. Sound waves do not propagate well through air, and therefore normal aerated lung generates an ultrasound pattern described as having an appearance similar to a "snowstorm". Blood vessels adjacent to the bronchial walls can also be identified. The density difference of non-aerated lung and abnormal solid tissue will produce hyperechoic findings at their interface on ultrasound. Non-solid lesions or ground-glass opacities will not have this distinct interface and may produce a diffuse hyperintense acoustic shadow. This has been referred to as the "blizzard" sign by some authors [7]. It is also important to identify image artifacts created when the radial EBUS probe is inadvertently withdrawn into the guide sheath catheter, as lesions can be missed if this occurs.

Several authors have proposed radial EBUS image classification systems which may help to differentiate malignant from benign lesions. Kurimoto and colleagues divided nodule appearances into three types: homogenous (type I), the presence of hyperechoic dots and arcs (type II), and heterogenous (type III) [8]. Each type was subdivided further based on the presence of blood vessels, bronchioles, and other characteristics resulting in a total of 6 categories. They noted that the type I pattern was benign in 23 of 25 cases (92.0%) while type II and III patterns were malignant in 98 of 99 cases (99.0%). Chao and colleagues graded the ultrasound

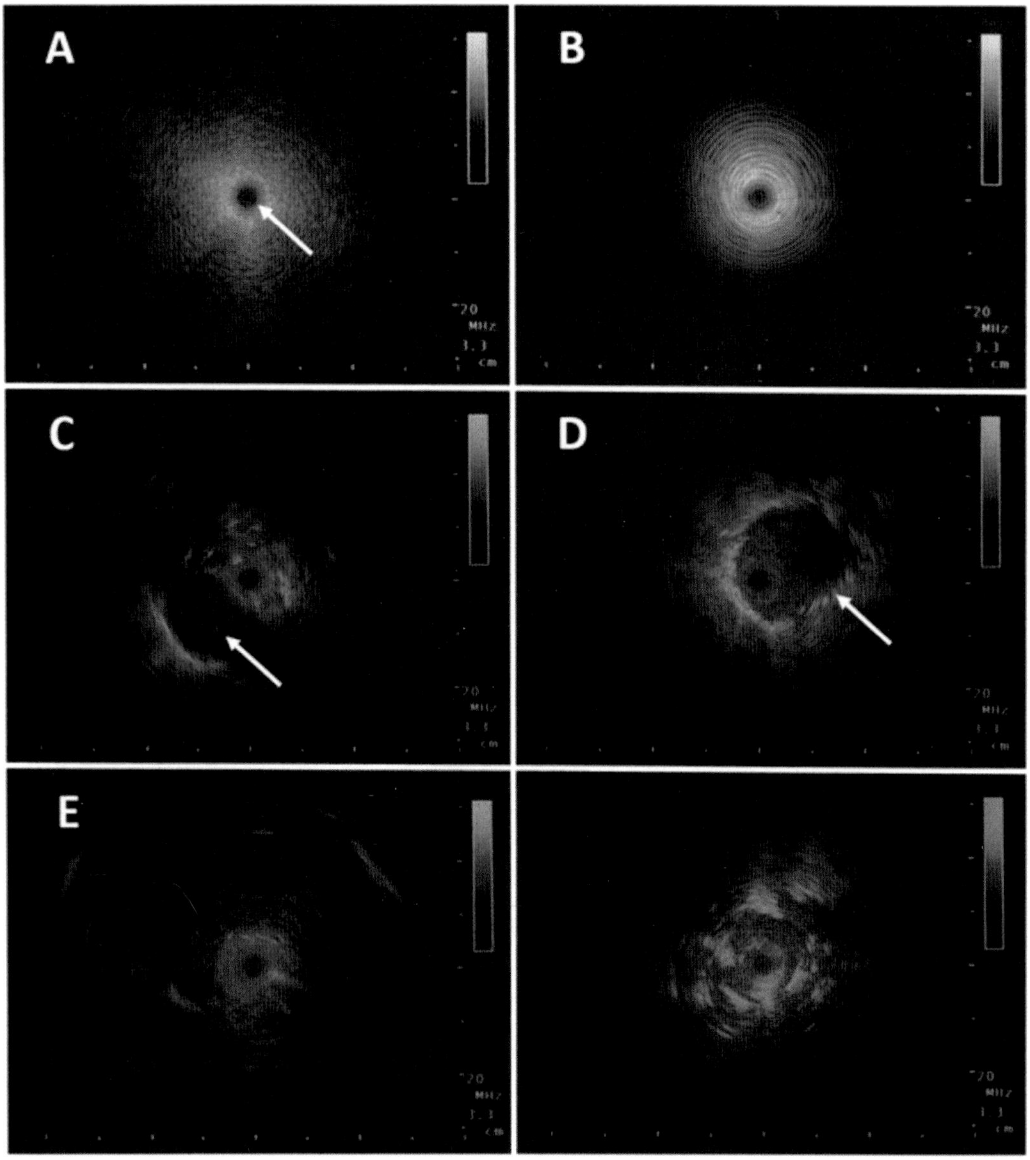

Fig. (3). Radial EBUS imaging. (A) Normal lung creates a "snowstorm" pattern due to poor propagation of ultrasound through air. The probe is located at the center of the image (arrow). (B) Artifact resulting from the probe being withdrawn into the guide sheath. (C) An adjacent blood vessel is indicated by the round, anechoic structure (arrow). (D) Lung nodule. The hyperechoic line represents the nodule edge (arrow). (E) Lung mass. Lesion size is indicated by the scale at the right and bottom of the display. (F) Heterogenous lung nodule with hyperechoic regions.

appearance of nodules based on 4 characteristics: continuous hyperechoic margins outside the lesion, homogenous or heterogeneous internal echoes, hyperechoic dots in the lesion, and concentric circles along the echo probe [9]. They found that homogenous internal echoes and concentric circles were associated with benign lesions in 94.7% and 87.5% of cases, respectively. The other two imaging patterns did not correlate significantly with benign or malignant lesions. They also reported that the evaluation of the ultrasound appearance of nodules took approximately 4 minutes of procedural time. At this time, classifying ultrasound image characteristics is primarily an academic exercise as no classification system is 100% sensitive or specific, and the complications from radial EBUS guided biopsy are low. In addition, classification based on predominant ultrasound patterns requires subjective evaluation by the bronchoscopist, which can result in variability in lesion classification. Biopsy remains the gold standard for diagnosis of benign and malignant lesions.

Diagnostic Yield and Factors Affecting Yield

The published diagnostic yield of bronchoscopy with radial probe EBUS directed biopsies is quite variable. However, reported studies also have significant heterogeneity in both patient and procedural variables. Some common limitations of published studies is that they are often retrospective evaluations, from single-centers, use limited numbers of bronchoscopists, and may have relatively small study populations. As a result, one must exercise caution when trying to generalize procedure performance characteristics to other settings or populations. Several meta-analyses have been performed to generate pooled analyses of these data to help overcome some of these study limitations. Diagnostic yield for radial probe EBUS guided biopsies is estimated to be 71% [10], while diagnostic sensitivity and specificity for lung cancer are 73% (95% CI, 70-76%) and 100% (95% CI, 99-100%), respectively [11]. However, studies included in these meta-analyses have significant variability for both diagnostic yield (range 53-86%) [10] and sensitivity for lung cancer (range 49-88%) [11]. Patient-related variables that may affect procedure performance characteristics and outcomes will be discussed in this section. In addition, other factors such as operator experience and use of additional guidance methods may also affect test performance.

Not surprisingly, lesion size is linked with procedural outcomes with a number of studies reporting improved diagnostic yield for larger lesions. Pooled data from 10 studies resulted in a diagnostic yield of 56.3% (95% CI, 51-61%) for lesions ≤2 cm compared to 77.7% (95% CI, 73-82%) for lesions >2 cm, with a total of 364 and 367 patients in each respective group [11]. A retrospective, single-center report of 467 patients similarly showed a direct correlation between diagnostic yield and lesion diameter, with yields of 58% (1-2 cm), 72% (2.1-3 cm), 77% (3.1-4 cm), 87% (4.1-5 cm), and 88% (>5.1 cm) [12]. In contrast, other studies evaluating only lung nodules <3 cm report no difference in yield based on nodule size, suggesting that other patient and procedural variables may play a more significant role in determining yield amongst smaller lesions [5, 13 - 15].

The diagnostic yield for malignant lesions is also likely to be higher than for benign lesions [11], making prevalence of malignancy in the study population an important consideration. It is also worthwhile to note that the specificity for malignant diagnoses is 100%, but is significantly lower for benign lesions. Histology specimens from transbronchial biopsy samples of benign lesions often demonstrates non-specific inflammatory changes. As a result, reported diagnostic yields often rely upon stability or regression of the lesion on subsequent radiographic imaging as an endpoint. Therefore, the pre-test probability for malignancy must be considered when interpreting the results of non-malignant biopsy findings in clinical use.

Another key factor affecting successful diagnostic biopsy is whether the target can be identified with the radial EBUS probe [5, 16 - 21]. The success rate of navigating the radial EBUS probe to the lesion ranges from 72-96% [5, 12, 17 - 21]. This variability likely reflects the heterogeneity in the respective study populations, lesion characteristics, as well as procedural techniques. In their retrospective series, Chen and colleagues noted that a directional curette was necessary to navigate to the target lesion in 21% of cases [12]. In addition, diagnostic yields are substantially higher if the radial EBUS probe can be positioned directly within the target lesion rather than adjacent or outside of the lesion [5, 12, 16]. Fig. (**4**) Diagnostic yields are reported to increase from approximately 42-48% to 84-87% when the probe is positioned within rather than adjacent to the lesion [5, 12].

Increasing the number of biopsies improves diagnostic yield, with optimization in yield after least five biopsy passes [16, 22]. Transbronchial biopsy has a higher diagnostic yield than other sampling modalities, but combination with brushing likely improves yield [5, 23]. The presence of an airway leading directly to the lesion, also known as the CT-bronchus sign, is less certain with reports of either no impact *versus* positive impact on diagnostic yield [15, 16, 24].

The significance of other factors are either not consistently demonstrated or reported in the medical literature. Lobar location of the lesion, use of fluoroscopy guidance, or the use of the guide-sheath technique have variable reported impact on yield. Other considerations such as the bronchoscopist experience, type of biopsy instrument used, distance to the lesion, and radiographic characteristics of the lesions (*e.g.* solid, part-solid, or non-solid) are not consistently reported in the medical literature making it difficult to assess the importance of these variables.

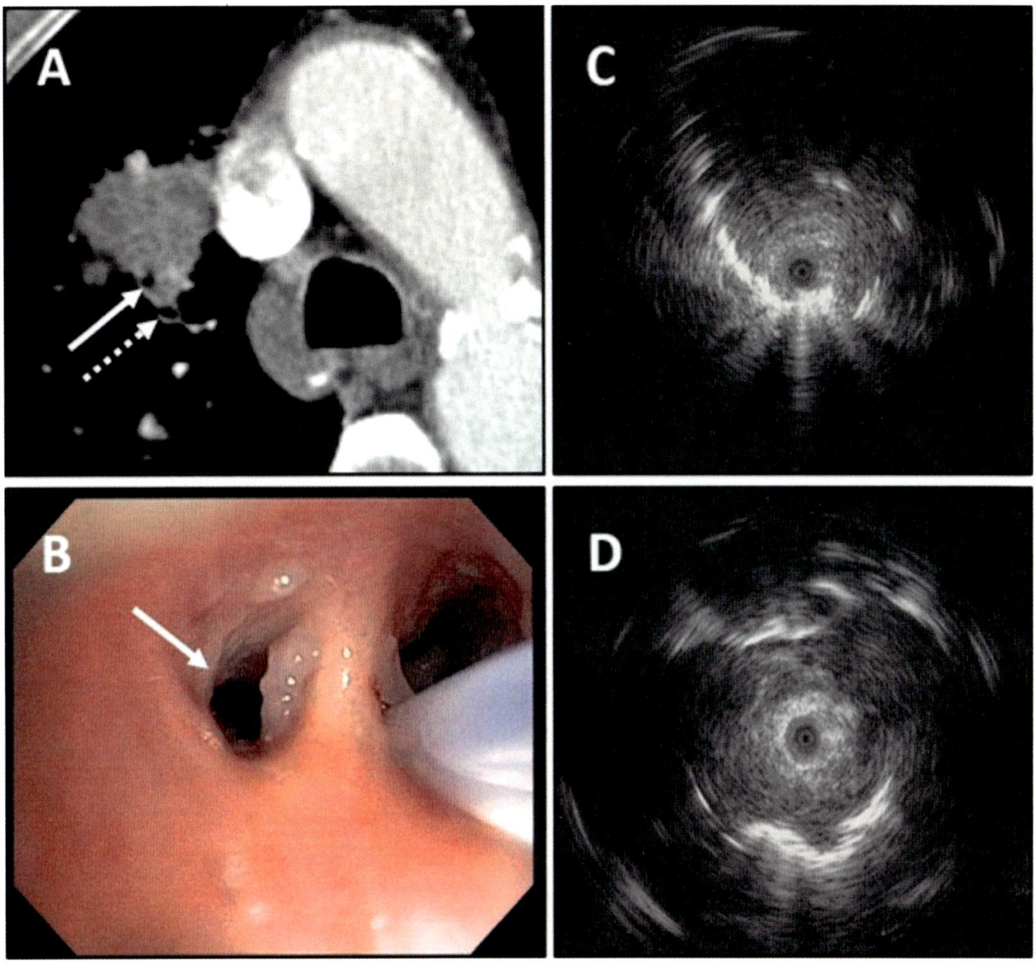

Fig. (4). Position of radial EBUS probe relative to the target lesion. (A) CT image of a mass in the right upper lobe, apical segment (RB1) with two proximal airways (solid and dotted arrows). (B) When the radial EBUS probe is inserted into the airway as shown (dotted arrow in panel A), an eccentric view is noted (C) indicating that the probe is positioned adjacent to the mass. When inserted into the airway indicated by the solid arrow (A and B), a concentric view is produced. (D) indicating positioning within the mass.

Procedure-related Complications

The principle complications related to the use of radial probe EBUS are similar to those from traditional transbronchial biopsy sampling. Pooled meta-analysis risk of pneumothorax following radial EBUS probe guided transbronchial biopsy is 1.0% [11]. In the included studies, the range of pneumothorax rates and total complication rates was 0-5.1% and 0-7.4%, respectively. The safety profile of radial EBUS probe guided sampling is therefore similar to traditional transbronchial biopsy. Routine post-procedure chest x-ray to evaluate for pneumothorax is not warranted in asymptomatic patients following traditional transbronchial biopsy [25] and that practice is commonly extended to radial EBUS probe guided procedures. Aside from pneumothorax, bleeding is an infrequent but significant procedure-specific complication occurring in only 1-2% of cases [12]. Other recommendations associated with pneumothorax and bleeding risk can be generalized from traditional transbronchial biopsy guidelines [25].

Comparison to Other Guided Bronchoscopy Methods

Physicians now have a variety of minimally-invasive methods by which to diagnose peripheral lung lesions. The historically poor diagnostic yields of traditional bronchoscopy have been improved significantly by new technologies such as radial probe EBUS, EMN, virtual bronchoscopy, and ultrathin bronchoscopy. Each of these modalities has unique procedural benefits that strengthen the physician's capability to diagnose peripheral lung lesions.

The primary benefit of radial probe EBUS is that it provides real-time confirmation that the target lesion has been located. Other guidance methods such as virtual bronchoscopy and EMN are dependent upon CT imaging to direct the biopsy accessories to the target location. However, limitations in CT acquisition will therefore limit the success of navigation by these methods. For example, if there have been interval changes in the size or location of a rapidly changing lesion, the bronchoscopist will be inadvertently guided to the wrong location based on data from the outdated image. Poor image quality due to respiratory motion artifact or secretions obscuring the airways will interfere with the EMN or virtual bronchoscopy technology to identify the bronchial anatomy. Ultrathin bronchoscopy can also provide real-time imaging into distal airways as far as eighth generation airways. But visualization is often limited in these very small airways, and some peripheral lesions lie beyond the visual reach of even ultrathin bronchoscopes. Ultrathin bronchoscopes also require smaller biopsy accessories to fit through the narrower working channel which can limit the diagnostic yield of biopsies or the amount of tissue available for specialized testing such as genetic marker testing for lung cancers.

In contrast, radial probe EBUS requires the bronchoscopist to have a good understanding of airway anatomy and be able to correlate precise anatomic locations from the CT scan with the bronchoscopic images during the procedure. It can be difficult to navigate the radial EBUS probe and guide-sheath catheter in distal airways, especially if airways are tortuous or distal branching is present. And lastly, the bronchoscopist needs to have expertise in interpreting the radial EBUS images to correctly identify when the radial EBUS probe has reached the target lesion. This can be especially challenging for non-solid or inflammatory lesions which often do not create an obvious hyperechoic border on radial probe EBUS imaging.

Equipment costs are also an important consideration when evaluating different navigation methods. Radial probe EBUS requires an ultrasound processor and a reusable EBUS probe. Virtual bronchoscopy and EMN both require specialized planning software and costly system hardware, and EMN also utilizes a disposable steerable guide catheter which adds considerably to procedure-related costs. And ultrathin bronchoscopy requires the purchase of specialized bronchoscopes which are ill-suited for routine bronchoscopy due to their narrow working channel diameter and limited optics.

Most data for diagnostic yields for guided bronchoscopy technologies stems from case series, making comparison between guidance methods problematic. Review of data calculates diagnostic yields of 67.0 (95% CI, 62.6-71.4%) for EMN, 70.0% (95% CI, 65.0-75.1%) for ultrathin bronchoscopy, and 72.0% (95% CI, 65.7-78.4%) for virtual bronchoscopy [10]. These data are comparable to the diagnostic yield of 71.1% (95% CI, 66.5-75.7%) for radial probe EBUS [10]. However, few studies directly compare navigation modalities. Direct comparison suggests that radial probe EBUS used in conjunction with traditional fluoroscopy guidance is better than fluoroscopy alone for lesions <3 cm [26]. And a prospective comparison between EMN and radial EBUS suggests that these are comparable technologies [27]. Diagnostic yield was 69% and 59% for radial probe EBUS and EMN, respectively, which were statistically similar. Performance characteristics were also similar between the two modalities for lesions ≤20 mm, 20-30 mm, and >30 mm.

Because no single technology is perfect, radial probe EBUS can be used in conjunction with either virtual bronchoscopy or EMN. After navigation is completed using either system, the radial EBUS probe can be inserted through the bronchoscope or EMN catheter to confirm successful navigation to the target lesion. In the previously mentioned comparison of radial probe EBUS to EMN, a third randomized group evaluated the combination of both modalities with a diagnostic yield of 88% which was statistically better than either modality used alone [27]. Diagnostic yield using both technologies was similarly improved for all sizes of lesions. The addition of radial EBUS to virtual bronchoscopy also improves diagnostic yields. Ishida and colleagues reported a diagnostic yield of 67.0% for radial probe EBUS alone compared to 80.4% when combined with virtual bronchoscopy for nodules ≤3 cm in size [28]. In contrast, the addition of radial probe EBUS to ultrathin bronchoscopy did not demonstrate any significant improvement over radial probe EBUS alone [29]. However, the relative paucity of prospective comparative data must be taken into account when generating conclusions about the respective performance characteristics of these different technologies.

Role of Radial Probe EBUS in Clinical Practice

Diagnosis of solitary pulmonary nodules is one obvious clinical application of radial probe EBUS technology. The emergence of CT imaging for routine workup of many clinical diseases leads to numerous incidentally identified lung nodules. Recent data and guidelines supporting CT screening for patients at high risk for lung cancer also leads to the discovery of many patients with lung nodules. The evaluation of lung nodules is a complex issue that cannot be adequately addressed in this forum. But in general, guidelines recommend that low risk nodules be followed with serial radiographs while higher risk nodules benefit from diagnostic surgical resection [30].

The evaluation of intermediate risk nodules, however, has been a difficult clinical problem for patients and physicians alike. Transthoracic needle aspiration (TTNA) has good sensitivity for lung lesions situated close to the pleura, with a meta-analysis pooled sensitivity of 90% (95% CI, 88-91%) [1]. Unfortunately, TTNA also is associated with a pooled risk for pneumothorax of 15%, and 7% risk of pneumothorax requiring a chest tube. Hemorrhage complicates TTNA only 1% of the time, but 18% of these cases require blood transfusion [1]. Despite these complications, TTNA remains clinically useful in the right situation. The emergence of improved diagnostic bronchoscopy methods, such as radial probe EBUS, has now enabled bronchoscopy to be incorporated into the evaluation algorithm for peripheral pulmonary nodules. Specific situations when radial probe EBUS guided bronchoscopy are appropriate for intermediate risk nodule evaluation include when clinical pretest probability and findings on imaging tests are discordant, in lesions with low to moderate probability for malignancy (~10-60%), when a benign diagnosis requiring specific medical treatment is suspected, and when a fully informed patient desires proof of a malignant diagnosis prior to surgery [1]. Guided diagnostic bronchoscopy can also be useful for high risk nodules in patients who are poor surgical candidates [30].

Other indications where radial probe EBUS may assist the bronchoscopist include staging of malignancies presenting with metastatic lesions to the lung and biopsy of infiltrates concerning for infectious or inflammatory processes. Radial probe EBUS can also be used for bronchoscopic placement of fiducial markers to guide radiation therapy for pulmonary malignancies in non-surgical candidates [31].

As previously noted, prevalence of malignancy influences the diagnostic sensitivity of radial probe EBUS bronchoscopy. It is therefore important to note that the incidence of malignancy in CT screening study patient populations are generally much lower than in studies examining performance characteristics of bronchoscopy with radial probe EBUS. And both of these study populations have important differences compared to patients encountered in clinical practice. Bronchoscopist experience is also likely to be vary in clinical practice compared to the medical literature. It is therefore likely that outcomes in a clinical patient population will differ from published data.

The role of radial probe EBUS and other navigation guidance techniques in algorithms for evaluating pulmonary lung nodules are currently limited by imperfect diagnostic yields coupled with the decreased survival outcomes of non-surgical therapies for early stage lung cancer. In the future, diagnostic algorithms will dramatically change if outcomes from less invasive therapies equal or outperform surgical resection. Improvements in therapeutic technologies, such as stereotactic body radiation therapy (SBRT) and bronchoscopy-delivered interventions, may one day transform our diagnostic approach to early stage lung cancers.

Procedural Training

As previously discussed, the impact of training experience on procedure outcomes has not been clearly demonstrated in the literature. Yamada and colleagues were unable to demonstrate any difference in diagnostic yields amongst operators with different levels of training and experience in bronchoscopy [16]. However, they theorized that this may have resulted from using at least two operators for each procedure to hold the bronchoscope and manipulate the guide sheath, radial EBUS probe, and biopsy accessories. It was likely that an experienced bronchoscopist would assist less experienced bronchoscopists, thereby influencing the procedure outcome. In addition, no studies looking at the learning curve of radial EBUS have been performed, so the effect of training for this procedure has not been well elucidated.

Nevertheless, generalization from other procedural data supports that all procedures have an associated learning curve. Therefore, standards have been created in the interest of maintaining appropriate diagnostic outcomes and ensuring patient safety. Several prominent societal guidelines were created by expert panel opinion for interventional pulmonology procedures. The purpose of these guidelines was to recommend a minimum number of procedures as a threshold for procedural competency. The American College of Chest Physicians recommends 50 radial probe EBUS cases for initial competency, while the European Respiratory Society and American Thoracic Society recommend 40 cases total for convex and radial probe EBUS [32, 33]. This volume of procedural experience is usually not encountered over the course of a traditional 3 year pulmonary/critical care subspecialty fellowship program, prompting the push for specialized intensive procedural training with a specific interventional pulmonology (IP) fellowship [34, 35]. Survey of participants in IP fellowship programs in the United States and Canada reported a mean of 75 radial probe EBUS cases during their additional one year of IP training [36]. However, it is unclear how this procedural volume compares to training sites outside of North America.

CONCLUSIONS

Radial probe EBUS guided bronchoscopy is an effective and safe method to obtain tissue in the diagnostic evaluation of peripheral lung lesions. Diagnostic yields and sensitivity for lung cancer are improved using radial probe EBUS compared to bronchoscopy with traditional transthoracic biopsy and brush sampling. Procedure performance characteristics are similar to other methods of guided navigation bronchoscopy, but improved when used as an adjunct with other complementary technologies. Radial probe EBUS has become a valuable tool for physicians in the evaluation of both malignant and benign peripheral lung lesions.

CONFLICT OF INTEREST

The authors declare no conflict of interest, financial or otherwise.

ACKNOWLEDGEMENTS

Declared none.

REFERENCES

[1] Rivera MP, Mehta AC, Wahidi MM. Establishing the diagnosis of lung cancer: Diagnosis and management of lung cancer, 3rd ed: American College of Chest Physicians evidence-based clinical practice guidelines. Chest 2013; 143(5) (Suppl.): e142S-65S.
[http://dx.doi.org/10.1378/chest.12-2353] [PMID: 23649436]

[2] Hürter T, Hanrath P. Endobronchial sonography: feasibility and preliminary results. Thorax 1992; 47(7): 565-7.
[http://dx.doi.org/10.1136/thx.47.7.565] [PMID: 1412103]

[3] Panchabhai TS, Mehta AC. Historical perspectives of bronchoscopy. Connecting the dots. Ann Am Thorac Soc 2015; 12(5): 631-41.
[http://dx.doi.org/10.1513/AnnalsATS.201502-089PS] [PMID: 25965540]

[4] Kikuchi E, Yamazaki K, Sukoh N, *et al.* Endobronchial ultrasonography with guide-sheath for peripheral pulmonary lesions. Eur Respir J 2004; 24(4): 533-7.
[http://dx.doi.org/10.1183/09031936.04.00138603] [PMID: 15459129]

[5] Kurimoto N, Miyazawa T, Okimasa S, *et al.* Endobronchial ultrasonography using a guide sheath increases the ability to diagnose peripheral pulmonary lesions endoscopically. Chest 2004; 126(3): 959-65.
[http://dx.doi.org/10.1378/chest.126.3.959] [PMID: 15364779]

[6] Hayama M, Izumo T, Matsumoto Y, Chavez C, Tsuchida T, Sasada S. Complications with endobronchial ultrasound with a guide sheath for the diagnosis of peripheral pulmonary lesions. Respiration 2015; 90(2): 129-35. Epub ahead of print. [http://dx.doi.org/10.1159/000431383] [PMID: 26112297]

[7] Izumo T, Sasada S, Chavez C, Matsumoto Y, Tsuchida T. Radial endobronchial ultrasound images for ground-glass opacity pulmonary lesions. Eur Respir J 2015; 45(6): 1661-8. [http://dx.doi.org/10.1183/09031936.00167914] [PMID: 25573408]

[8] Kurimoto N, Murayama M, Yoshioka S, Nishisaka T. Analysis of the internal structure of peripheral pulmonary lesions using endobronchial ultrasonography. Chest 2002; 122(6): 1887-94. [http://dx.doi.org/10.1378/chest.122.6.1887] [PMID: 12475821]

[9] Chao TY, Lie CH, Chung YH, Wang JL, Wang YH, Lin MC. Differentiating peripheral pulmonary lesions based on images of endobronchial ultrasonography. Chest 2006; 130(4): 1191-7. [http://dx.doi.org/10.1378/chest.130.4.1191] [PMID: 17035455]

[10] Wang Memoli JS, Nietert PJ, Silvestri GA. Meta-analysis of guided bronchoscopy for the evaluation of the pulmonary nodule. Chest 2012; 142(2): 385-93. [http://dx.doi.org/10.1378/chest.11-1764] [PMID: 21980059]

[11] Steinfort DP, Khor YH, Manser RL, Irving LB. Radial probe endobronchial ultrasound for the diagnosis of peripheral lung cancer: systematic review and meta-analysis. Eur Respir J 2011; 37(4): 902-10. [http://dx.doi.org/10.1183/09031936.00075310] [PMID: 20693253]

[12] Chen A, Chenna P, Loiselle A, Massoni J, Mayse M, Misselhorn D. Radial probe endobronchial ultrasound for peripheral pulmonary lesions. A 5-year institutional experience. Ann Am Thorac Soc 2014; 11(4): 578-82. [http://dx.doi.org/10.1513/AnnalsATS.201311-384OC] [PMID: 24635641]

[13] Paone G, Nicastri E, Lucantoni G, *et al.* Endobronchial ultrasound-driven biopsy in the diagnosis of peripheral lung lesions. Chest 2005; 128(5): 3551-7. [http://dx.doi.org/10.1378/chest.128.5.3551] [PMID: 16304312]

[14] Yoshikawa M, Sukoh N, Yamazaki K, *et al.* Diagnostic value of endobronchial ultrasonography with a guide sheath for peripheral pulmonary lesions without X-ray fluoroscopy. Chest 2007; 131(6): 1788-93. [http://dx.doi.org/10.1378/chest.06-2506] [PMID: 17565021]

[15] Hsia DW, Jensen KW, Curran-Everett D, Musani AI. Diagnosis of lung nodules with peripheral/radial endobronchial ultrasound-guided transbronchial biopsy. J Bronchology Interv Pulmonol 2012; 19(1): 5-11. [http://dx.doi.org/10.1097/LBR.0b013e31823fcf11] [PMID: 23207256]

[16] Yamada N, Yamazaki K, Kurimoto N, *et al.* Factors related to diagnostic yield of transbronchial biopsy using endobronchial ultrasonography with a guide sheath in small peripheral pulmonary lesions. Chest 2007; 132(2): 603-8. [http://dx.doi.org/10.1378/chest.07-0637] [PMID: 17573504]

[17] Shirakawa T, Imamura F, Hamamoto J, *et al.* Usefulness of endobronchial ultrasonography for transbronchial lung biopsies of peripheral lung lesions. Respiration 2004; 71(3): 260-8. [http://dx.doi.org/10.1159/000077424] [PMID: 15133346]

[18] Dooms CA, Verbeken EK, Becker HD, Demedts MG, Vansteenkiste JF. Endobronchial ultrasonography in bronchoscopic occult pulmonary lesions. J Thorac Oncol 2007; 2(2): 121-4. [http://dx.doi.org/10.1097/JTO.0b013e31802fbc96] [PMID: 17410026]

[19] Chung YH, Lie CH, Chao TY, *et al.* Endobronchial ultrasonography with distance for peripheral pulmonary lesions. Respir Med 2007; 101(4): 738-45. [http://dx.doi.org/10.1016/j.rmed.2006.08.014] [PMID: 17015004]

[20] Huang CT, Ho CC, Tsai YJ, Yu CJ, Yang PC. Factors influencing visibility and diagnostic yield of transbronchial biopsy using endobronchial ultrasound in peripheral pulmonary lesions. Respirology 2009; 14(6): 859-64.
[http://dx.doi.org/10.1111/j.1440-1843.2009.01585.x] [PMID: 19703067]

[21] Eberhardt R, Ernst A, Herth FJ. Ultrasound-guided transbronchial biopsy of solitary pulmonary nodules less than 20 mm. Eur Respir J 2009; 34(6): 1284-7.
[http://dx.doi.org/10.1183/09031936.00166708] [PMID: 19460785]

[22] Asahina H, Yamazaki K, Onodera Y, *et al.* Transbronchial biopsy using endobronchial ultrasonography with a guide sheath and virtual bronchoscopic navigation. Chest 2005; 128(3): 1761-5.
[http://dx.doi.org/10.1378/chest.128.3.1761] [PMID: 16162785]

[23] Boonsarngsuk V, Kanoksil W, Laungdamerongchai S. Comparison of diagnostic performances among bronchoscopic sampling techniques in the diagnosis of peripheral pulmonary lesions. J Thorac Dis 2015; 7(4): 697-703.
[PMID: 25973236]

[24] Evison M, Crosbie PA, Morris J, Martin J, Barber PV, Booton R. Can computed tomography characteristics predict outcomes in patients undergoing radial endobronchial ultrasound-guided biopsy of peripheral lung lesions? J Thorac Oncol 2014; 9(9): 1393-7.
[http://dx.doi.org/10.1097/JTO.0000000000000249] [PMID: 25122434]

[25] Du Rand IA, Blaikley J, Booton R, *et al.* British Thoracic Society Bronchoscopy Guideline Group. British Thoracic Society guideline for diagnostic flexible bronchoscopy in adults: accredited by NICE. Thorax 2013; 68 (Suppl. 1): i1-i44.
[http://dx.doi.org/10.1136/thoraxjnl-2013-203618] [PMID: 23860341]

[26] Sánchez-Font A, Giralt L, Vollmer I, Pijuan L, Gea J, Curull V. Endobronchial ultrasound for the diagnosis of peripheral pulmonary lesions. A controlled study with fluoroscopy. Arch Bronconeumol 2014; 50(5): 166-71.
[http://dx.doi.org/10.1016/j.arbr.2014.03.014] [PMID: 24439465]

[27] Eberhardt R, Anantham D, Ernst A, Feller-Kopman D, Herth F. Multimodality bronchoscopic diagnosis of peripheral lung lesions: a randomized controlled trial. Am J Respir Crit Care Med 2007; 176(1): 36-41.
[http://dx.doi.org/10.1164/rccm.200612-1866OC] [PMID: 17379850]

[28] Ishida T, Asano F, Yamazaki K, *et al.* Virtual Navigation in Japan Trial Group. Virtual bronchoscopic navigation combined with endobronchial ultrasound to diagnose small peripheral pulmonary lesions: a randomised trial. Thorax 2011; 66(12): 1072-7.
[http://dx.doi.org/10.1136/thx.2010.145490] [PMID: 21749984]

[29] Oki M, Saka H, Kitagawa C, *et al.* Randomized study of endobronchial ultrasound-guided transbronchial biopsy: thin bronchoscopic method *versus* guide sheath method. J Thorac Oncol 2012; 7(3): 535-41.
[http://dx.doi.org/10.1097/JTO.0b013e3182417e60] [PMID: 22198427]

[30] Gould MK, Donington J, Lynch WR, *et al.* Evaluation of individuals with pulmonary nodules: when is it lung cancer? Diagnosis and management of lung cancer, 3rd ed: American College of Chest Physicians evidence-based clinical practice guidelines. Chest 2013; 143(5) (Suppl.): e93S-e120S.
[http://dx.doi.org/10.1378/chest.12-2351] [PMID: 23649456]

[31] Steinfort DP, Siva S, Kron T, *et al.* Multimodality guidance for accurate bronchoscopic insertion of fiducial markers. J Thorac Oncol 2015; 10(2): 324-30.
[http://dx.doi.org/10.1097/JTO.0000000000000389] [PMID: 25616177]

[32] Ernst A, Silvestri GA, Johnstone D. American College of Chest Physicians. Interventional pulmonary procedures: guidelines from the American College of Chest Physicians. Chest 2003; 123(5): 1693-717.
[http://dx.doi.org/10.1378/chest.123.5.1693] [PMID: 12740291]

[33] Bolliger CT, Mathur PN, Beamis JF, *et al.* European Respiratory Society/American Thoracic Society. ERS/ATS statement on interventional pulmonology. Eur Respir J 2002; 19(2): 356-73. [http://dx.doi.org/10.1183/09031936.02.00204602] [PMID: 11866017]

[34] Pastis NJ, Nietert PJ, Silvestri GA. American College of Chest Physicians Interventional Chest/Diagnostic Procedures Network Steering Committee. Variation in training for interventional pulmonary procedures among US pulmonary/critical care fellowships: a survey of fellowship directors. Chest 2005; 127(5): 1614-21. [http://dx.doi.org/10.1378/chest.127.5.1614] [PMID: 15888836]

[35] Lamb CR, Feller-Kopman D, Ernst A, *et al.* An approach to interventional pulmonary fellowship training. Chest 2010; 137(1): 195-9. [http://dx.doi.org/10.1378/chest.09-0494] [PMID: 20051404]

[36] Yarmus L, Feller-Kopman D, Imad M, Kim S, Lee HJ. Procedural volume and structure of interventional pulmonary fellowships: a survey of fellows and fellowship program directors. Chest 2013; 144(3): 935-9. [http://dx.doi.org/10.1378/chest.12-3028] [PMID: 23558929]

CHAPTER 7

Simplistic Approach to Mediastinal Lymph Node Staging - What a Pulmonary Interventionist Needs to Know

Nishant Gupta[1], **Dhiraj Baruah**[2] and **Kaushik Shahir**[2,*]

[1] *Department of Radiology, Columbia University Medical Center, New York, NY, USA*

[2] *Department of Radiology, Medical College of Wisconsin, WI, USA*

Abstract: Lymph node staging is a critical part in management of lung cancer, which can directly affect the patient treatment and outcomes. It is imperative that the interventional pulmonologist to not only be aware of the up-to-date nodal classification proposed by the International Association for the Study of Lung Cancer (IASLC), but should also have a basic understanding of the station identification on Computed Tomography(CT) scans performed for staging. This review article will provide a simplistic approach to mediastinal nodal staging based on CT scan which an interventional pulmonologist can routinely use and incorporate it effectively in their daily practice.

Keywords: Clinical trials, Interventional pulmonologist, Lung cancer, Lymph node, Lymph nodal map.

INTRODUCTION

Intrapulmonary, hilar and mediastinal lymphadenopathy detection and assessment is the critical factor in the staging and management of primary lung cancer. The nodal (N) portion of TNM staging is an integral part of any staging system. In past years, thoracic lymph nodal mapping has been described using both numerical and anatomical descriptors, leading to discrepancies and preventing a universal nomenclature. In 2009, the International Association for the Study of Lung Cancer (IASLC) proposed a new lymph nodal map to provide a precise lymph nodal station anatomy as well as to reconcile the differences between previously used maps. The overall goal for a universally accepted lymph nodal map is to assess outcomes, compare inter-institutional results, plan clinical trials, and, most importantly, select appropriate therapies and predictions prognoses.

* **Corresponding author Kaushik Shahir:** Department of Radiology (Cardiothoracic Division), Medical College of Wisconsin, 9200 W Wisconsin Ave, Milwaukee, WI – 53226, USA; Tel: 414-805-3120; Fax: 414-259-9290; E-mail: Kshahir@mcw.edu

Ali I. Musani (Ed.)

Prior Lymph Nodal Classifications

In 1960, Naruke proposed the first lymph nodal map, which was then widely accepted in Japan, North America and Europe [1]. The American Thoracic Society (ATS) then proposed a revised lymph nodal map in 1980-1990. In 1996, the Mountain-Dressler modification of the ATS classification was proposed, combining both the ATS and Naruke maps and referred to as the MD-ATS map [2]. Even after the modification, the MD-ATS map was rarely used in Europe, while Japan continued to use Naruke map; however, it was a widely accepted in North America.

International Association for the Study of Lung Cancer (IASLC) Lymph Node Map

IASLC started working on a lung cancer staging project in 1998. They found divergences in the nodal (N) descriptions of the MD-ATS and Naruke classifications, leading to significant differences in the staging of individual lung cancers. These factors motivated the IASLC to develop an improved lymph node classification system to resolve discrepancies between the MD-ATS and Naruke classifications, as well as propose anatomically definite lymph node stations. After approximately one decade, a new IASLC map was proposed, with seven specific anatomical zones for the thoracic lymph nodes: supraclavicular, upper, aortopulmonary, subcarinal, lower, hilar-interlobar and peripheral. Additionally, 14 numbered stations (station 1-14) were assigned to the thoracic lymph nodes. Right-sided and left-sided nodes were now described using the descriptors "R" or "L," respectively [3]. Figs. (**1** & **2**) present chest radiographs illustrating the diagrammatic representation of the IASLC lymph node map.

The seventh edition of the TNM in 2009 included the new IASLC lymph nodal classification. This TNM edition proposed N0 to designate patients without lymph node involvement. N1 disease designated patients with metastatic lymph nodes involving ipsilateral peripheral or hilar zones (stations 10-14). N2 disease additionally included metastatic extension to either subcarinal zones (stations 2-9) or ipsilateral mediastinal (upper, aortopulmonary and lower zones). The N3 label referred to the ipsilateral or contralateral supraclavicular zones (Station 1) or any nodal involvement in the contralateral mediastinal, hilar-interlobar, and peripheral zones.

CT Based Approach and Description to Define Mediastinal Lymph Node Status (Figs. 3 and 4)

Station 1: Supraclavicular zone lymph nodes (also known as "highest mediastinal nodes" in the MD-ATS classification system) are bounded superiorly by the lower margin of cricoid cartilage. The inferior border is formed laterally by both clavicles and in midline by the upper border of the manubrium. The midline of the trachea divides the nodes into RIGHT or LEFT side and is denoted by 1R or 1L (for RIGHT or LEFT, respectively).

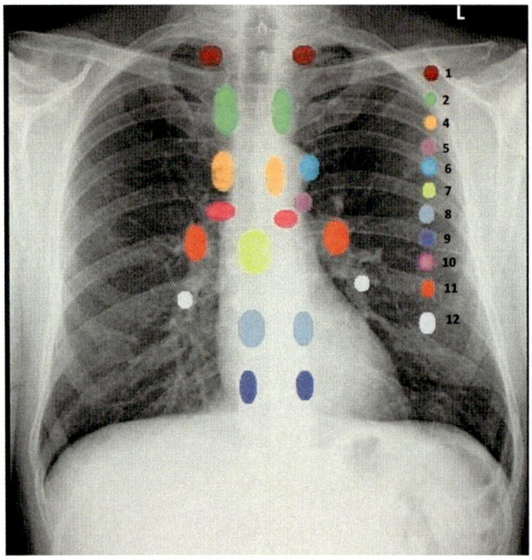

Fig. (1). Lymph node stations projected on chest PA. 1 – Highest Mediastinal. 2 – Upper Paratracheal. 4 – Lower Paratracheal. 5 – Subaortic (Aortopulmonary window). 6 – Paraaortic (Ascending aorta and phrenic). 7 – Subcarinal. 8 – Paraesophageal (Below the level of Carina). 9 – Pulmonary Ligament. 10 – Hilar. 11 – Interlobar. 12 – Lobar.

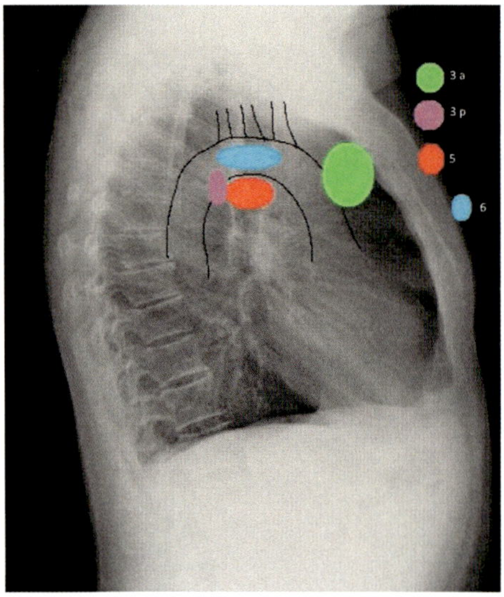

Fig. (2). Lymph node stations projected on lateral chest radiograph. 3 – Prevascular (3a) and Retrotracheal (3b). 5 – Subaortic (Aortopulmonary window). 6 – Paraaortic (Ascending aorta and phrenic).

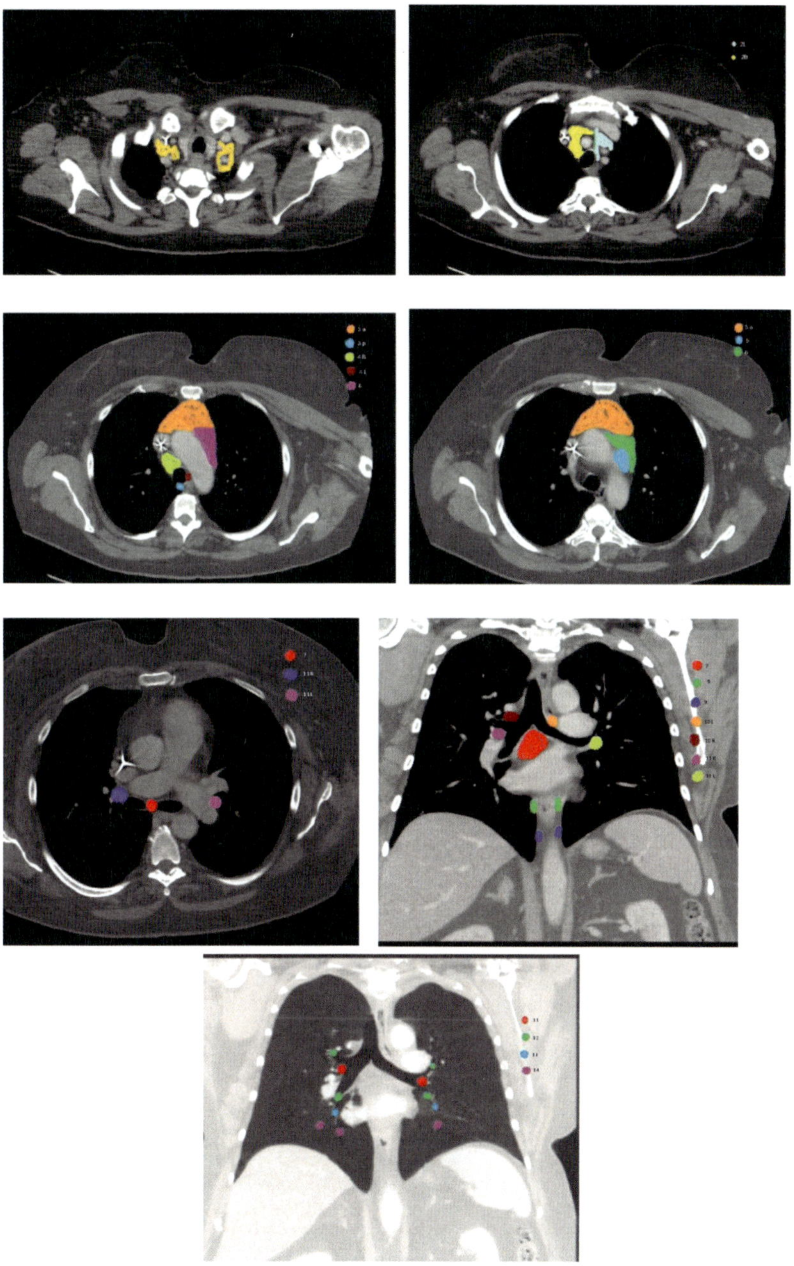

Fig. (3). Axial CT images in mediastinal window and Coronal image in lung window showing the lymph nodal stations. 1 – Highest Mediastinal. 2 – Upper Paratracheal. 3 – Prevascular (3a) and Retrotracheal (3b). 4 – Lower Paratracheal. 5 – Subaortic (Aortopulmonary window). 6 – Paraaortic (Ascending aorta and phrenic). 7 – Subcarinal. 8 – Paraesophageal (Below the level of Carina). 9 – Pulmonary Ligament. 10 – Hilar. 11 – Interlobar. 12 – Lobar. 13 – Segmental. 14 – Subsegmental.

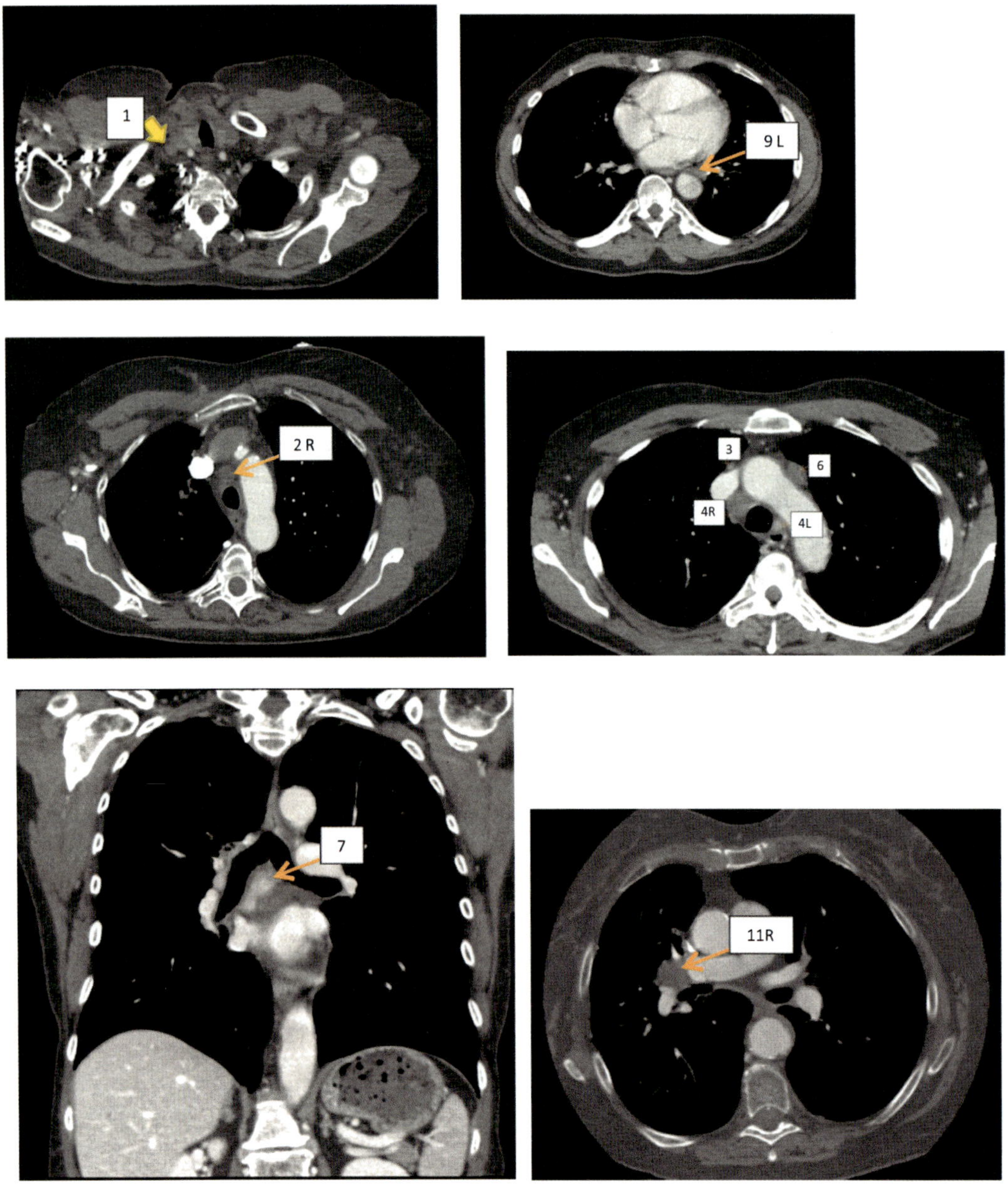

Fig. (4). Axial and coronal CT images in mediastinal window showing a few abnormal lymph nodes in different stations. 1 – Highest Mediastinal. 2 – Upper Paratracheal. 3 – Prevascular (3a) and Retrotracheal (3b). 4 – Lower Paratracheal. 6 – Paraaortic (Ascending aorta and phrenic). 7 – Subcarinal. 9 – Pulmonary Ligament. 11 – Interlobar.

Station 2: Upper paratracheal lymph nodes (2R and 2L). The superior margin is formed laterally by lung apices and medially by the superior border of the manubrium on both sides. The lower margin on the RIGHT side (2R) is formed at the level of the intersection of the caudal margin of the innominate vein with the trachea. On the LEFT side (2L), it is formed by the upper border of the aortic arch. However, it is sometimes difficult to identify the intersection of the innominate vein and the trachea on a CT scan [4, 5]. At station 2, the left tracheal border is identified as the border dividing 2R and 2L.

Station 3: Prevascular (3a) and retrotracheal (3b) lymph nodes. The boundaries are as follows:

3a- Right Side: The right lung apex forms the superior border, with the inferior border at the level of the carina. The posterior aspect of the sternum forms the anterior border, while the anterior border of the superior vena cava forms the posterior border.

3a- Left Side: The right lung apex forms the superior border, with the inferior border at the level of the carina. The posterior aspect of the sternum forms the anterior border, while the LEFT common carotid artery forms the posterior border.

Special Note for 3a Station: Both the superior vena cava on the right side and the left common carotid artery on the left side can be difficult to evaluate in axial CT images, as the structures are not continuous along the craniocaudal aspect.

3p- Retrotracheal lymph node zone: The upper border is formed by the lung apex, while the lower border is at the level of the carina.

Station 4: Lower paratracheal lymph nodes (4R and 4L) borders are clearly identified on CT scans; therefore, one can distinctly differentiate between station 4 and station 10 lymph nodes.

Right Lower Paratracheal Nodes (4R) consist of RIGHT paratracheal nodes and pretracheal nodes up to the LEFT lateral border of the trachea. They are bounded superiorly by the intersection between the trachea and the caudal margin of the innominate vein and inferiorly by the lower border of the azygos vein.

Left Lower Paratracheal Nodes (4L) consist of lymph nodes LEFT of the LEFT lateral tracheal border, and medial to the ligamentum arteriosum. They are bounded superiorly by the superior margin of the aortic arch and inferiorly by the superior rim of the LEFT main pulmonary artery.

Station 5: Subaortic lymph nodes (aortopulmonary window). They extend from the inferior margin of the aortic arch to the superior margin of the left main pulmonary artery. Station 5 nodes and 4L nodes are separated by the ligamentum arteriosum.

Station 6: Paraaortic lymph nodes (ascending aorta or phrenic nodes) consist of lymph nodes anterior and lateral to the ascending aorta and aortic arch. These lymph nodes are bounded superiorly by a line drawn tangential to the superior border of the aortic arch and inferiorly along the lower margin of the aortic arch.

Station 7: Subcarinal lymph nodes are bounded superiorly by the carina and inferiorly by the superior border of lower lobe bronchus on the LEFT side and the bronchus intermedius on the RIGHT side.

Station 8: Paraesophageal nodes (below the level of carina) consist of nodes along the esophageal wall, as well as on either side of the midline. Please note that paraesophageal nodes do not include subcarinal nodes, which are included in Station 7. Station 8 is bounded superiorly by the upper border of the lower lobe bronchus on the LEFT, the lower border of the bronchus intermedius on the RIGHT and inferiorly by the diaphragm.

Station 9: Pulmonary ligament nodes include nodes within the pulmonary ligament and are bounded superiorly by the inferior pulmonary vein and inferiorly by the diaphragm.

Station 10 Hilar nodes consist of nodes near the main stem bronchus and hilar vessels, including the proximal portions of the pulmonary veins and main pulmonary artery. These are bounded superiorly by the lower rim of the azygos vein on the RIGHT and the superior rim of the pulmonary artery on the LEFT. They are bounded inferiorly by the interlobar region on both sides.

Station 11: Interlobar lymph nodes are located between the origins of the lobar bronchi and consist of 11s and 11i lymph nodes. 11s lymph nodes lie between the upper lobe bronchus and the bronchus intermedius on the right. 11i lymph nodes lie between the middle and the lower lobe bronchi on the right.

Stations 12, 13 & 14: Station 12, 13 and 14 lymph nodes are adjacent to the lobar, segmental or subsegmental bronchi, respectively.

CONCLUSION

Mediastinal lymph node staging is important for the staging and treatment of patients with lung cancer. We described a simplified approach to identify these lymph nodes on CT scans following the IASLC system.

CONFLICT OF INTEREST

The authors declare no conflict of interest, financial or otherwise.

ACKNOWLEDGEMENTS

Declared none.

REFERENCES

[1] Naruke T, Suemasu K, Ishikawa S. Lymph node mapping and curability at various levels of metastasis in resected lung cancer. J Thorac Cardiovasc Surg 978(76): 833-9. [PMID: 713589]

[2] Mountain CF, Dresler CM. Regional lymph node classification for lung cancer staging. Chest 1997; 111(6): 1718-23. [http://dx.doi.org/10.1378/chest.111.6.1718] [PMID: 9187199]

[3] Rusch VW, Asamura H, Watanabe H, *et al.* The IASLC lung cancer staging project: a proposal for a new international lymph node map in the forthcoming seventh edition of the TNM classification for lung cancer. J Thorac Oncol 2009; 4(5): 568-77.

[4] Ichimura H, Kikuchi S, Ishikawa H. Caudal border of level 2R in the new international lymph node map for lung cancer. J Thorac Oncol 2010; 5(4): 579. [http://dx.doi.org/10.1097/JTO.0b013e3181d3cd08] [PMID: 20357628]

[5] Rusch VW, Asamura H. Response: a critique of the international association for the study of lung cancer lymph node map. J Thorac Oncol 2012; 7(3): 481. [http://dx.doi.org/10.1097/JTO.0b013e318249a9dd] [PMID: 22334009]

CHAPTER 8

EBUS TBNA for Diagnosis and Staging of Lung Cancer

David Fielding[1,*] and **Noriaki Kurimoto**[2]

[1] *Department of Thoracic Medicine, Royal Brisbane and Women's Hospital, Butterfield St & Bowen Bridge Rd, Herston QLD 4029, Australia*

[2] *St. Marianna University, Kanagawa Prefecture, Japan*

Abstract: Endobronchial Ultrasound Guided Transbronchial Needle Aspiration (EBUS TBNA) is the accepted first test in the pretreatment staging of lung cancer suitable for curative therapy. Virtually all patients having Surgery or Radical Radiotherapy should undergo the procedure, with the exception of clinical Stage 1A patients. Even cases with tumors larger than 3cm (Stage 2 and greater) who have a CT and PET clear mediastinum should have EBUS TBNA staging. Clinical (CT and PET) negative mediastinal nodes have an incidence of occult metastatic disease of over 20%.

Technical aspects of EBUS TBNA are becoming standardized given its now over 10 years of use in the clinical setting. Rapid on site examination of EBUS TBNA samples can be extremely helpful in the performance of staging procedures particularly to allow curtailment of the procedure once malignant cells are detected.

EBUS TBNA can be used to make the diagnosis of lung cancer especially where the mass is adjacent a proximal airway. EBUS TBNA material is ideally suited to be used for genetic analysis of malignant cases and this feature alone ensures EBUS TBNA will continue to have a central role in the management of lung cancer patients.

Keywords: Bronchoscopy, Endobronchial Ultrasound Guided Transbronchial Needle Aspiration (EBUS TBNA), Lung cancer, Mediastinal nodes, Occult metastatic disease, Radical Radiotherapy, Rapid-on-site-evaluation (ROSE).

INTRODUCTION

Lung cancer is the commonest cause of cancer-related death [1]. Many patients present with enlarged mediastinal lymph nodes. EBUS TBNA (Endobronchial ultrasound transbronchial needle aspiration) is a highly sensitive and specific way to make the diagnosis of primary and secondary lung malignancy at bronchoscopy

* **Corresponding author David Fielding:** Department of Thoracic Medicine, Royal Brisbane and Women's Hospital, Butterfield St & Bowen Bridge Rd, Herston QLD 4029, Australia; Tel: +617 36468111;
E-mail: david.fielding@health.qld.gov.au

Ali I. Musani (Ed.)

[2, 3]. Mediastinal lymph nodes sampling can make the diagnosis of up to 65% of all lung cancer patients, with a sensitivity of 95% [4]. Lung cancer often presents at an advanced stage and hence small biopsies are the only samples available as opposed to large surgical specimens [5, 6]. Further it is an important way to re-biopsy in the setting of relapse after therapy [4, 7]. In lung cancer, the decision on which node(s) to sample rests on a range of factors. Most important is whether the procedure is for diagnosis, or being used for staging after the diagnosis of lung cancer has already been made. Typically in diagnostic cases there is a large tumour mass and patients having stage 3B or 4 disease. Here there is obvious metastatic disease such as bony or CNS disease and EBUS TBNA provides a simple, rapid and accurate way to make a tissue diagnosis and obtain tissue for genetic analysis. Typically the lymph nodes in this situation are large and readily accessible. Conversely in staging EBUS TBNA, lymph nodes are often small and need to be systematically sampled starting at the highest lymph node group (N3) working back towards N1 node groups with the use of Rapid –on –site-evaluation (ROSE).

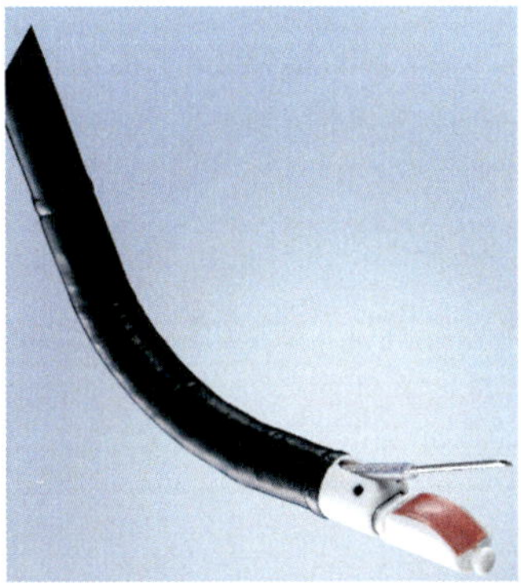

Fig. (1). EBUS-TBNA scope (BF-UC260FW, Olympus) Photo provided by Olympus.

EBUS TBNA Procedure

EBUS TBNA is performed either as a conscious sedation or general anaesthetic outpatient procedure. The purpose-designed combined white light and ultrasound scope allows simultaneous airway visualisation with a white light fibre bundle, with real time ultrasound images of lymph nodes adjacent the major airways (Fig. **1**). To locate a particular node, first of all the scope is sited against the wall using surface anatomical landmarks, then characteristic ultrasound appearances of each individual lymph node are checked for confirmation. Then with the scope held in position a dedicated EBUS TBNA needle (Fig. **2**) is passed through the wall of the trachea or main bronchus into the lymph node. Usually, suction is applied and the needle is gently moved in and out inside the node (Fig. **3A and B**). The needle is then removed and samples are then extruded, usually onto cytology slides and into saline pots for subsequent cell block preparation.

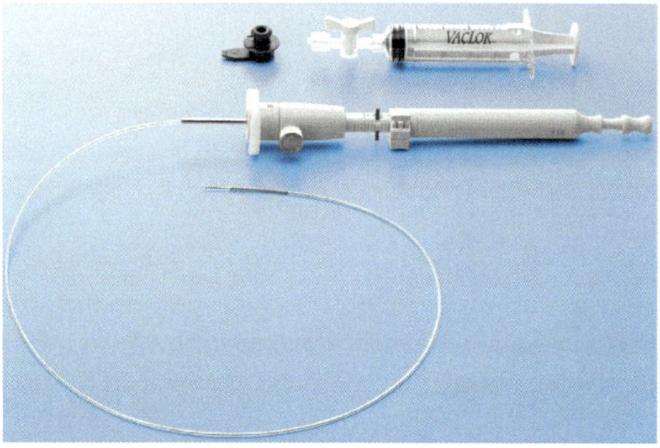

Fig. (2). EBUS-TBNA needle photo provided by Olympus.

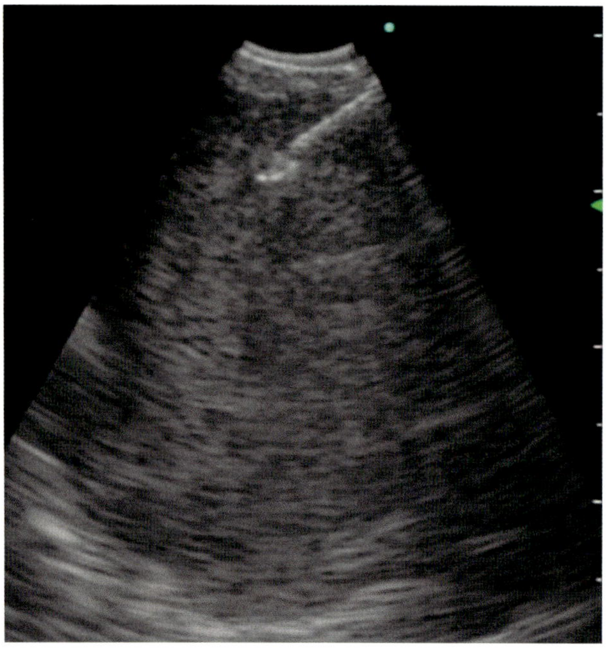

Fig. (3A). EBUS-TBNA with needle in a large node.

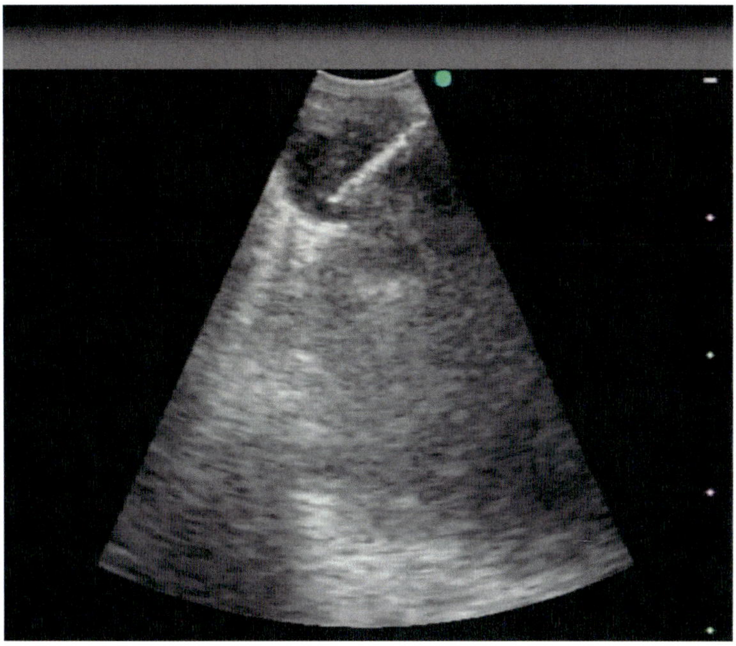

Fig. (3B). EBUS-TBNA with needle in a small node.

After aspiration the needle is removed from the scope and node material is extruded onto slides for cytology and into saline for cell block to allow histology and genetic analysis [8]. Usually 3-4 passes into a node is adequate to confirm malignancy. On-site cytology (ROSE) provides accurate assessment of the tumour in the bronchoscopy suite to advise the bronchoscopist that adequate material is being obtained [9]. In addition aspirates in saline for cell block process (paraffin embedding for sectioning) and tissue fragments in formalin allow for histology, and immunohistochemistry [2]. Additional cell block material is sent for genetic testing, particularly for EGFR mutation in adenocarcinomas [8, 10 - 12].

Technical Aspects Including Balloons, Stylet, Use of the Sheath

EBUS TBNA utilises a dedicated bronchoscope fitted with a balloon which can be filled with fluid to allow ultrasound imaging across the bronchus wall. It also uses a dedicated needle with a stylet and a tip for application for suction. There is some variation in how these various parts of the apparatus are applied. For example some operators always use a balloon, always leave the stylet in when they enter the lymph node, and always apply suction. Conversely other operators do none of the things, finding the procedure more inexpensive and streamlined without them. These factors have recently been reviewed in a guideline paper by Wahidi and co-authors [13]. Many proceduralists vary their practice to suit conditions. For example if an initial aspirate is bloody many proceduralists would perform the subsequent aspirates without suction. Regarding balloons some node stations (10R, 4L) require more angulation to oppose the ultrasound surface of the scope onto the bronchial wall. Experience suggests that where such nodes are the focus of a procedure balloon application on the scope tip would be warranted.

Needle Size

Needle size is of some relevance in the diagnosis of lung cancer. Typically a 21Guage needle has been marginally favoured over a 22 Gauge needle in previous studies. One relatively small series divided 56 cases into having either 21 or 22 Gauge needle sampling [14]. In malignant cases sensitivities for cytology were 88.9% *versus* 52.2% (P=0.01), and for histology were100% *versus* 82.6% (P=0.09). In another study of 45 lesions [10] tumour cells abundance was equal between 21G and 22G needles. However, with the pathologists blinded to needle type, histology was better preserved in five lesions from the 21G needle, hence it was considered the 21G might be better for sampling nodes of unknown aetiology. Conversely, there was more blood contamination with the 21G needle (P <0.0001).

New core needles are available in 22 and 25 Gauge sizes and their place in lung cancer diagnosis remains to be determined. It is unclear whether these needles truly deliver a core sample or simply provide more material which is better for creation of a cell block. For cell block preparation material is collected in a saline pot and spun down, with the cell pellet being embedded in paraffin and subsequent "histological" sections being cut. Some proceduralists manually select what appear to be cores from the saline pot and place these directly in formalin, leaving the remainder for cell block preparation. It is unclear at this time whether there is any need to do this, as generally cell block preparations are highly sensitive for the diagnosis of lung cancer. In a study of 270 lung cancer samples, cell lock was compared to cytology analysis [15]. Cell blocks could be obtained from 48% of aspirates and added diagnostic material to that from cytology smears in 8%. Importantly, Cell blocks obtained during EBUS-TBNA also allowed EGFR mutation testing in 60%.

Recently a 19 Gauge EBUS TBNA needle has become available which combines a large calibre with flexibility (due to nitinol construction) [16]. Initial reports suggest the accessibility of all node positions and sizes is excellent with this large needle and further studies are awaited to determine its efficacy.

Needle Techniques

As mentioned below EBUS TBNA is a highly sensitive test; however the procedure will be of course be negative if the node in question cannot be accessed. In the early experience of operators a common reason is inability to pass the needle through the cartilages in a lymph node. Many authorities have described the basic principles of the use of the sheath to facilitate the placement of the apparatus between cartilage rings, so the sharp needle can be advanced unopposed. A very elegant refinement of this aspect of the procedure described by Inoue *et al* ("the outer sheath method") starts with the plastic outer sheath extended and in view in the top of the ultrasound image. The scope is very slowly pulled back and the sheath is carefully watched for a "drop" into a space between cartilages [17]. In a comparative study of 340 patients divided into before and after introduction of this outer sheath method, there was a significant improvement in diagnostic yield from 93% to 98%. Other reasons for false negative tests include bloody aspirates (particularly in metastatic malignancies such as renal cell carcinoma and melanoma) as well as large necrotic nodes. In the latter cases some authorities paradoxically recommend sampling the more vascular parts of a node as these are more viable. Finally it is important for the needle to not be passed distal to the node, so early training focuses on starting the needle insertion at the near (head) end of the node.

EBUS TBNA and Lung Cancer Diagnosis

Many series have reported the utility of EBUS TBNA in confirming the diagnosis of lung cancer (Table **1**) [17]. In the largest single group prospective study of 502 patients published by Herth *et al*, results of EBUS TBNA for hilar or mediastinal adenopathy of unknown origin were presented. These were nodes of more than 1 cm diameter in short axis. This series did include some staging cases. Adequate cellular material was obtained in 94% of cases [18]. In a 2013 meta-analysis [19], 9 studies were reviewed, 7 of which were prospective. The mean time for the EBUS TBNA procedure was 24 minutes.

Table 1. Summary of studies of Diagnostic Yield of EBUS TBNA for lung cancer.

	Studies	Patients	Mean Age	Sens	Spec	PPV	NPV
Herth 2006 (18)	1	502		94	100		0.11
Dong 2013 (19)	9	1066	62.3	90 (0.84-0.96)	99	0.99	0.93

Diagnosing Primary Masses

EBUS TBNA can also be used to make the diagnosis on primary lung cancers and masses situated centrally in a peribronchial position in the inner third of the lung. In one retrospective study of 32 cases, there was 94% diagnostic yield for malignancy overall for EBUS-TBNA. Thirteen patients had a transbronchial lung biopsy, yield 61%, and 8 patients could have endobronchial biopsy, yield 75%. In another study of 60 patients [20], EBUS TBNA was able to make the diagnosis of the primary central lung cancer in 46 cases (77%) after a prior negative standard bronchoscopy. Other diagnostic procedures such as CT FNA or surgical biopsy could be cancelled in 47% and 30% of patients, respectively.

In patients presenting with superior vena cava syndrome, EBUS TBNA provides an effective rapid means of making a tissue diagnosis. One review series of 17 patients with this problem showed malignancy was confirmed in 16 patients in procedures under conscious sedation with local anesthetic. There was no major complications in any patients.

Rapid on Site Examination (ROSE)

With ROSE a cytologist or technician examines smears of TBNA material after each pass. The rationale is so that the proceduralist gets immediate feedback on sample quality and diagnostic success. It is particularly important for staging procedures. Most authorities recommend the Diff Quik method (Fig. **4**). Suggested adequacy of smears has been published [21] and includes the following: 1. identifiable pathology (*e.g.* malignancy or granuloma), 2.smears with presence of > 5 low power fields (×100) 3. Each with ≥ 100 lymphocytes and 4 < 2 groups of bronchial cells/low power field (×100) 5. The presence of germinal center fragments, irrespective of the above mentioned criteria. Many centres use ROSE however it is not always available due to cost and organisational issues.

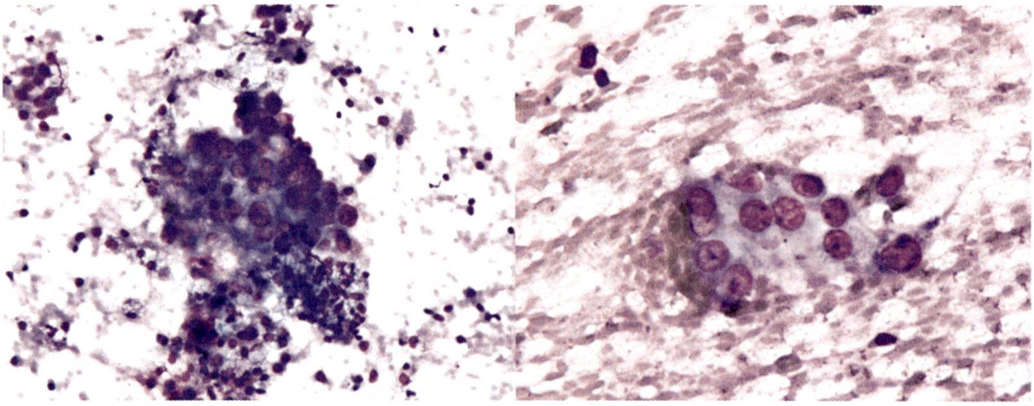

Fig. (4). ROSE: Diff quik method: slides demonstrating adenocarcinoma.
(Courtesy Akihiro Bessho, Okayama Red Cross General Hospital, Okayama, Japan).

One prospective randomized study of 108 patients [22] showed that the ROSE group could stop the procedure after sampling just one site in significantly higher numbers (58.9% vs 44.1%, P = .01) These authors also showed that there were fewer instances where the samples were insufficient for molecular analysis (0 cases vs 6 in the non ROSE group, P = .05). Another prospective study of 108 patients showed a significant reduction in the ROSE group of the requirement for intra-procedural extra steps such as transbronchial lung biopsy. Also there was a significant reduction in the number of passes required to make a diagnosis: in the ROSE group (2.2 *vs.* 3.1 punctures in the non-ROSE group, p < 0.001) [23]. Although ROSE is widely used during EBUS-TBNA, this study did not show a significant reduction in procedure time.

ROSE facilitates the division of EBUS TBNA samples into that which is used for pathologic diagnosis and that for molecular testing, without limiting the ability to make a pathologic diagnosis [13, 24]. ROSE is regarded as essential for staging EBUS TBNA by most authorities, because of the unnecessary length of procedures if all node stations are sampled- see below.

Method of Performing an EBUS TBNA Staging Procedure

Fig. (**5**) shows the present version of the Thoracic Lymph node stations as they appear to a proceduralist. The advantages of EBUS TBNA over mediastinoscopy in terms of reach are that it can ample low mediastinal nodes such as low station 7 and 10 nodes, and has easier access to low left paratracheal nodes (4L). Hilar nodes can be reached which clearly cannot be sampled by mediastinoscopy. Stations 5 and 6 are not accessible. Stations 8 and 9 are not accessible by EBUS TBNA but can be reached by EUS FNA- see below. The main principle of the staging procedure is that the highest most group of nodes (N3) need to have cancer excluded first, as management decisions clearly are dramatically changed by such a diagnosis. N3 nodes are contralateral to the primary tumour; for right sided tumours an N3 node is on the left of the tracheal edge (not merely to the left of the midline). After that, sequential sampling of N2 and then N1 nodes is performed. It is important to sample in this order because going back to an N3 node after sampling an N2 node can result in cells from the previous pass contaminating the N3 sample; it is not possible to completely remove malignant cells from a needle by saline flushing. Within each nodal group (N3/N2/N1) it is optimal to sample from distal to proximal to the tumour. For example, N2 sampling on the right would start at 2R then proceed to a high 4 R location then a low 4R location, depending on where the abnormal nodes are situated. Adequate exclusion of N2 disease requires thorough assessment of possibly involved stations: The ERS guidelines stipulate:" A complete assessment of mediastinal and hilar nodal stations, and sampling of at least three different mediastinal nodal stations (4R, 4L, 7) is suggested in patients with NSCLC and an abnormal mediastinum by CT or CT-PET (recommendation grade D)".

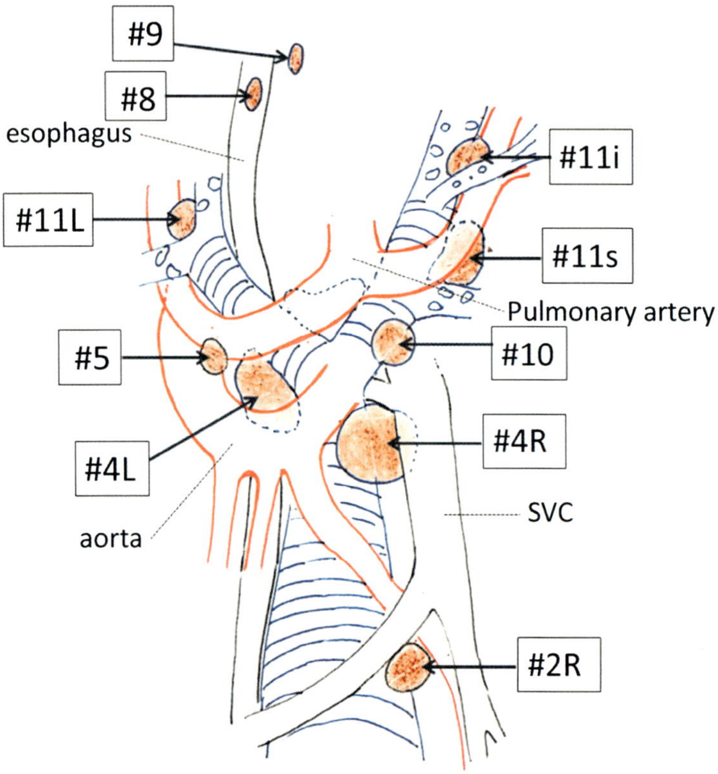

Fig. (5). Diagram of anatomy of the nodal stations as they appear to a proceduralist. Key landmarks include the Right main pulmonary artery, the Brachiocephalic vessels, and the right tracheobronchial angle.

Which Patients should have EBUS TBNA Staging?

The 2013 ACCP guidelines state that a staging procedure is regarded as unnecessary where there is extensive bilateral mediastinal involvement, although this may represent a site for tissue confirmation of disease if not obtained by other means. These guidelines stipulate EBUS TBNA (and or EUS) as the first test to perform this task as opposed to surgical biopsy [24]. "In patients with high suspicion of N2, 3 involvement, either by discrete mediastinal lymph node enlargement or PET uptake (and no distant metastases), a needle technique ([EBUS]-needle aspiration [NA], Endoscopic Ultrasound Needle Aspiration (EUS-NA) or combined EBUS/EUS-NA) is recommended over surgical staging as a best first test. In cases where the clinical suspicion of mediastinal node involvement remains high after a negative result using a needle technique, surgical staging (*e.g.,* mediastinoscopy, video-assisted thoracic surgery [VATS], *etc.*) should be performed".

It is however mandatory in lung cancer surgical cases to sample all nodes of more than 1cm in short axis and all PET positive nodes, particularly ipsilateral nodes, even where the PET positive nodes are less than 1 cm on CT. In such cases with pre- procedure radiological abnormalities, experts in the field sample every node which is visible even to as small as 5mm. It is acknowledged that this requires considerable expertise, and may not always be possible. If the mediastinum is CT and PET negative EBUS TBNA sampling is still recommended where there is a central tumour or there is N1 disease. Usually, EBUS TBNA staging is not required for patients with a CT negative and PET CT negative mediastinum [24]. "For patients with a peripheral clinical stage IA tumor (negative nodal involvement by CT and PET), it is suggested that invasive preoperative evaluation of the mediastinal nodes is not required". However for Stage 2 tumours with a normal mediastinum (larger than 3 cm) recent ERS staging guidelines [25] stipulate EBUS TBNA or EUS FNA should be performed (Recommendation class C).

Other scenarios where EBUS TBNA staging should be performed have been iterated by the ATS and ERS guidelines and include cases where the primary tumour has low PET avidity, cases where the primary tumour is close to the hilum and in cases of radiologic N1 disease [25]. Despite the above comments there is still an incidence of cancer positivity in CT and PET CT negative mediastinal cases (see below).

The landmark study on EBUS TBNA staging was published by Yasufuku and colleagues [26]. Here all patients having resection for lung cancer had pre-procedure CT and PET. EBUS TBNA was performed on 102 patients immediately prior to surgery, and surgical pathology on resected nodes was used as the study gold standard, unless detailed surgical node mapping was not performed in those that were found to have inoperable N3 or extensive N2 disease. A total of 147 mediastinal and 53 hilar lymph nodes were sampled. EBUS-TBNA showed malignancy in 37 lymph node stations. CT was abnormal ("positive") for 92 lymph nodes, and PET was abnormal ("positive") for 89 lymph nodes, both considerably more than were ultimately proven to be malignant. Table **2** shows the summary of results from this paper, demonstrating the superior performance of EBUS TBNA.

Table 2. Summary of results of comparative study of CT, PET and EBUS TBNA staging prior to surgery, by Yasufuku and co-authors [26].

	CT	**PET**	**EBUS TBNA**
Sensitivity	76.9%	80.0%	92.3%
Specificity	55.3%	70.1%	100%

(Table 2) contd.....

	CT	PET	EBUS TBNA
Diagnostic Accuracy	60.8%	72.5%	98.0%

A Meta-analysis of staging analysed over 5000 patients having sonographic staging procedures for lung cancer [27]. Table 3 shows the results of that review, including comparisons to previous reports of surgical and other staging modalities.

Table 3. Summary of combined studies of EBUS TBNA staging, combined from reference [27].

	Number of Patients	Prevalence of Malignancy	Sensitivity	Specificity	PPV	NPV
CT Staging	7368	30	55	81	58	83
PET/CT	2014	22	62	90	63	90
Mediastinoscopy	9267	33	78	100	100	91
All forms of surgical mediastinal staging	10648	34	81	100	100	91
EBUS	2756	58	89	100	100	91
EUS	2443	58	89	100	100	86
EUS+EBUS	811	33	91	100	100	96

EBUS TBNA for N0 Disease

A retrospective review of EBUS-TBNA for N0 disease has been performed [28]. N0 disease was defined as nodes ≤1 cm in the short axis and PET-CT maximum standardized uptake value ≤2.5 Two hundred twenty patients with radiographic N0 disease underwent EBUS-TBNA was used to sample 734 nodes in 220 patients. The median node diameter was 0.72 cm. N status was up-staged in 49 patients (22.3%): 18 by EBUS-TBNA, 27 by surgery, and 4 by imaging follow-up. EBUS clearly cannot reach all node stations, so when only including nodes which could be accessed, the overall false-negative rate of EBUS-TBNA was only 5.5% (sensitivity, 60%; specificity, 100%; and Negative predictive value 93.4%).; These authors pointed out the high false negative rate of standard image modalities, and hence the importance of EBUS TBNA staging in N0 patients where non-surgical curative therapies such as Radiotherapy are planned.

EBUS TBNA is also useful for distinguishing clinical N0 from N1 disease which is clearly important for patients undergoing induction therapies [29]. A retrospective review of patients having lung cancer resection was performed with a focus on those patients who did not have clinical N2 or N3 disease. Of 163 patients, 94 were clinical N0 and 69 were clinical N1. A total of 453 lymph nodes were sampled including 338 mediastinal and 115 N1 nodes. The sensitivity, specificity, diagnostic accuracy, and negative predictive value of EBUS-TBNA to accurately differentiate between N0 and N1 disease was 76.2%, 100%, 96.6%, and 96.2%, respectively.

Combined Staging and Diagnostic Procedure with EBUS TBNA

It is not uncommon for patients to present with small peripheral pulmonary nodules and an ipsilateral hilar or mediastinal node, particularly if presenting in an asymptomatic relatively early stage. The node in this situation represents an easier target than the primary itself (Fig. **6**). Sampling can be done in combination with the staging principles highlighted above. ROSE is particularly helpful here not only for staging but to obviate the need to go on and sample the primary mass [4].

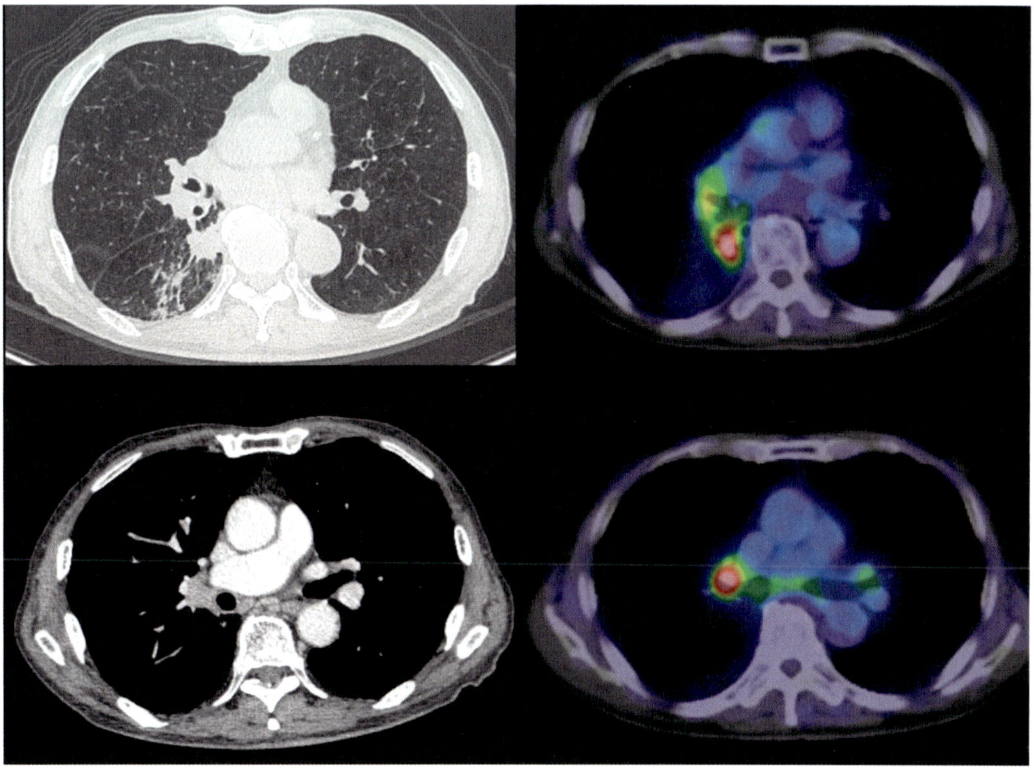

Fig. (6). PET/CT scans of primary lesion and #11s LN. Here the #11 node represents an easy target to allow diagnosis and staging in one procedure.
(Courtesy Katsuhiko Morita, Shimonoseki Medical Center, Shimonoseki, Japan).

Other Causes of PET Positive Nodes with Negative EBUS TBNA (False Positive PET)

Anthracosis or anthracosilicosis of nodes is well described as a false positive cause of PET positivity [30]. Microscopic anthracotic pigment (MAP) obtained from EBUS TBNA aspirates is the cytologic corrollary of this radiologic finding. In a series of 133 patients having EBUS TBNA staging for lung cancer 279 mediastinal lymph nodes were sampled, including 100 malignant nodes. MAP was seen in 61 (21.7%) lymph nodes, and among these only 3 had malignant cells ($P < 0.001$). The nodes with MAP were slightly smaller on average (9.0 vs 10.8 mm, $P = 0.001$). The MAP nodes had only slightly lower (non-significant). SUV values on FDG-PET (4.4 vs 4.7, $P = 0.256$). MAP was negatively associated with malignancy on multivariate analysis (adjusted OR, 0.12; 95% CI, 0.03-0.42; $P < 0.001$). Therefore where there is a question about the final N status of a particular station after PET CT and EBUS TBNA, the presence of MAP can help in confirming benign disease.

Sarcoidosis can cause PET positive nodes and may occur at any age although would be clinically more suspected in younger patients. Detection of non caseating granulomas on EBUS TBNA smears and cell blocks is a key plank in the diagnosis of sarcoidosis [31]. Tuberculosis tends to have more asymmetric PET positivity but can be a cause of false positive nodes [32].

Genetics on EBUS TBNA Lung Cancer Samples

During the past decade, substantial progress has been made in the characterization of molecular abnormalities in non-small cell carcinoma (NSCLC) tumors that are being used as molecular targets and predictive biomarkers for selection of targeted therapy [5, 33]. These recent advances in NSCLC targeted therapy require the analysis of a panel of molecular abnormalities in tumor specimens, including gene mutations (*e.g.,* EGFR, KRAS, BRAF, DDR2), gene amplifications (*e.g.,* MET, FGFR1), and fusions (*e.g.,* EML4-ALK) by applying different methods to tumor tissue (biopsy) and cell (cytology) samples.

Formalin Fixed Paraffin Embedded (FFPE) Samples

Studies have reported single gene mutation detection from EBUS derived samples for EGFR p53, BRAF, PIK3CA, RET and ROS1, as well as multigenic analyses for defined numbers of genes [34 - 36]. Adenocarcinomas are the best studies with well-known mutations in EGFR, KRAS and ALK fusions [5]. Present sampling methods for DNA use FFPE material in lung cancer are usually single gene approaches, mostly for KRAS, EGFR and ALK [4]. FFPE retrieval of specimens is a highly specialized process and involves dissection of material identified on slides by specialist pathologists. Material is retrieved from the paraffin block in a lengthy process. Furthermore, formalin fixation and paraffin embedding of specimens damages DNA, reducing the utility of the specimens. Also this process is heavily dependent on the quantity of tumour tissue within the specimens, which varies greatly, for example due to the amounts of non-informative stromal tissue.

One study analysed data from 204 procedures which proved carcinoma [37] including small cell 43, squamous cell 64, adenocarcinoma 40, adenosquamous 2, large cell 12, NSCLC-NOS 31 and non-lung primary 12. From cell block material, subtyping could be obtained in 118 (79.2%) with the remainder being NSCLC Not Otherwise specified (NOS). EGFR testing was done in 36 patients with an excellent test success rate of 88.8% (95%CI 74.7-95.6%). However squamous cell mutations are also well reported now and include EGFR II, DDR2 and FGFR 1 mutations [38]. Lockwood *et al.,* have determined the different genetic pathways responsible for the differential development and clinical phenotypes of adenocarcinomas and squamous cell carcinomas [39].

Next Generation Sequencing

Targeted Next Generation Sequencing (NGS) however allows for the detection of multiple gene mutations on the same material in a manner which is highly reproducible with existing single gene approaches [40]. Wide experience across a range of tumours including breast, prostate, colon and lung has demonstrated the detection of multiple genes in addition to those already commonly known [41]. NGS allows for rapid turn-around of specimens to facilitate timely treatment decisions. The result is clinicians get broad information quickly. NGS can be done with tiny amounts of material without the need for extra biopsies (Li). Fresh samples can undergo genetic testing [42] and may yield more DNA than the FFPE processed samples, however snap freezing for this purpose is usually only available in academic centres including for gene discovery purposes [38]. A number of authors have reported NGS findings from FFPE samples of NSCLC. Takeda studied transbronchial lung biopsy and resected tumour specimens from 110 patients with NSCLC using a gene sequencing panel which covered 22 mutational hotspots as well as 72 major variants of ALK, RET, ROS1, and NTRK1 transcripts [43]. The most common mutations were TP53 (42 patients), EGFR (25 patients), STK11 (12 patients) and KRAS (10 patients). Potentially actionable mutations were found in 50% of those with adenocarcinomas and 14% of those with Squamous cell carcinomas. Deeb *et al* reported NGS on FFPE material from 23 primary and metastatic lung cancers with known EGFR and KRAS mutations from previous routine diagnostic evaluation [44]. When needed micro or macro dissection of blocks was performed to achieve at least 25% tumour cell content. Of the 25 EGFR and KRAS mutations detected by 454 deep sequencing test, 24 (96%) were correctly identified by pyrosequencing. In addition 4 other non- synonymous mutations were detected including 1 sample with multiple EGFR mutations and a PIK 3CA mutation.

Qiu reported NGS findings from percutaneous fine needle aspiration cytology of 89 metastatic lymph nodes in adenocarcinoma [45]. In this cohort of Chinese patients, NGS on tumour DNA retrieved from FFPE blocks showed 34% of samples had EGFR mutations.

Recently Roy-Chodhuri *et al*. examined cytology preparations for DNA yield and NGS in 207 samples from a range of sites including EBUS TBNA samples [46]. NGS was possible in over 70% of cases. As expected NGS success was related to DNA yield from the samples, but surprisingly was not related to cellularity of the smears. This may relate to the study only selecting cases with high cellularity prior to performing NGS, which meant that all cases in their study had high cellularity (60-70% tumour percentage on slides). An earlier study from the same group reported 61 tumour FNA specimens for adequacy of DNA yield for NGS [47]. From 33 smears and 28 FFPE cell blocks they found 31 specimens yielded sufficient DNA (10ng, for a 46 gene Ion PGM sequencer). This was after excluding specimens with estimated <20% tumour percentage.

Karnes *et al*. reported a comparison of multiplex genetic sampling of paired FFPE cell block and cytology smear samples from FNA samples in 5 lung adenocarcinoma [48]. Extremely high concordance was observed – the average concordance of single nucleotide variants was 99.5%. These authors therefore recommended that NGS methods be incorporated into the use of cytology specimen workflows.

CONCLUSION

In conclusion, numerous authors have demonstrated the potential of NGS when applied to samples from fine needle aspiration and the potential for this to be applied to EBUS TBNA specimens is high and would be a great step forward.

CONFLICT OF INTEREST

The authors declare no conflict of interest, financial or otherwise.

ACKNOWLEDGEMENTS

Declared none.

REFERENCES

[1] Coleman MP, Forman D, Bryant H, *et al.* ICBP Module 1 Working Group. Cancer survival in Australia, Canada, Denmark, Norway, Sweden, and the UK, 1995-2007 (the International Cancer Benchmarking Partnership): an analysis of population-based cancer registry data. Lancet 2011; 377(9760): 127-38.
[http://dx.doi.org/10.1016/S0140-6736(10)62231-3] [PMID: 21183212]

[2] Nakajima T, Yasufuku K, Suzuki M, *et al.* Assessment of epidermal growth factor receptor mutation by endobronchial ultrasound-guided transbronchial needle aspiration. Chest 2007; 132(2): 597-602. [http://dx.doi.org/10.1378/chest.07-0095] [PMID: 17573511]

[3] Fielding D, Windsor M. Endobronchial ultrasound convex-probe transbronchial needle aspiration as the first diagnostic test in patients with pulmonary masses and associated hilar or mediastinal nodes. Intern Med J 2009; 39(7): 435-40. [http://dx.doi.org/10.1111/j.1445-5994.2008.01731.x] [PMID: 19371395]

[4] Czarnecka-Kujawa K, Yasufuku K. Molecular alterations in non-small-cell lung cancer: perspective for targeted therapy and specimen management for the bronchoscopist. Respirology 2014; 19(8): 1117-25. [http://dx.doi.org/10.1111/resp.12377] [PMID: 25302756]

[5] Reck M, Heigener DF, Mok T, Soria J-C, Rabe KF. Management of non-small-cell lung cancer: recent developments. Lancet 2013; 382(9893): 709-19. [http://dx.doi.org/10.1016/S0140-6736(13)61502-0] [PMID: 23972814]

[6] Morton ML, Bai X, Merry CR, *et al.* Identification of mRNAs and lincRNAs associated with lung cancer progression using next-generation RNA sequencing from laser micro-dissected archival FFPE tissue specimens. Lung Cancer 2014; 85(1): 31-9. [http://dx.doi.org/10.1016/j.lungcan.2014.03.020] [PMID: 24735754]

[7] Anraku M, Pierre AF, Nakajima T, *et al.* Endobronchial ultrasound-guided transbronchial needle aspiration in the management of previously treated lung cancer. Ann Thorac Surg 2011; 92(1): 251-5. [http://dx.doi.org/10.1016/j.athoracsur.2011.03.007] [PMID: 21592457]

[8] Nakajima T, Yasufuku K. How I do it--optimal methodology for multidirectional analysis of endobronchial ultrasound-guided transbronchial needle aspiration samples. J Thorac Oncol 2011; 6(1): 203-6. [http://dx.doi.org/10.1097/JTO.0b013e318200f496] [PMID: 21178716]

[9] Cameron SE, Andrade RS, Pambuccian SE. Endobronchial ultrasound-guided transbronchial needle aspiration cytology: a state of the art review. Cytopathology 2010; 21(1): 6-26. [http://dx.doi.org/10.1111/j.1365-2303.2009.00722.x] [PMID: 20015257]

[10] Nakajima T, Yasufuku K, Takahashi R, *et al.* Comparison of 21-gauge and 22-gauge aspiration needle during endobronchial ultrasound-guided transbronchial needle aspiration. Respirology 2011; 16(1): 90-4. [http://dx.doi.org/10.1111/j.1440-1843.2010.01871.x] [PMID: 20920141]

[11] Mohamed S, Yasufuku K, Nakajima T, *et al.* Analysis of cell cycle-related proteins in mediastinal lymph nodes of patients with N2-NSCLC obtained by EBUS-TBNA: relevance to chemotherapy response. Thorax 2008; 63(7): 642-7. [http://dx.doi.org/10.1136/thx.2007.090324] [PMID: 18390633]

[12] Mitsudomi T, Morita S, Yatabe Y, *et al.* West Japan Oncology Group. Gefitinib *versus* cisplatin plus docetaxel in patients with non-small-cell lung cancer harbouring mutations of the epidermal growth factor receptor (WJTOG3405): an open label, randomised phase 3 trial. Lancet Oncol 2010; 11(2): 121-8. [http://dx.doi.org/10.1016/S1470-2045(09)70364-X] [PMID: 20022809]

[13] Wahidi MM, Herth F, Yasufuku K, *et al.* Technical Aspects of Endobronchial Ultrasound-Guided Transbronchial Needle Aspiration: CHEST Guideline and Expert Panel Report. Chest 2016; 149(3): 816-35. [http://dx.doi.org/10.1378/chest.15-1216] [PMID: 26402427]

[14] Saji J, Kurimoto N, Morita K, *et al.* Comparison of 21-gauge and 22-gauge Needles for Endobronchial Ultrasound-Guided Transbronchial Needle Aspiration of Mediastinal and Hilar Lymph Nodes. J Bronchology Interv Pulmonol 2011; 18(3): 239-46. [http://dx.doi.org/10.1097/LBR.0b013e3182273b41] [PMID: 23208567]

[15] Sanz-Santos J, Serra P, Andreo F, Llatjós M, Castellà E, Monsó E. Contribution of cell blocks obtained through endobronchial ultrasound-guided transbronchial needle aspiration to the diagnosis of lung cancer. BMC Cancer 2012; 12: 34-4.
[http://dx.doi.org/10.1186/1471-2407-12-34] [PMID: 22264305]

[16] Felix JH, Daniela G, Pallav LS, Ralf E. Endobronchial Ultrasound-Guided TBNA (EBUS-TBNA) with a 19 Gauge Needle - First Experience B103 fixing a hole: Advances in diagnostic and therapeutic bronchoscopy. American Thoracic Society 2015; pp. A3726-6.

[17] Inoue T, Kurimoto N, Furuya N, *et al.* New technique for endobronchial ultrasound-guided transbronchial needle aspiration to improve diagnostic yield. J Bronchology Interv Pulmonol 2013; 20(1): 28-32.
[http://dx.doi.org/10.1097/LBR.0b013e3182834028] [PMID: 23328138]

[18] Varela-Lema L, Fernández-Villar A, Ruano-Ravina A. Effectiveness and safety of endobronchial ultrasound-transbronchial needle aspiration: a systematic review. Eur Respir J 2009; 33(5): 1156-64.
[http://dx.doi.org/10.1183/09031936.00097908] [PMID: 19407050]

[19] Dong X, Qiu X, Liu Q, Jia J. Endobronchial ultrasound-guided transbronchial needle aspiration in the mediastinal staging of non-small cell lung cancer: a meta-analysis. Ann Thorac Surg 2013; 96(4): 1502-7.
[http://dx.doi.org/10.1016/j.athoracsur.2013.05.016] [PMID: 23993894]

[20] Tournoy KG, Rintoul RC, van Meerbeeck JP, *et al.* EBUS-TBNA for the diagnosis of central parenchymal lung lesions not visible at routine bronchoscopy. Lung Cancer 2009; 63(1): 45-9.
[http://dx.doi.org/10.1016/j.lungcan.2008.04.004] [PMID: 18514365]

[21] Nayak A, Sugrue C, Koenig S, Wasserman PG, Hoda S, Morgenstern NJ. Endobronchial ultrasound-guided transbronchial needle aspirate (EBUS-TBNA): a proposal for on-site adequacy criteria. Diagn Cytopathol 2012; 40(2): 128-37.
[http://dx.doi.org/10.1002/dc.21517] [PMID: 22246929]

[22] Trisolini R, Cancellieri A, Tinelli C, *et al.* Randomized Trial of Endobronchial Ultrasound-Guided Transbronchial Needle Aspiration With and Without Rapid On-site Evaluation for Lung Cancer Genotyping. Chest 2015; 148(6): 1430-7.
[http://dx.doi.org/10.1378/chest.15-0583] [PMID: 26158441]

[23] Oki M, Saka H, Kitagawa C, *et al.* Rapid on-site cytologic evaluation during endobronchial ultrasound-guided transbronchial needle aspiration for diagnosing lung cancer: a randomized study. Respiration 2013; 85(6): 486-92.
[http://dx.doi.org/10.1159/000346987] [PMID: 23571718]

[24] Silvestri GA, Gonzalez AV, Jantz MA, *et al.* Methods for staging non-small cell lung cancer: Diagnosis and management of lung cancer.American College of Chest Physicians evidence-based clinical practice guidelines Chest. 3rd ed. 2013; 143: pp. e211S-50S.

[25] Vilmann P, Clementsen PF, Colella S, *et al.* Combined endobronchial and oesophageal endosonography for the diagnosis and staging of lung cancer. European Society of Gastrointestinal Endoscopy (ESGE) Guideline, in cooperation with the European Respiratory Society (ERS) and the European Society of Thoracic Surgeons (ESTS). Eur Respir J 2015; 46(1): 40-60.
[http://dx.doi.org/10.1183/09031936.00064515] [PMID: 26034128]

[26] Yasufuku K, Nakajima T, Motoori K, *et al.* Comparison of endobronchial ultrasound, positron emission tomography, and CT for lymph node staging of lung cancer. Chest 2006; 130(3): 710-8.
[http://dx.doi.org/10.1378/chest.130.3.710] [PMID: 16963667]

[27] Gu P, Zhao Y-Z, Jiang L-Y, Zhang W, Xin Y, Han B-H. Endobronchial ultrasound-guided transbronchial needle aspiration for staging of lung cancer: a systematic review and meta-analysis. European Journal Of Cancer (Oxford, England: 1990) 2009; 45: 1389-96.

[28] Ong P, Grosu H, Eapen GA, *et al.* Endobronchial ultrasound-guided transbronchial needle aspiration

for systematic nodal staging of lung cancer in patients with N0 disease by computed tomography and integrated positron emission tomography-computed tomography. Ann Am Thorac Soc 2015; 12(3): 415-9.
[http://dx.doi.org/10.1513/AnnalsATS.201409-429OC] [PMID: 25584815]

[29] Yasufuku K, Nakajima T, Waddell T, Keshavjee S, Yoshino I. Endobronchial ultrasound-guided transbronchial needle aspiration for differentiating N0 *versus* N1 lung cancer. Ann Thorac Surg 2013; 96(5): 1756-60.
[http://dx.doi.org/10.1016/j.athoracsur.2013.05.090] [PMID: 23953728]

[30] Park YS, Lee J, Pang JC, *et al.* Clinical implication of microscopic anthracotic pigment in mediastinal staging of non-small cell lung cancer by endobronchial ultrasound-guided transbronchial needle aspiration. J Korean Med Sci 2013; 28(4): 550-4.
[http://dx.doi.org/10.3346/jkms.2013.28.4.550] [PMID: 23580351]

[31] Plit M, Pearson R, Havryk A, Da Costa J, Chang C, Glanville AR. Diagnostic utility of endobronchial ultrasound-guided transbronchial needle aspiration compared with transbronchial and endobronchial biopsy for suspected sarcoidosis. Intern Med J 2012; 42(4): 434-8.
[http://dx.doi.org/10.1111/j.1445-5994.2011.02446.x] [PMID: 21299786]

[32] Hata Y, Sakamoto S, Otsuka H, *et al.* EBUS-TBNA-related complications in a patient with tuberculous lymphadenopathy. Intern Med 2013; 52(22): 2553-9.
[http://dx.doi.org/10.2169/internalmedicine.52.9273] [PMID: 24240796]

[33] Rosell R, Bivona TG, Karachaliou N. Genetics and biomarkers in personalisation of lung cancer treatment. Lancet 2013; 382(9893): 720-31.
[http://dx.doi.org/10.1016/S0140-6736(13)61715-8] [PMID: 23972815]

[34] Nakajima T, Yasufuku K, Nakagawara A, Kimura H, Yoshino I. Multigene mutation analysis of metastatic lymph nodes in non-small cell lung cancer diagnosed by endobronchial ultrasound-guided transbronchial needle aspiration. Chest 2011; 140(5): 1319-24.
[http://dx.doi.org/10.1378/chest.10-3186] [PMID: 21527506]

[35] van Eijk R, Licht J, Schrumpf M, *et al.* Rapid KRAS, EGFR, BRAF and PIK3CA mutation analysis of fine needle aspirates from non-small-cell lung cancer using allele-specific qPCR. PLoS One 2011; 6(3): e17791-1.
[http://dx.doi.org/10.1371/journal.pone.0017791] [PMID: 21408138]

[36] Sakairi Y, Sato K, Itoga S, *et al.* Transbronchial biopsy needle rinse solution used for comprehensive biomarker testing in patients with lung cancer. J Thorac Oncol 2014; 9(1): 26-32.
[http://dx.doi.org/10.1097/JTO.0000000000000024] [PMID: 24346091]

[37] Esterbrook G, Anathhanam S, Plant PK. Adequacy of endobronchial ultrasound transbronchial needle aspiration samples in the subtyping of non-small cell lung cancer. Lung Cancer 2013; 80(1): 30-4.
[http://dx.doi.org/10.1016/j.lungcan.2012.12.017] [PMID: 23312886]

[38] Wu K, Huang RS, House L, Cho WC. Next-generation sequencing for lung cancer. Future Oncol 2013; 9(9): 1323-36.
[http://dx.doi.org/10.2217/fon.13.102] [PMID: 23980680]

[39] Lockwood WW, Wilson IM, Coe BP, *et al.* Divergent genomic and epigenomic landscapes of lung cancer subtypes underscore the selection of different oncogenic pathways during tumor development. PLoS One 2012; 7(5): e37775-5.
[http://dx.doi.org/10.1371/journal.pone.0037775] [PMID: 22629454]

[40] Wistuba II. Molecular testing of non-small cell lung carcinoma biopsy and cytology specimens. Am Soc Clin Oncol Educ Book 2012; 459-64.
[PMID: 24451780]

[41] Banerji S, Cibulskis K, Rangel-Escareno C, *et al.* Sequence analysis of mutations and translocations across breast cancer subtypes. Nature 2012; 486(7403): 405-9.
[http://dx.doi.org/10.1038/nature11154] [PMID: 22722202]

[42] Coco S, Truini A, Vanni I, *et al.* Next generation sequencing in non-small cell lung cancer: new avenues toward the personalized medicine. Curr Drug Targets 2015; 16(1): 47-59.
[http://dx.doi.org/10.2174/1389450116666141210094640] [PMID: 25495923]

[43] Takeda M, Sakai K, Terashima M, *et al.* Clinical application of amplicon-based next-generation sequencing to therapeutic decision making in lung cancer. Annals Of Oncology: Official Journal Of The European Society For Medical Oncology / ESMO 2015; 26: 2477-2482.2015;

[44] Deeb KK, Hohman CM, Risch NF, Metzger DJ, Starostik P. Routine Clinical Mutation Profiling of Non-Small Cell Lung Cancer Using Next-Generation Sequencing. Arch Pathol Lab Med 2015; 139(7): 913-21.
[http://dx.doi.org/10.5858/arpa.2014-0095-OA] [PMID: 26125431]

[45] Qiu T, Guo H, Zhao H, Wang L, Zhang Z. Next-generation sequencing for molecular diagnosis of lung adenocarcinoma specimens obtained by fine needle aspiration cytology. Sci Rep 2015; 5: 11317-7.
[http://dx.doi.org/10.1038/srep11317] [PMID: 26066407]

[46] Roy-Chowdhuri S, Chow C-W, Kane MK, *et al.* Optimizing the DNA yield for molecular analysis from cytologic preparations. Cancer Cytopathol 2015.
[PMID: 26630358]

[47] Kanagal-Shamanna R, Portier BP, Singh RR, *et al.* Next-generation sequencing-based multi-gene mutation profiling of solid tumors using fine needle aspiration samples: promises and challenges for routine clinical diagnostics. Modern Pathology: An Official Journal Of The United States And Canadian Academy Of Pathology Inc 2014; 27: 314-27.

[48] Karnes HE, Duncavage EJ, Bernadt CT. Targeted next-generation sequencing using fine-needle aspirates from adenocarcinomas of the lung. Cancer Cytopathol 2014; 122(2): 104-13.
[http://dx.doi.org/10.1002/cncy.21361] [PMID: 24227699]

CHAPTER 9

Percutaneous Tracheostomy: Indications, Complications and Techniques

Rahul Nanchal*

Division of Pulmonary and Critical Care Medicine, Medical College of Wisconsin, Wisconsin, WI 53226, USA

Abstract: Percutaneous Tracheostomy has become the preferred method of tracheostomy placement in critically ill patients. The most common indications are prolonged mechanical ventilation and inability to protect the airway. The procedure is safe, simple and is easily performed by non-surgical providers. It has advantages over surgical tracheostomy in terms of fewer stoma infections and decreased costs. The most widely used method of performing percutaneous dilatational tracheostomy is the single dilator method (Ciaglia Blue Rhino). Although there are several other techniques, the single dilator method has the most experience and best safety profile. The use of bronchoscopy and ultrasound as adjuncts facilitates placement of the tracheostomy tube, minimizes complications and enhances patient safety.

Keywords: Bleeding, Bronchoscopy, Ciaglia Blue Rhino, Complications of Tracheostomy, Percutaneous Dilatational Tracheostomy, Posterior Tracheal Injury, Prolonged Mechanical Ventilation, Respiratory Failure, Single Dilation Technique, Surgical Tracheostomy, Tracheal Stenosis, Ultrasound.

INTRODUCTION AND EPIDEMIOLOGY

Tracheostomy is one of the most commonly performed procedures in critically ill patients who require prolonged mechanical ventilation [1 - 4]. Although difficult to demonstrate mortality differences between tracheostomy or prolonged translaryngeal intubation [5], known benefits of tracheostomy include lesser need for sedation, easier participation in physical therapy, better oral and pulmonary hygiene, enhanced patient comfort, shorter weaning times and shorter lengths of intensive care unit (ICU) and hospital stay. Approximately 10% or mechanically ventilated patients receive a tracheostomy [6, 7]. The average number of tracheostomies performed in the United States exceeds 100,000 [8] and up to 34% of patients ventilated for more than 48 hours receive a tracheostomy for prolonged

* **Corresponding author Rahul Nanchal:** Division of Pulmonary and Critical Care Medicine, Medical College of Wisconsin, Wisconsin, WI 53226, USA; Tel: 414-955-7042; Fax: 414-955-6211; E-mail: Rnanchal@mcw.edu

Ali I. Musani (Ed.)

mechanical ventilation [9]. Traditionally, tracheostomies were performed surgically by surgeons or otolaryngologists, however, increasingly, the percutaneous method is now preferred for placement. Techniques to perform percutaneous tracheostomy are easily learned even by individuals who do not have extensive surgical training or experience. Thus in the modern era percutaneous tracheostomies are frequently performed by non-surgical intensivists and interventional pulmonologists. In this chapter, we review the indications, complications, techniques and outcomes of percutaneous tracheostomy.

History

The first report of percutaneous dilatational tracheostomy (PDT) appeared in 1955, when Sheldon *et al.* described a method of obtaining a rapid and stable airway in patients with severe traumatic brain injury [10]. They used a fixation needle, finder needle and a cutting trocar to place the tracheostomy. However, reports of tracheal and aortic injuries using this technique suggested that excessive force was required to place the tracheostomy and resulted in suboptimal outcomes. The current techniques of serial dilation over a wire to place the tracheostomy tube emerged in 1985 when Ciaglia *et al.* first reported their experiences [11].

Comparison to Surgical Tracheostomy

PDT has become the favored approach to insertion of a tracheostomy tube because several lines of evidence have shown superiority over conventional surgical tracheostomy [12 - 15]. The most recent Cochrane review found that although there were no differences in mortality and serious life threatening procedure related events, PDT significantly reduced the rate of wound infection/stomatitis and unfavorable scarring [16]. Further, in contradiction to previously published meta-analyses, rates of accidental decannulation and tracheostomy tube occlusion/obstruction were also similar [16]. There are other intuitive advantages of PDT over surgical tracheostomy – beside performance that eliminates risks associated with patient transport, lesser resource utilization and expense in contrast to performing the procedure in the operating room and avoidance of delays in performing the procedure once the decision to perform tracheostomy is reached. In support several investigations have suggested lower costs associated with PDT; the majority of cost savings occurring as result of avoiding the operating room [17, 18]. Thus the preponderance of evidence suggests that compared to surgical tracheostomy; PDT is safe and associated with lesser complications, procedure time and costs.

Indications for Percutaneous Tracheostomy

The proportion of patients receiving PDT in comparison to surgical tracheostomies varies greatly from country, hospital and practice setting [19, 20]. Nonetheless, PDT has become the technique of choice in intensive care units across the globe. Traditionally thought to be contraindicated in conditions such as severe obesity, emergency situations, enlarged thyroid, head and neck cancer and coagulopathy, with growing experience the indications of PDT have expanded and those for which surgical tracheostomy is mandated have diminished [21, 22]. There are no randomized controlled trials for indications of PDT. The risk, benefits and timing of PDT should be evaluated on an individual basis. The indications for percutaneous tracheostomy are listed in Table **1**.

Table 1. Indications for Percutaneous.

1. Prolonged Mechanical Ventilation
2. Facilitation of ventilation support/ventilator weaning
3. Airway Protection (aspiration syndromes, traumatic brain injury, neuromuscular weakness or bulbar dysfunction)
4. Prolonged need for intra-tracheal suctioning and pulmonary hygiene
5. Upper airway obstruction
6. Trauma or infection of oral cavity, pharynx or larynx
7. Minimization of sedation

Contraindications to Percutaneous Tracheostomy

As the experience with PDT techniques has advanced, many of the traditionally thought contraindications to PDT have abated. PDT has become the preferred modality of tracheostomy placement in the majority of critically ill patients. A careful risk/benefit evaluation should be performed with consideration of the following factors – 1) Anatomic feasibility (ability to hyperextend the neck and identify important landmarks) 2) Presence of aberrant blood vessels 3) Ability to re-intubate at bedside in case of accidental extubation 4) Tolerance to transient hypoxemia and hypercarbia. A list of relative contraindications to PDT appears in Table **2**.

Table 2. Relative Contraindications for Percutaneous Tracheostomy.

1. Need for Emergency Airway Access
2. Unfavorable Anatomy (Short neck, unidentifiable landmarks, limited neck movement, morbid obesity)
3. Cervical spine injury/Unstable neck
4. Uncorrectable coagulopathy
5. Thyroid or tracheal pathology
6. Aberrant blood vessels
7. Evidence of soft tissue infection in the neck
8. Significant ventilator requirements (Non tolerance of transient hypoxia and hypercarbia)

Complications of Percutaneous Tracheostomy

Complications of tracheostomy tube placement though infrequent may be life threatening. Complications are arbitrarily classified as early and late, with the ones categorized as early occurring within one week of tracheostomy tube placement. The tracheostomy stoma requires approximately one week to mature and inadvertent decannulation during this period may occur. Attempts to replace a tracheostomy tube in an immature stoma may be difficult and lead to creation of a false lumen and loss of airway. In addition to complications related to the tracheostomy, difficulties may arise secondary to mucous plugging of the inner cannula and inappropriate tracheostomy tube cuff pressures. Care should be taken to ensure tracheostomy tube patency and maintenance of suitable cuff pressures. Early complications of PDT include bleeding, stomal infections, subcutaneous emphysema, posterior tracheal wall injury, tracheostomy tube obstruction and tracheostomy tube dislodgement. In comparison to surgical tracheostomy, PDT carries a significantly lesser risk of stomal infections [16]. Prophylactic antibiotics are not recommended before tracheostomy placement and appropriate wound care is usually adequate for treating minor infections.

Bleeding represents the most common early complication following PDT [13]. Major bleeding is rare, but minor bleeding may be life threatening if it leads to airway obstruction. Bleeding during the first 48 hours is most often from injury to the superficial veins and is almost all cases easily controlled by local measures such as packing, surgical, gel foam, silver nitrate or injection of lidocaine with epinephrine. Evaluation of the neck vasculature with ultrasound prior to tracheostomy can help reduce the incidence of early bleeding [23]. Bleeding that occurs after the first 48 hours of tracheostomy placement should be investigated carefully as it may be the result of erosion of the tracheostomy tube into major vessels such as the innominate artery.

Posterior tracheal wall injury during tracheostomy is a potentially fatal complication. It occurs most frequently secondary to poor control of the guide-wire and guiding catheter [24]. Most injuries are small and heal spontaneously, however larger tears may cause significant airway bleeding and leakage of air around the tube or into the mediastinum. When injury is significant it may require surgical repair or placement of self-expanding metallic stents.

Tracheostomy tube obstruction can lead to rapid respiratory deterioration and death [25]. It is imperative this complication is promptly recognized and addressed. Tube obstruction may result from plugging secondary to mucous, clotted blood or passage of the tube into a false lumen. Suctioning and changing of the inner cannula usually are enough to relieve obstruction. Use of bronchoscopy during placement helps prevent the formation of false passages.

Tracheostomy tube dislodgement before the tract matures is another potential life threatening complication. The tracheostomy tube in these circumstances should never be replaced blindly; replacement under guidance with bronchoscopy is recommended. However securing an airway should not be delayed, if replacement with bronchoscopy cannot be done promptly, oro-tracheal intubation should be performed. Experts recommend suturing the phalange of the tracheostomy tube to the skin as well as the use of tracheostomy ties to minimize this complication.

Late complications are often classified in relation to the stoma [26 - 29] – suprastomal, stomal and infrastomal. Suprastomal complications are generally secondary to inappropriately high tracheostomy tube placement or cricothyroidotomy. These include subglottic stenosis, tracheal stenosis and granulation tissue formation. Stomal stenosis can occur if the anterior tracheal wall is fractured during PDT. The anterior tracheal wall invaginates and causes a fixed obstruction. Infrastomal complications include tracheal stenosis, tracheomalacia, trachea-esophageal fistulas and trachea-innominate fistulas. Tables **3a** and **3b** list potential early and late complication of PDT with their approximate incidence.

Table 3a. Early Tracheostomy Complications.

1. Bleeding (2%-5%)
2. Infection (0.5%)
3. Posterior membrane injury (0.2%-12.5%)
4. Tracheostomy tube obstruction (0% - 3.5%)
5. Subcutaneous Emphysema (0% - 5%)
6. Tracheal Tube Dislodgment (1%)

Table 3b. Late Tracheostomy Complications.

1. **Suprastomal** – Subglottic Stenosis, tracheal stenosis, granulation tissue formation
2. **Stomal** – Anterolateral stenosis, anterior tracheal fracture
3. **Infrastomal** – Tracheo-esophageal fistula, Tracheo-innominate fistula, tracheomalacia, tracheal stenosis

Percutaneous Dilatational Tracheostomy in the High Risk Patient

Bleeding diatheses and obesity are two main factors driving preference of surgical tracheostomy over PDT. A few small retrospective studies of percutaneous tracheostomy in high risk patients with coagulopathy, thrombocytopenia and other bleeding disorders have shown low complication rates. Although small, these studies suggest that careful correction of coagulopathy in the peri-procedure period allows for safe PDT [30 - 32]. Similarly, small studies have failed to demonstrate any differences in complication rates with PDT in obese patients [33 - 35]. In large prospective, single center evaluation of over 1000 percutaneous tracheostomies, the investigators identified coagulopathy and thrombocytopenia as major risk factors for bleeding; however rates of complications in obese patients were not increased [36]. This suggests that the decision to perform PDT in high risk patients can be individualized. Success likely depends on factors such as operator experience, degree and correction of coagulopathy and favorable surface anatomy.

Percutaneous Dilatational Tracheostomy Procedure

Several commercial kits are available for PDT. A brief description of these appears later in the chapter. The basic contents of the kits are similar and include an introducing needle, a guide wire, a bolstering catheter and one or more dilators. Evidence to suggest benefit of one technique over the other is absent, however single step dilatation is most often use secondary to fewer minor complications and ease of insertion compared to other techniques [37]. There are minor variations in the procedure itself dependent on the kit used; however basic common steps [38] are outlined below:

Preparation

1. NPO overnight as vomitus may be provoked by direct tracheal or indirect pharyngeal or esophageal stimulation
2. Hold anticoagulation if applicable
3. Ensure adequate anesthesia/analgesia and neuromuscular blockade

Instruments

1. Applicable PDT kit
2. Intubation equipment including equipment for handling a difficult airway should be at hand should accidental extubation occur
3. Fiber optic bronchoscope
4. Ultrasound machine

Procedure

1. We recommend that at least two operators be involved with the procedure. One performing the percutaneous tracheostomy and one guiding with bronchoscopy
2. Ensure optimal patient positioning – maximal cervical spine extension (caution with cervical injuries and unstable neck) with optimal presentation of the anterior neck. A pillow placed under the shoulders facilitates this positioning

3. Identification of landmarks – The cricoid cartilage and tracheal rings should be palpated and the ideal site for tracheostomy determined and marked. Placement of the tracheostomy should always occur beneath the cricoid cartilage and ideally between the second and third tracheal rings. Proximal placement increases the risk of tracheal stenosis and more distal placement the risk of erosion into the great vessels of the mediastinum
4. Adequate sterilization of site and provision of local anesthesia. The local anesthetic should contain epinephrine to minimize bleeding from the site
5. A skin incision approximately one centimeter in length in the vertical direction should be made at the site of tracheostomy placement. The incision should be as small as possible to reduce the risk of bleeding, infection and ensure a tight fitting stoma. In the plane of the incision, dissection of soft tissue and fascia should be performed down to the trachea. Through the incision the cricoid cartilage and tracheal rings should then be palpated and landmarks confirmed.
6. Under guidance with bronchoscopy the endotracheal tube should be then retracted just above the site of placement of tracheostomy. Trans-illumination with bronchoscopy through the anterior tracheal wall facilitates optimum placement of the endotracheal tube and confirms ideal site for tracheostomy placement.
7. The trachea should then be punctured through the incision ideally between the second and third tracheal rings and the guide-wire introduced through the needle. Confirmation of needle position and unhindered passage of the guide-wire and are made *via* visualization through the bronchoscope.
8. The stoma is then then dilated with one or more dilators over the guide-wire.
9. The tracheostomy tube is then placed then placed through the stoma. Confirmation of placement of tracheostomy tube in the trachea and optimum positioning is confirmed *via* insertion of the bronchoscope through the tracheostomy tube. The cuff of the tracheostomy tube is then inflated and the ventilator is connected to the tube. The bronchoscope may be now reintroduced through the endotracheal tube to asses for any bleeding above the tracheostomy tube and to visualize optimum tracheostomy tube cuff position within the trachea. The endotracheal tube is then withdrawn
10. The tracheostomy should be secured using a combination of tracheal ties and suturing the phalange.

Percutaneous Dilatational Tracheostomy Techniques

Table **4** lists the various techniques of PDT currently in use. The single dilator technique has the best safety profile is probably most commonly employed. A brief description of techniques appears below

Table 4. Percutaneous Dilatational Tracheostomy Techniques.

Procedure	**Technique**
Sequential Dilation (Ciaglia)	Multistep dilation with sequential dilators
Single Dilation (Ciaglia Blue Rhino)	Single step dilation with one tapered dilator
Translaryngeal (Fantoni)	Retrograde passage with cannula as dilator
Griggs guide-wire dilating forceps (GGWDF)	Dilation with specific forceps
PercuTwist	Dilation with PercuTwist Kit (hydrophilic coating)
Balloon dilation (Ciaglia Blue Dolphin)	Single Step Dilation with a balloon
Rezende-Neto	Combination of GGWDF and PercuTwist

Sequential Dilation Technique

After passage of the guide-wire into the tracheal lumen, an 8F Teflon catheter guide in threaded over the guide-wire and the stoma is dilated serially using dilators ranging from 12F to 28F. The tracheostomy tube fitted over an appropriately sized dilator is then inserted into the stoma over the guide-wire [11].

Single Dilation Technique (Ciaglia Blue Rhino)

A single tapered dilator is used instead of serial dilation. The single dilator has a hydrophilic coating which makes insertion rapid and easy. Since this dilator is softer, it is less likely to damage the posterior tracheal wall [39].

Translaryngeal Percutaneous Tracheostomy (Fantoni)

In this technique, the trachea is cannulated under bronchoscopic guidance, however the guide-wire is passed retrograde out through the mouth. Then a specialized long narrow tube with a low pressure cuff is inserted through the mouth and used to ventilate the patient. This specialized tube leaves enough room for a specialized translarygeal tracheostomy tube to be passed over the guide-wire emerging from the mouth. The tracheostomy tube is passed from the mouth along the guide-wire and pushed through the trachea and out from the incision site. The specialized tracheostomy tube is then rotated such that the intra-tracheal portion points towards the carina [40].

Griggs Guide-Wire Dilating Forceps Technique

This technique involves using modified forceps called guide-wire dilator forceps which are advanced over the wire into the trachea and used for dilatation. The forceps are then opened to the same diameter as the skin incision to split the tracheal membrane between the tracheal rings to the desired diameter. The tracheostomy tube is fitted over a trocar and advanced into the trachea [41].

PercuTwist

The PercuTwist dilator is a screw like dilator that is advanced over the guide-wire and rotated like a screw to achieve dilatation. The maneuver is facilitated by a hydrophilic coating of the dilator. Once dilation is complete, the dilator is removed by rotating it in the opposite direction [42].

Balloon Dilatation (Ciaglia Blue Dolphin)

This technique is very similar to single step dilation, except that in efforts to minimizing tracheal ring fracture, rather than applying inward pressure towards the tracheal lumen using a tapered dilator, radial force is applied to the tracheal wall with a balloon. A balloon tipped catheter loading assembly with prepared tracheostomy tube is advanced into the trachea under bronchoscopic guidance. The balloon is next filled with saline with an inflation pump to a maximum pressure of 11 atmospheres. Then the balloon is completely deflated and tracheostomy tube advanced over the guide-wire into the trachea [43].

Rezende-Neto Technique

This technique is a combination of the PercuTwist and Griggs technique. In this method after the endotracheal tube is pulled back under ultrasound guidance until the cuff is at the level of the thyroid cartilage. The tracheal wall is punctured with an intravenous catheter after incision and pre-tracheal fascia dissection. After guide-wire insertion, dilation is achieved with a threaded dilator as described in the PercuTwist method. After removal of the dilator, a self-retaining retractor forceps is passed over the guide-wire into the trachea and then opened to enlarge the tracheal opening laterally and maintain an open tracheal orifice. A flexible tip introducer is inserted into the airway with facilitation by the retractor. The retractor is then removed and a tracheostomy tube is then placed in the airway [44].

Comparison of Various Techniques of Percutaneous Dilatational Tracheostomy

The majority of the data surrounding techniques for PDT compare serial dilation to single dilation technique. Kost *et al.* in a study of 500 consecutive patients undergoing PDT demonstrated a higher complication rate for serial dilation (13.6%) than single dilation (6.5%) [45]. While no other study was able to reproduce a complication or mortality difference, several unequivocally found time and cost saving with the single dilation (Blue Rhino) method [46, 47]. Fantoni's technique has been compared in 3 randomized control trials to Grigg's, multiple dilator and single dilator techniques respectively. None of these trials showed a clear benefit of one technique over the other. The PercuTwist technique was found to be inferior to the single step dilation method in two trials both in terms of complications and operative time. Similarly the Griggs technique when compared to single step dilation was found to be inferior. Bynahn *et al.* in their description of a single center 5 year experience with five different PDT techniques found that Fantoni's technique and single step dilation were associated with fewest complications. They went on to recommend single step dilation as the procedure of choice due to its simplicity [48]. In a meta-analysis, Cabrini *et al.* concluded that single dilation and Griggs method were equivalent in terms of safety and success, however single step dilation had lesser minor complications [49]. Studies comparing single step dilation and balloon dilation techniques are limited by small sample sizes; however they have all concluded that single step dilation is the favored approach secondary to shorter execution times, fewer complications and ease of use. From the available evidence it appears that single step dilation (Ciaglia Blue Rhino) is the preferred modality for placement of percutaneous tracheostomy [50].

Bronchoscopy during Percutaneous Dilatational Tracheostomy

Although there are no randomized controlled trials comparing performance of PDT with and without bronchoscopy one systematic review of all published deaths related to PDT identified the lack of bronchoscopic guidance as a major risk factor [51]. The use of bronchoscopy during PDT offers several advantages – 1) Identification of correct tracheostomy site (midline placement, level at tracheal rings, and light at anterior tracheal wall) 2) confirmation of intra-tracheal guide-wire placement 3) confirmation of proper introduction of dilator 3) prompt identification of tracheal wall injury or tracheal ring fracture 4) optimal positioning of the tracheal tube post procedure. We therefore use and recommend routine use of bronchoscopic guidance during placement of percutaneous tracheostomy tubes.

Ultrasound during Percutaneous Dilatational Tracheostomy

In one small study the use of ultrasound to guide placement of PDT was associated with less hypoxia and shorter procedure times than the use of bronchoscopy [52], however the majority of studies have used both. A recent systematic review that examined published data regarding the safety and efficacy of ultrasound before and/or during PDT concluded that a prospective randomized trial comparing ultrasound and traditional landmark guided technique is required to establish a role in clinical practice [53]. Prior to the procedure the use of ultrasound allows the evaluation of anatomy of the major vessels and the thyroid gland in relation to the tracheostomy site. It also allows for the identification of any small vessels anterior to the tracheostomy site [23]. Further, ultrasound can be used to identify the position of tracheal rings and midline even in obese patients. In a prospective study, ultrasound guided percutaneous tracheostomy was found to be feasible and safe in obese patients. The study demonstrated that ultrasound provided information on cervical anatomy that modified and guided the specific choice of the puncture site for percutaneous tracheostomy [54]. Potential advantages to using real time ultrasound to perform PDT include decreased hypercarbia and avoidance of potential rises in intracranial pressure in neurologically injured patients because of no bronchoscope in the airway, avoidance of vascular structures in the anterior neck and optimal selection of site particularly in obese patients with difficult surface anatomy for landmarks. We routinely use ultrasound prior to tracheostomy to identify vascular structures in the anterior neck as well as cervical anatomy.

SUMMARY

PDT is a common procedure performed in intensive care units worldwide. As experience with PDT is growing the indications are expanding. The procedure appears safe, relatively simple and can be performed easily by non-surgical providers. A variety of commercial kits and techniques are available, however the wealth of experience is with the single dilator (Ciaglia Blue Rhino) technique. This technique has fewer associated complications and costs. The use of bronchoscopy and ultrasound as adjuncts seems to enhance patient safety and minimizes complications. Although easy to perform, patient selection is extremely important; consideration should be given to traditional surgical tracheostomy when complications are anticipated.

CONFLICT OF INTEREST

The authors declare no conflict of interest, financial or otherwise.

ACKNOWLEDGEMENTS

Declared none.

REFERENCES

[1] Cools-Lartigue J, Aboalsaud A, Gill H, Ferri L. Evolution of percutaneous dilatational tracheostomy--a review of current techniques and their pitfalls. World J Surg 2013; 37(7): 1633-46. [http://dx.doi.org/10.1007/s00268-013-2025-6] [PMID: 23571862]

[2] Durbin CG Jr. Tracheostomy: why, when, and how? Respir Care 2010; 55(8): 1056-68. [PMID: 20667153]

[3] Kollef MH, Ahrens TS, Shannon W. Clinical predictors and outcomes for patients requiring tracheostomy in the intensive care unit. Crit Care Med 1999; 27(9): 1714-20. [http://dx.doi.org/10.1097/00003246-199909000-00003] [PMID: 10507588]

[4] Wood DE. Tracheostomy. Chest Surg Clin N Am 1996; 6(4): 749-64. [PMID: 8934006]

[5] Siempos II, Ntaidou TK, Filippidis FT, Choi AM. Effect of early *versus* late or no tracheostomy on mortality and pneumonia of critically ill patients receiving mechanical ventilation: a systematic review and meta-analysis. Lancet Respir Med 2015; 3(2): 150-8. [http://dx.doi.org/10.1016/S2213-2600(15)00007-7] [PMID: 25680911]

[6] Fischler L, Erhart S, Kleger GR, Frutiger A. Prevalence of tracheostomy in ICU patients. A nation-wide survey in Switzerland. Intensive Care Med 2000; 26(10): 1428-33. [http://dx.doi.org/10.1007/s001340000634] [PMID: 11126252]

[7] Frutos-Vivar F, Esteban A, Apezteguía C, *et al.* International Mechanical Ventilation Study Group. Outcome of mechanically ventilated patients who require a tracheostomy. Crit Care Med 2005; 33(2): 290-8. [http://dx.doi.org/10.1097/01.CCM.0000150026.85210.13] [PMID: 15699830]

[8] Yu M. Tracheostomy patients on the ward: multiple benefits from a multidisciplinary team? Crit Care 2010; 14(1): 109. [http://dx.doi.org/10.1186/cc8218] [PMID: 20156313]

[9] Quality of Life After Mechanized Ventilation in the Elderly Study Investigators. 2-month mortality and functional status of critically ill adult patients receiving prolonged mechanical ventilation. Chest 2002; 121(2): 549-58. [http://dx.doi.org/10.1378/chest.121.2.549] [PMID: 11834671]

[10] Shelden CH, Pudenz RH, Freshwater DB, Crue BL. A new method for tracheotomy. J Neurosurg 1955; 12(4): 428-31. [http://dx.doi.org/10.3171/jns.1955.12.4.0428] [PMID: 14392499]

[11] Ciaglia P, Firsching R, Syniec C. Elective percutaneous dilatational tracheostomy. A new simple bedside procedure; preliminary report. Chest 1985; 87(6): 715-9. [http://dx.doi.org/10.1378/chest.87.6.715] [PMID: 3996056]

[12] Freeman BD, Isabella K, Lin N, Buchman TG. A meta-analysis of prospective trials comparing percutaneous and surgical tracheostomy in critically ill patients. Chest 2000; 118(5): 1412-8. [http://dx.doi.org/10.1378/chest.118.5.1412] [PMID: 11083694]

[13] Delaney A, Bagshaw SM, Nalos M. Percutaneous dilatational tracheostomy *versus* surgical tracheostomy in critically ill patients: a systematic review and meta-analysis. Crit Care 2006; 10(2): R55. [http://dx.doi.org/10.1186/cc4887] [PMID: 16606435]

[14] Higgins KM, Punthakee X. Meta-analysis comparison of open *versus* percutaneous tracheostomy. Laryngoscope 2007; 117(3): 447-54. [http://dx.doi.org/10.1097/01.mlg.0000251585.31778.c9] [PMID: 17334304]

[15] Dulguerov P, Gysin C, Perneger TV, Chevrolet JC. Percutaneous or surgical tracheostomy: a meta-analysis. Crit Care Med 1999; 27(8): 1617-25. [http://dx.doi.org/10.1097/00003246-199908000-00041] [PMID: 10470774]

[16] Brass P, Hellmich M, Ladra A, Ladra J, Wrzosek A. Percutaneous techniques *versus* surgical techniques for tracheostomy. Cochrane Database Syst Rev 2016; 7: CD008045. [PMID: 27437615]

[17] Freeman BD, Isabella K, Cobb JP, *et al.* A prospective, randomized study comparing percutaneous with surgical tracheostomy in critically ill patients. Crit Care Med 2001; 29(5): 926-30. [http://dx.doi.org/10.1097/00003246-200105000-00002] [PMID: 11378598]

[18] Cobean R, Beals M, Moss C, Bredenberg CE. Percutaneous dilatational tracheostomy. A safe, cost-effective bedside procedure. Arch Surg 1996; 131(3): 265-71. [http://dx.doi.org/10.1001/archsurg.1996.01430150043008] [PMID: 8611091]

[19] Kluge S, Baumann HJ, Maier C, *et al.* Tracheostomy in the intensive care unit: a nationwide survey. Anesth Analg 2008; 107(5): 1639-43.
[http://dx.doi.org/10.1213/ane.0b013e318188b818] [PMID: 18931225]

[20] Krishnan K, Elliot SC, Mallick A. The current practice of tracheostomy in the United Kingdom: a postal survey. Anaesthesia 2005; 60(4): 360-4.
[http://dx.doi.org/10.1111/j.1365-2044.2004.04106.x] [PMID: 15766339]

[21] Deppe AC, Kuhn E, Scherner M, *et al.* Coagulation disorders do not increase the risk for bleeding during percutaneous dilatational tracheotomy. Thorac Cardiovasc Surg 2013; 61(3): 234-9.
[http://dx.doi.org/10.1055/s-0032-1322608] [PMID: 23344764]

[22] Takahashi M, Itagaki S, Laskaris J, Filsoufi F, Reddy RC. Percutaneous tracheostomy can be safely performed in patients with uncorrected coagulopathy after cardiothoracic surgery. Innovations (Phila) 2014; 9(1): 22-6.
[http://dx.doi.org/10.1097/IMI.0000000000000041] [PMID: 24534764]

[23] Rajajee V, Fletcher JJ, Rochlen LR, Jacobs TL. Real-time ultrasound-guided percutaneous dilatational tracheostomy: a feasibility study. Crit Care 2011; 15(1): R67.
[http://dx.doi.org/10.1186/cc10047] [PMID: 21342494]

[24] Trottier SJ, Hazard PB, Sakabu SA, *et al.* Posterior tracheal wall perforation during percutaneous dilational tracheostomy: an investigation into its mechanism and prevention. Chest 1999; 115(5): 1383-9.
[http://dx.doi.org/10.1378/chest.115.5.1383] [PMID: 10334157]

[25] Trottier SJ, Ritter S, Lakshmanan R, Sakabu SA, Troop BR. Percutaneous tracheostomy tube obstruction: warning. Chest 2002; 122(4): 1377-81.
[http://dx.doi.org/10.1378/chest.122.4.1377] [PMID: 12377868]

[26] Koitschev A, Graumueller S, Zenner HP, Dommerich S, Simon C. Tracheal stenosis and obliteration above the tracheostoma after percutaneous dilational tracheostomy. Crit Care Med 2003; 31(5): 1574-6.
[http://dx.doi.org/10.1097/01.CCM.0000065189.64560.A8] [PMID: 12771635]

[27] Walz MK, Schmidt U. Tracheal lesion caused by percutaneous dilatational tracheostomy--a clinico-pathological study. Intensive Care Med 1999; 25(1): 102-5.
[http://dx.doi.org/10.1007/s001340050794] [PMID: 10051086]

[28] Epstein SK. Late complications of tracheostomy. Respir Care 2005; 50(4): 542-9.
[PMID: 15807919]

[29] Fernandez-Bussy S, Mahajan B, Folch E, Caviedes I, Guerrero J, Majid A. Tracheostomy Tube Placement: Early and Late Complications. J Bronchology Interv Pulmonol 2015; 22(4): 357-64.
[http://dx.doi.org/10.1097/LBR.0000000000000177] [PMID: 26348694]

[30] Al Dawood A, Haddad S, Arabi Y, Dabbagh O, Cook DJ. The safety of percutaneous tracheostomy in patients with coagulopathy or thrombocytopenia. Middle East J Anaesthesiol 2007; 19(1): 37-49.
[PMID: 17511181]

[31] Auzinger G, O'Callaghan GP, Bernal W, Sizer E, Wendon JA. Percutaneous tracheostomy in patients with severe liver disease and a high incidence of refractory coagulopathy: a prospective trial. Crit Care 2007; 11(5): R110.
[http://dx.doi.org/10.1186/cc6143] [PMID: 17922915]

[32] Kluge S, Meyer A, Kühnelt P, Baumann HJ, Kreymann G. Percutaneous tracheostomy is safe in patients with severe thrombocytopenia. Chest 2004; 126(2): 547-51.
[http://dx.doi.org/10.1378/chest.126.2.547] [PMID: 15302743]

[33] Byhahn C, Lischke V, Meininger D, Halbig S, Westphal K. Peri-operative complications during percutaneous tracheostomy in obese patients. Anaesthesia 2005; 60(1): 12-5.
[http://dx.doi.org/10.1111/j.1365-2044.2004.03707.x] [PMID: 15601266]

[34] Romero CM, Cornejo RA, Ruiz MH, *et al.* Fiberoptic bronchoscopy-assisted percutaneous tracheostomy is safe in obese critically ill patients: a prospective and comparative study. J Crit Care 2009; 24(4): 494-500.
[http://dx.doi.org/10.1016/j.jcrc.2008.06.001] [PMID: 19327297]

[35] Blankenship DR, Kulbersh BD, Gourin CG, Blanchard AR, Terris DJ. High-risk tracheostomy: exploring the limits of the percutaneous tracheostomy. Laryngoscope 2005; 115(6): 987-9.
[http://dx.doi.org/10.1097/01.MLG.0000163107.80668.12] [PMID: 15933506]

[36] Rosseland LA, Laake JH, Stubhaug A. Percutaneous dilatational tracheotomy in intensive care unit patients with increased bleeding risk or obesity. A prospective analysis of 1000 procedures. Acta Anaesthesiol Scand 2011; 55(7): 835-41.
[http://dx.doi.org/10.1111/j.1399-6576.2011.02458.x] [PMID: 21615346]

[37] Sanabria A. Which percutaneous tracheostomy method is better? A systematic review. Respir Care 2014; 59(11): 1660-70.
[http://dx.doi.org/10.4187/respcare.03050] [PMID: 25185145]

[38] Mallick A, Bodenham AR. Tracheostomy in critically ill patients. Eur J Anaesthesiol 2010; 27(8): 676-82.
[PMID: 20523214]

[39] Durbin CG Jr. Techniques for performing tracheostomy. Respir Care 2005; 50(4): 488-96.
[PMID: 15807911]

[40] Fantoni A, Ripamonti D. A non-derivative, non-surgical tracheostomy: the translaryngeal method. Intensive Care Med 1997; 23(4): 386-92.
[http://dx.doi.org/10.1007/s001340050345] [PMID: 9142576]

[41] Griggs WM, Worthley LI, Gilligan JE, Thomas PD, Myburg JA. A simple percutaneous tracheostomy technique. Surg Gynecol Obstet 1990; 170(6): 543-5.
[PMID: 2343371]

[42] Westphal K, Maeser D, Scheifler G, Lischke V, Byhahn C. PercuTwist: a new single-dilator technique for percutaneous tracheostomy. Anesth Analg 2003; 96(1): 229-32.
[PMID: 12505957]

[43] Zgoda MA, Berger R. Balloon-facilitated percutaneous dilational tracheostomy tube placement: preliminary report of a novel technique. Chest 2005; 128(5): 3688-90.
[http://dx.doi.org/10.1378/chest.128.5.3688] [PMID: 16304334]

[44] Rezende-Neto JB, Oliveira AJ, Neto MP, Botoni FA, Rizoli SB. A technical modification for percutaneous tracheostomy: prospective case series study on one hundred patients. World J Emerg Surg 2011; 6: 35.
[http://dx.doi.org/10.1186/1749-7922-6-35] [PMID: 22047013]

[45] Kost KM. Endoscopic percutaneous dilatational tracheotomy: a prospective evaluation of 500 consecutive cases. Laryngoscope 2005; 115(10 Pt 2): 1-30.
[http://dx.doi.org/10.1097/01.MLG.0000163744.89688.E8] [PMID: 16227862]

[46] Johnson JL, Cheatham ML, Sagraves SG, Block EF, Nelson LD. Percutaneous dilational tracheostomy: a comparison of single- *versus* multiple-dilator techniques. Crit Care Med 2001; 29(6): 1251-4.
[http://dx.doi.org/10.1097/00003246-200106000-00036] [PMID: 11395616]

[47] Byhahn C, Wilke HJ, Halbig S, Lischke V, Westphal K. Percutaneous tracheostomy: ciaglia blue rhino *versus* the basic ciaglia technique of percutaneous dilational tracheostomy. Anesth Analg 2000; 91(4): 882-6.
[http://dx.doi.org/10.1097/00000539-200010000-00021] [PMID: 11004042]

[48] Byhahn C, Westphal K, Meininger D, Gürke B, Kessler P, Lischke V. Single-dilator percutaneous tracheostomy: a comparison of PercuTwist and Ciaglia Blue Rhino techniques. Intensive Care Med

2002; 28(9): 1262-6.
[http://dx.doi.org/10.1007/s00134-002-1405-4] [PMID: 12209274]

[49] Cabrini L, Monti G, Landoni G, *et al.* Percutaneous tracheostomy, a systematic review. Acta Anaesthesiol Scand 2012; 56(3): 270-81.
[http://dx.doi.org/10.1111/j.1399-6576.2011.02592.x] [PMID: 22188176]

[50] Cianchi G, Zagli G, Bonizzoli M, *et al.* Comparison between single-step and balloon dilatational tracheostomy in intensive care unit: a single-centre, randomized controlled study. Br J Anaesth 2010; 104(6): 728-32.
[http://dx.doi.org/10.1093/bja/aeq087] [PMID: 20413380]

[51] Simon M, Metschke M, Braune SA, Püschel K, Kluge S. Death after percutaneous dilatational tracheostomy: a systematic review and analysis of risk factors. Crit Care 2013; 17(5): R258.
[http://dx.doi.org/10.1186/cc13085] [PMID: 24168826]

[52] Chacko J, Brar G, Kumar U, Mundlapudi B. Real time ultrasound guided percutaneous dilatational tracheostomy - with and without bronchoscopic control: an observational study. Minerva Anestesiol 2014.
[PMID: 25057932]

[53] Rudas M, Seppelt I. Safety and efficacy of ultrasonography before and during percutaneous dilatational tracheostomy in adult patients: a systematic review. Crit Care Resusc 2012; 14(4): 297-301.
[PMID: 23230879]

[54] Guinot PG, Zogheib E, Petiot S, *et al.* Ultrasound-guided percutaneous tracheostomy in critically ill obese patients. Crit Care 2012; 16(2): R40.
[http://dx.doi.org/10.1186/cc11233] [PMID: 22390815]

CHAPTER 10

Tracheobronchomalacia (TBM) and Excessive Dynamic Airway Collapse (EDAC)

Tayfun Caliskan[1], **Gaurav Kumar**[2] and **Septimiu Murgu**[3,*]

[1] *Department of Pulmonology, University of Health Sciences, Tibbiye Ave, Selimiye Street, 34668, Uskudar, Istanbul, Turkey*

[2] *Department of Pulmonary & Critical Care, 9200 West Wisconsin Avenue, Specialty Clinics Building, Suite E52000, Milwaukee, WI53226, USA*

[3] *Interventional Pulmonology Fellowship Program Director, The University of Chicago Medicine, 5841 S Maryland Ave, MC 6076, Chicago, IL 60637, USA*

Abstract: Expiratory central airway collapse has been better understood within the recent years due to development in computed tomography, bronchoscopic imaging and physiologic measurements of flow dynamics in the central airways. This article is a comprehensive narrative review of tracheobronchomalacia (TBM) and excessive dynamic airway collapse (EDAC). We address in detail their pathophysiology and treatment options. The current literature supports the fact that EDAC is essentially distinct from TBM, caused by different factors and may not represent a true central airway disorder that needs invasive treatment such as surgery or stent insertion. Intermittent positive pressure ventilation could function as pneumatic stenting, which helps the selected patients recover from chronic cough and inability to raise secretions. Symptomatic patients with true TBM (crescent type) may need silicone stent insertion, followed by membranous tracheoplasty if symptoms improve. Future research will clarify the flow limitation in EDAC and TBM and assist in determining the appropriate therapy for individual patients.

Keywords: Airway collapse, Choke points, Excessive dynamic airway collapse, Excessive central airway collapse, Flow limiting segments, Tracheobroncho-malacia, Tracheomalacia.

DEFINITION AND CLASSIFICATIONS

Clarifying the “cut off” values for abnormal dynamic airway narrowing and morphologic types of excessive central airway collapse (ECAC).

* **Corresponding author Septimiu Murgu:** Interventional Pulmonology Fellowship Program Director, The University of Chicago Medicine, 5841 S Maryland Ave, MC 6076, Chicago, IL 60637, USA; Tel: 773-834-3892; E-mail: smurgu@medicine.bsd.uchicago.edu

Ali I. Musani (Ed.)

Central airways are dynamic structures as their cross-sectional area (CSA) changes with each phase of respiration. During normal expiration, the posterior membranous wall of central airways invaginates, leading to narrowing of the airway lumen (without tracheal cartilage deformation), hence leading to a normal, physiologic dynamic airway collapse (DAC) [1]. These changes are due to an increase in pleural pressures during exhalation [2]. Older studies suggest that DAC leads to a reduction in CSA of the airway lumen by maximum 40% [3]. Excessive central airway collapse (ECAC), is the excessive narrowing of the airway lumen during exhalation which leads to the reduction of the CSA of more than 50% [4]. ECAC can either be due to Tracheobronchomalacia (TBM) or Excessive Dynamic Airway Collapse (EDAC). TBM is characterized solely by the weakness of cartilaginous structures of the tracheobronchial wall, whereas EDAC is due to posterior membrane invagination into the airway lumen during expiration without associated cartilage collapse [5].

Regarding the definition of "excessive" collapse, the site at which the CSA is measured in tracheobronchial tree or the modality used to measure the collapse varies widely in the published literature. A study which used multi-detector computed tomography (MDCT) to assess forced expiratory tracheal collapsibility of 51 healthy volunteers with normal pulmonary function demonstrated a wide range of expiratory tracheal collapsibility, which frequently exceeds the current diagnostic threshold for tracheomalacia (TM) (*i.e.* >50% expiratory reduction in CSA). The mean percentage of expiratory reduction in tracheal lumen CSA was 54.34% ±18.6 in the upper trachea and 56.14% ±19.3 in the lower trachea [6]. Mean percentage of the expiratory collapse was 66.9% ± 19.0 for the right main bronchus and 61.4% ± 16.7 for the left main bronchus [7]. In another study of 100 patients with chronic obstructive pulmonary disease (COPD), the tracheal collapse was evaluated by using low-dose, paired inspiratory-dynamic expiratory computed tomography (CT). The mean percentage of expiratory reduction in mid-tracheal lumen CSA was 59% ± 19% and 61% ± 18% expiratory reduction in lower trachea [8]. Also, the different studies have used different threshold to define dynamic collapse in COPD and asthma patients. For example, one study defined excessive collapse as greater than 80% [8], whereas others have defined 50% expiratory reduction in luminal CSA [9].

The terms "TBM" and "EDAC" are often used interchangeably, but they are pathophysiologically and morphologically distinct, although at times, they can co-exist in the same patient. There has been increasing acceptance of the differences between TBM and EDAC [10 - 12]. Based on morphology (*i.e.* airway shape), TBM can further be classified into three sub-categories: *saber sheath-type*, in which there is a collapse of the *lateral* tracheal walls during expiration; *crescent-type*, in which there is a collapse of the *anterior* cartilaginous airway wall during expiration and *circumferential-type,* in which there is a collapse of *both the anterior and lateral* airway walls.

A multidimensional, comprehensive classification system (FEMOS) has been proposed to incorporate previously described severity and extent criteria but also to add the morphology, the origin and functional status of patients with ECAC (Table **1**) [13 - 15]. This classification allows for comprehensive assessment of ECAC, to plan treatment and follow patient`s progress during their follow-up visits.

Table 1. FEMOS Classification of expiratory central airway collapse.

Function	Modified World Health Organization functional classification	Class I (F1)	No limitation of usual physical activity
		Class II (F2)	Mild limitation of physical activity
		Class III (F3	Marked limitation of physical activity
		Class IV (F4)	Unable to perform any physical activity at rest
Extent	Location and distribution of the abnormal airway segment	Normal (E1)	No airway abnormality
		Focal (E2)	Abnormality is present in one main or lobar bronchus or one tracheal
		Multifocal (E3)	Abnormality is present in two contiguous or at least two non-contiguous regions
		Diffuse (E4)	Abnormality is present in more than two contiguous regions
Morphology	Morphology of the airway lumen assessed during dynamic bronchoscopy in the sitting and in the supine position	Sabre-sheath type	Reduction in the transverse or coronal diameter
		Crescent type	Reduction in the anteroposterior or sagittal diameter
		Circumferential type	Reduction in both the transverse and sagittal diameters
Origin	Etiology of the airway abnormality	Idiopathic	No underlying etiology is identified
		Secondary	Result of an illness or other pathological process
Severity	Degree of reduction in airway lumen during expiration as seen during bronchoscopy	Normal (S1)	No abnormal airway collapse
		Mild (S2)	Expiratory airway collapse is 50–75%
		Moderate (S3)	Expiratory airway collapse is 75–100%
		Severe (S4)	Expiratory airway collapse is 100% and the airway walls make contact

Etiology

Etiology of TBM and EDAC can be divided into two categories: a. Congenital (primary) and b. Acquired disease (secondary) and most cases of adult TBM or EDAC belong to the latter group (Table **2**). A congenital etiology that can be seen in adulthood is Mounier-Kuhn syndrome or congenital tracheobronchomegaly, a disease process characterized by atrophy of the myoelastic fibers of the large airways resulting in tracheobronhomegaly, tracheal diverticuli, EDAC, and bronchiectasis. Acquired or secondary causes of TBM can be due to chronic airway inflammation or mechanical causes (injury and chronic compression). Examples of chronic airway inflammation are relapsing polychondritis, recurrent respiratory infections, prolonged intubation and indwelling tracheostomy. Examples of mechanical causes of TBM are blunt chest trauma, post-pneumonectomy or lobectomy, tracheostomy, endobronchial electrosurgery (high power of 40-60 Watts can destroy bronchial cartilage). It can also be seen in situations where there is long standing extrinsic compression of the airways like lung or airway tumors, thyroid masses, aortic or pulmonary artery aneurysm, bronchogenic cysts, pulmonary artery sling, or aberrant right subclavian artery [4, 16, 17]. EDAC, on the other hand, is mainly seen in patients suffering from morbid obesity, COPD, and asthma, especially if they have two or more of these co-morbidities.

Histopathology of TBM and EDAC

There is a paucity of information regarding histology of TBM or EDAC, with most information coming from case reports. When due to radiation therapy, destruction of cartilage with infiltration of T-lymphocyte and macrophages could be seen [18]. In relapsing polychondritis, there is empty lacunae and erosion of the cartilage by a mixed population of inflammatory cells [19]. Atrophy of the longitudinal elastic fibers in the posterior membranous wall has been noted in acquired TBM, although this report likely describes EDAC [13].

Table 2. Etiology of TBM and EDAC.

Etiology of TBM/EDAC	Associated Conditions	Potential Mechanisms
A. Congenital /Primary		
	Mounier-Kuhn syndrome	Congenital atrophy of elastic fibers
B. Acquired/Secondary		
1. Chronic airway Inflammation	Recurrent infections, prolonged intubation	Cartilage inflammation
	COPD, Asthma	Small airway inflammation
	Relapsing polychondritis	Auto-immune condition causing recurrent episodes of chondritis and inflammation of the connective tissue tracheobronchial tree

(Table 2) contd.....

Etiology of TBM/EDAC	Associated Conditions		Potential Mechanisms
2. Mechanical	Manipulation of the airways - post pneumectomy or lobectomy		Impaired blood supply and necrosis
	Tracheostomy		Chronic inflammation of the airway walls
	Closed chest trauma		Unidentified cartilage fractures of the trachea
	Endobronchial electrosurgery		Thermal energy destruction of the cartilaginous wall
	Long standing extrinsic compression of the airways	Malignant - Carcinoma, Teratoma, Lymphoma, Neuroblastoma	Direct tumor invasion of the cartilaginous wall
		Non-Malignant 1. Vascular anomalies- innominate artery, aortic arch ring, pulmonary artery sling, aberrant Right subclavian) 2. Cysts: Thymic cyst, bronchogenic cyst	Chronic extrinsic compression and secondary weakness of the cartilage

Physiology and Pathophysiology

Two main theories that can explain the expiratory flow limitation and these two theories can be applied to understand the flow dynamics in TBM and EDAC- Equal pressure point (EPP) theory and Wave speed theory.

Equal Pressure Point Theory

This theory is based on the "Starling resistor" model of the lung (Fig. **1**). The pressure in the alveoli is the sum total of elastic recoil pressure and pleural pressure. During inspiration, the pleural pressure and the alveolar pressure are negative relative to the atmospheric pressure (pressure at the mouth); hence, air flows from the atmosphere to the alveoli. Whereas during quiet expiration, the pleural pressure remains negative, the alveolar pressure rises above atmospheric pressure. Therefore, the air flows from the alveoli to the atmosphere. During the airflow from alveoli to the atmosphere, mainly due to friction losses, the intraluminal airway pressure decreases from the alveoli to the mouth. At the beginning of expiration, the intraluminal pressure is equal to the sum of alveolar pressure and pleural pressure, but later in expiration, the intraluminal pressure decreases, and it eventually becomes equal to the pleural pressure (Fig. **1**). The point in the airway at which this process occurs is known as the equal pressure point (EPP). Airways from the site of EPP towards the mouth will collapse during the expiratory phase as the intraluminal pressure is less than the pleural pressure. This region of dynamic airway compression in the vicinity of the EPP is referred to as a flow-limiting segment (FLS). EPP has Starling resistor effect on the airflow in the airways; the driving pressure for airflow is the difference between alveolar pressure and pleural pressure, rather than the pressure difference between the alveoli and the mouth. Any increased expiratory effort will increase both alveolar pressure and the pleural pressure and the difference between the two will remain the same. Therefore, the driving pressure will continue to be the same, effort independent and the airflow reached its maximum value for that particular lung volume [20]. It is noted in healthy adults that FLS have a tracheal location at total lung capacity (*i.e.* early in expiration), but as lung volume decreases during exhalation, FLS move peripherally but still stay in the central airways in the lobar, segmental, and at the most sub-segmental bronchi (Fig. **1**).

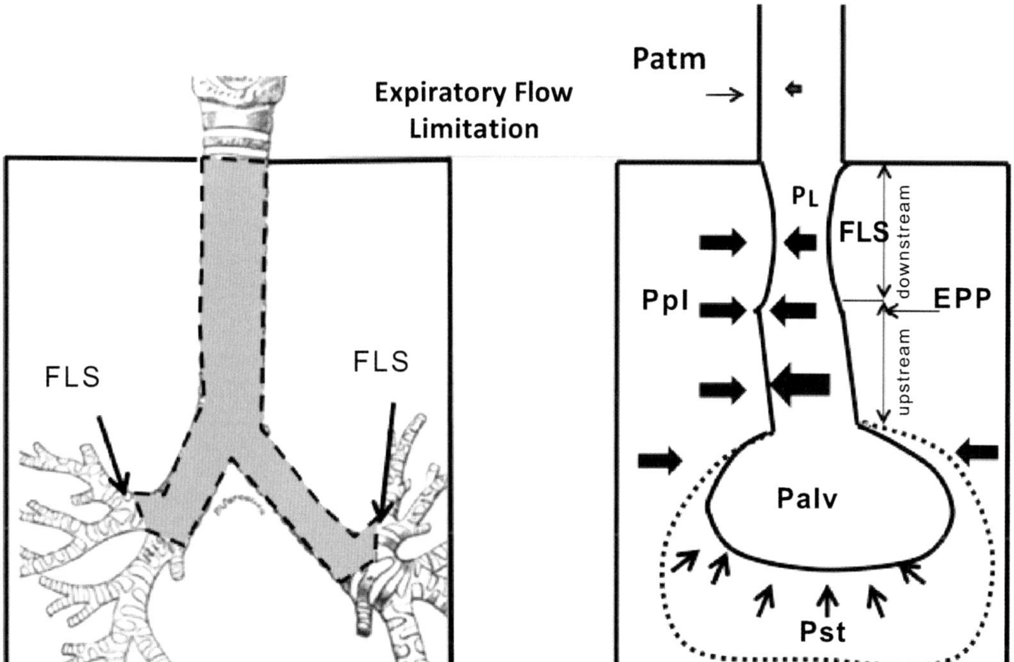

Fig. (1). Expiratory flow limitation theory and impact on EDAC. **Right panel.** Airflow during expiration is determined by the alveolar pressure (Palv) which is approximately equal to the recoil pressure of the lungs (Pst) plus the pleural pressure (Ppl): P alv = P pl + Pst. During forced expiration, the intraluminal pressure (PL) becomes equal to pleural pressure (Ppl) at a point called the equal pressure point (EPP). The upstream segment (alveolarward from the EPP) the transmural pressure (Ptm=PL-Ppl) is positive, but in the downstream segment (mouthward from the EPP) is negative within the intrathoracic airways. At a given lung volume, driving pressure upstream from the EPP would be equal to lung elastic recoil (Pst), while downstream from the EPP, airways would be compressed during expiration. This region of compression of intraluminal caliber is referred to as a flow-limiting segment (FLS) or "choke point". In emphysema, the reduced Pst and increased Rus result in decreased transluminal pressure EDAC; in morbid obesity the reduced Pst from restriction and increased Ppl will also result in EDAC . **Left panel.** The EPP migrate upstream as the lung volume decrese during exhalation (decreasing the Pst), resulting in a lengthening of the increasingly narrow downstream segment see as EDAC on dynamic CT or bronchoscopy. This increases airway resistance and prevents further increases in expiratory airflow, causing the EPP to become fixed when airflow becomes constant. FLS move peripherally during exhalation to the lobar/ segmental and at most subsegmental bronchi.

Wave Speed Theory

Airflow induces a propagating wave in the walls of the airways, as a result of the interaction of recoil force of the elastic airway wall and the axial inertial force of the flowing gas (*i.e.* air). The wave speed theory states that the velocity of this wave that is generated in the conduit is dependent on the characteristics of the conduit and the density of the gas; and that the velocity of the air in the tube cannot exceed the velocity of the pressure wave. Maximal expiratory flow is thus reached when the velocity of air matches the speed of wave propagation at some point in the intrathoracic airways, and this site is the FLS [21] where the flow becomes independent of the downstream pressure [22]. This is usually described by the following equation:

$$V_{ws} = A\ [A/\rho X C_{aw})]$$

Where V_{ws}: Wave-speed flow; A: Cross-sectional area, Caw (dA/dP_{tm}): airway compliance; ρ: density of fluid within the system

The flow of the wave speed is directly proportional to the CSA and inversely proportional to compliance of the airways. Hence, two characteristics determine the location of the FLS–area and compliance [23]. At high lung volumes, FLS are observed in the second or third generation bronchi but as the lung volume decreases during expiration, the airway caliber decreases, and the FLS move towards the alveoli [24].

These two theories are supported by experiments [25], which proved that once flow limitation has occurred at the FLS, proximal airway resistance does not affect the airflow. FLS in adult humans are often located at the level of the lobar bronchi. Thus, the tracheal collapsibility noted as EDAC on chest CT or bronchoscopy, should not impede flow, as the trachea and main stem bronchi are downstream from the choke points (aka flow limiting segments). EDAC that is seen in patients with COPD, asthma, and morbid obesity represents the airway downstream from the choke points and is not responsible for flow limitation, and thus stenting of EDAC is not expected to improve airflow or dyspnea [11]. From a physiological standpoint the difference between EDAC and TBM is that in patients with TBM, the FLS are in the central airways, whereas in EDAC, they are in the peripheral airways [16]. The FLS could be measured by the degree of pressure drop along with the collapsing segment. This measurement could help to identify which patients with ECAC will benefit from interventions [26].

Diagnostic Strategies

Pulmonary Function Tests (PFTs)

Pulmonary function tests (PFTs) may be useful in evaluating a patient with suspected ECAC but they are typically not specific for TBM or EDAC diagnoses [27]. In fact, only 44.4% of the patients with TBM show an obstructive ventilatory defect, 17.8% have a definite or highly likely restrictive ventilatory defect, 16.7% have a mixed defect, and 21.1% have normal results by PFTs [28]. Recent survey-based data shows that 38% of clinicians do not perform further work up for in patients suspected to have TBM if the PFTs are normal and 73% of respondents in this study used PFTs to influence their diagnostic plan [29]. Some studies show that in EDAC (although called TBM in the original paper), central airway collapse is not closely related to airflow obstruction, and expiratory flow limitation at rest often occurs in peripheral airways without central airway collapse [30]. Also, in the patients with COPD, there is no significant correlation between percentage expiratory tracheal collapse and PFTs [8]. In fact, COPD patients demonstrate a wide range of end-expiratory tracheal collapse [31]. Central airway stabilization with stent insertion or tracheoplasty, however, benefits some patients with COPD and ECAC, with meaningful improvement in the quality of life and functional status [32]. Thus spirometry measurements are not necessarily representative of symptomatic improvement. This suggests that central airway stabilization (either with sent insertion or tracheoplasty) either improve cough and secretion management or improve pulmonary mechanics but not the airflow as measured by forced expiratory volume in 1 second (FEV_1) % predicted [4]. Recently, even comprehensive pulmonary physiologic testing like PFTs and impulse oscillometry (IOS) measurements failed to show a correlation with the degree of EDAC during exercise in symptomatic military personnel [33].

On spirometry, flow-volume loop (FVL) might show notching, maximum forced expiratory flow, biphasic expiratory curve or flow oscillations [34].

The Notch which is noted on volume time curve is considered to reflect a sudden decrease in the air flow at the beginning of expiration when the airway collapses. It is due to an initial phase in which a small volume of air is rapidly exhaled, followed by an upward deflection in the spirogram and then the continuation of exhalation.

Low Maximal Flow on FVL has also been noted. Maximal flow is reached quickly after the expiration of a small volume of air. Following the maximal airflow, there is a large fall in airflow although only a small volume of air is exhaled. There is subsequently a phase in which flow rate falls very little during the remainder of expiration. This phase causes the long plateau seen on the FVL such that FVL from patients with TBM or EDAC may be biphasic, with a linear phase of sharply falling velocity followed by an almost linear phase of slow velocity.

Flow Oscillations or saw–tooth pattern, defined as a reproducible sequence of alternating decelerations and accelerations of airflow, can be seen in patients with TBM and EDAC on the expiratory limb of the FVL. When saw tooth pattern is present on the inspiratory arm of the FVL, it suggests obstructive sleep apnea, structural or functional disorders of the larynx, neuromuscular diseases, Parkinson's disease, or tumors of the upper airway [34].

The shape of the expiratory flow-volume tracing is, however, neither sensitive nor specific for either TBM or EDAC. Among subjects with TBM, the most frequent findings are a below-predicted maximum forced expiratory flow (81.6%), biphasic morphology (19.7%), followed by a notched expiratory loop and expiratory oscillations (2.6%) [28]. PFTs and flow-volume loops can be normal in 17.1% of patients with moderate to severe TBM, and they should not be used to diagnose TBM or EDAC or classify its severity [28, 35].

Dynamic Chest Computed Tomography

Unlike routine CT imaging, in which the airways are evaluated at maximum end-inspiration, dynamic imaging involves obtaining CT during or after provocative maneuvers such as expiration or coughing. TBM and EDAC are not detected with routine end-inspiratory CT imaging. Since dynamic CT is a noninvasive diagnostic method compared with bronchoscopy, it can be used as the initial test when TBM and EDAC are suspected.

Visual and quantitative analysis of the central airways provides a comprehensive assessment by allowing the accurate diagnosis of TBM, determining its extent, assessing for predisposing conditions, and helping in the evaluating candidates who might benefit from stent placement or tracheoplasty procedures. This technique can also be helpful for assessing the response of airway dynamics following therapeutic intervention. Scout images are captured to determine the area of coverage (trachea, main stem bronchi, and bronchus intermedius). Scanning is performed in a craniocaudal direction during both end-inspiratory (imaging during suspended end inspiration) and dynamic expiratory phases (imaging during forceful exhalation) (Fig. **2**), the percentage of airway collapse (AC) is calculated by subtracting the dynamic expiratory CSA from the end-inspiratory CSA, divided by the end-inspiratory CSA [4]. Some protocols capture images at three different time points during the respiratory cycle: at the end of inspiration, at the end of expiration, and during dynamic exhalation [36]. Image acquisition performed during dynamic exhalation accentuates airway collapse because images are captured during forced expiratory maneuver, not tidal expiration. The abnormal collapse detected does not reflect the patient's airway dynamics during tidal respiration. Supervision and coaching of patients are necessary, which are not always feasible with very dyspneic, uncooperative, or critically ill patients. If patients start coughing, the degree of AC is accentuated even further [4].

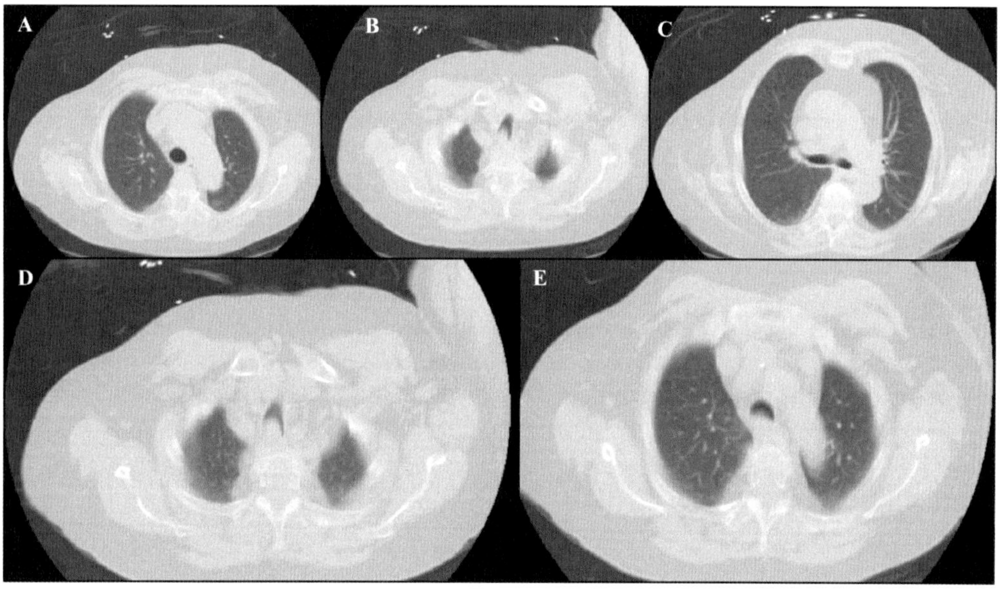

Fig. (2). Chest computed tomography images of a patient with TBM. Normal tracheal lumen, right main bronchus and left main bronchus during inspiration (**A, C**). Tracheal collapse at the end of expiration (**B**). The tracheal collapse during dynamic expiration (**D, E**).

The major concerns for CT are radiation exposure and the ability to perform provocative maneuvers, especially in pediatric patients. In addition, patient cooperation is essential as the imaging is captured during a single forced expiratory maneuver. The use of end-inspiratory CT images alone is not useful for detecting TBM or EDAC, because after closing the vocal cords for a breath-hold, the intraluminal airway pressure can become positive, the transmural pressure increases and the airways will be distended [4]. End-expiratory CT images at suspended exhalation may also be misleading for similar reasons; the intraluminal pressure may be higher than during dynamic expiration, and because the expiratory effort has ceased, the pleural pressure is not maximal, and the degree of collapse may be diminished. In fact, studies of patients with COPD show that the degree of tracheal collapse at end expiration does not predict the degree of collapse during dynamic exhalation [37]. Paired end-inspiratory and end-expiratory MDCT may be a suitable alternative for the assessment of infants and children younger than five years of age who are unable to cooperate with dynamic expiratory breathing instructions [38, 39]. The radiation dose of paired inspiratory-expiratory CT imaging can be reduced by 23% while maintaining similar diagnostic confidence for the assessment of the tracheal lumen compared to a standard-dose technique in pediatric patients [40]. Thus, a reduced-dose technique is recommended for evaluating TBM in children.

Dynamic expiratory imaging shows a significantly greater degree and extent of airway collapse than standard end-expiratory imaging in patients suspected of TBM or EDAC. In fact, MDCT dynamic expiratory imaging was compared with the suspended end-expiratory imaging in patients with suspected TBM [37]. In the study, the mean percentage of airway collapse was significantly greater with dynamic expiratory imaging than with the end-expiratory imaging at three different levels in the central airways: lower thoracic trachea (26% *vs.* 16.6%, $p<0.009$), right bronchi (25.2% *vs.* 14%, $p<0.01$) and left main (24.7% *vs.* 13.3%, $p<0.01$) bronchi. Regardless of the threshold value for defining TBM or EDAC, dynamic expiratory imaging results in diagnosing TBM in more patients than end-expiratory imaging. CT imaging with dynamic expiration, or forceful exhalation, is thus preferred over imaging at end-expiration because higher intrathoracic pressures are generated by the former maneuver, leading to a greater degree of airway collapse in patients with TBM [41, 42].

Dynamic CT is used in the assessment of TBM and EDAC as a complementary test for dynamic bronchoscopy [43]. Dynamic CT is a highly sensitive method for detecting TBM [44], but it can also be used for the preoperative evaluation of patients with TBM who are referred for tracheoplasty and for monitoring progress post therapy [45]. In the preoperative stage, dynamic CT helps with localization and determination of the degree of AC. CT measurements of forced expiratory tracheal collapse are reproducible over time in healthy volunteers and thus can be used for monitoring and assessment of progression of disease [4]. In addition, dynamic CT can also be used to assess the degree of airway collapse, craniocaudal extent of AC, and to define intrinsic (*e.g.*, cartilage thickening in relapsing polychondritis) or extrinsic (*e.g.* Compression by mediastinal masses or vascular structures) abnormalities. It also allows for measurement of the airway caliber to plan stent insertion if needed [46]. The postoperative evaluation after tracheoplasty can be performed using CT, which can reveal changes in the degree of expiratory airway collapse and can potentially detect complications of such as airway dehiscence, mediastinal hematoma, or abscess [47]. CT has been used to follow up patients after stent airway placement to assess stent patency, detect complications *such as* migration, formation of granulation tissue, mucus obstruction, or choke point migration.

Also, CT can help evaluate for associated conditions and other pathology that would require different interventions. It also allows to assess-the changes of lung parenchyma that may cause or be associated with ECAC (*i.e.* emphysema, bronchiolitis, air trapping). TBM was demonstrated in 69% of the adult patients with cystic fibrosis during forced expiratory maneuvers using dynamic CT and in 29% of the adult patients with cystic fibrosis during coughing [48]. Apart from noninvasiveness, the other advantage of CT over bronchoscopy is its ability to evaluate for structures around the airways that could be potential-etiology for TBM (*i.e.,* goiter, aortic aneurysm, double aortic arch). The disadvantages of CT are that it does not provide details about the airway mucosa, exposure to ionizing radiation and requires patient cooperation with respiratory maneuvers.

Recent survey based data show that 80% of clinicians do not diagnose TBM solely on dynamic CT and only 39% identify TBM on CT [29]. The most widely accepted diagnostic criterion for TBM on CT imaging is the same as that is applied in bronchoscopy which is defined as ≥50% expiratory reduction in the CSA of the airway lumen [41]. Studies have shown, however, that the normal, physiologic range of airway collapsibility may exceed this threshold [6, 49]. Forced-expiratory bronchial collapsibility in healthy volunteers was assessed by using MDCT and 73% of the participants exceeded the diagnostic threshold level (>50% expiratory reduction in CSA) for bronchomalacia [15]. Recent dynamic CT studies are in agreement with the physiologic understanding of EDAC based on the flow limitation theories. Although the previous definition of abnormal collapse greater than 50% cross-sectional luminal collapse is still used by some investigators, symptomatic collapse, which may require interventions, is usually observed when cross-sectional luminal collapses greater than 95% to 100% [50]. The different degrees of AC noted on imaging studies led to radiologic subtyping according to severity [15].

Because there is overlap in the degree of expiratory collapse among healthy volunteers and patients with ECAC, hence % expiratory decrease in CSA should not be the only criterion for defining this disease process or for deciding specific treatment strategies. Until a new physiology based criterion can be established, the finding of greater than 50% airway collapsibility on dynamic expiratory CT imaging should be correlated clinically with respiratory symptoms and pulmonary function tests to determine its physiologic significance [41]. Excessive expiratory tracheal collapse, in fact, has been observed in 20% of patients with COPD, but the magnitude of collapse is independent of disease severity and does not correlate significantly with physiologic parameters [8, 31]. The correlations of tracheal volume and collapsibility on inspiratory and end-expiratory CT were evaluated with lung volume and with lung function in smokers [51]. Significant correlation between the tracheal volume and collapsibility, and the lung volume and collapsibility was noted. In addition, the highly collapsed trachea did not indicate more severe airflow limitation or air-trapping in smokers because only weak correlation was found with FEV_1/FVC or RV/TLC ratios, respectively. These findings add to the body of evidence that the collapsed trachea on end-expiratory scans in the form of EDAC may not be a morbid finding and it should be distinguished from the abnormally collapsed trachea in TBM.

Advances in CT technology now allows for faster image acquisition. Cine MDCT requires the use of a 64-row or greater. MDCT scanner combined with a coughing maneuver is used for the diagnosis of TBM. 64-MDCT has advantages for functional imaging because it has high spatial and temporal resolution, and has large anatomic coverage. This method is technically feasible and offers a promising alternative to previous cine CT methods for diagnosing TM [52]. Three-dimensional reconstruction images are useful for obtaining a perspective on the extent and degree of collapse, and the axial images can be used for accurate measurements of CSA. A novel MDCT with 320 x 0.5 detector rows with a dynamic expiratory low-dose is another viable technique for the comprehensive evaluation of TBM [53]. With 320-MDCT scanner, 16 cm of craniocaudal coverage can be achieved with a single gantry rotation, thereby covering the entire intrathoracic trachea in the majority of adults (41). The patients referred for a clinical suspicion of TM were studied on a 320-row MDCT unit by using the following parameters: 120 kVp, 40-50 mA, 0.5-second gantry rotation, and z-axis coverage of 160 mm sufficient to cover the thoracic trachea to the proximal bronchi. Image acquisition occurred during a forceful exhalation. The image data set was subject to the following analyses: CSA of airway lumen at 4 predefined locations (thoracic inlet, aortic arch, carina, and bronchus intermedius) and measurement of airway volume [53]. In another study, measurements of expiratory collapse obtained using 64 MDCT system (120 kVp, 40 mAs, 0.625 mm collimation) with spirometric monitoring at end-inspiration and during forced expiration of the central airways on routine axial and multiplanar reformatted (MPR) images were compared [54]. Measurements of the trachea, right main and left main bronchus were obtained on axial and MPR images. Differences in mean % collapse for axial *versus* MPR images were small and unlikely to influence clinical management. This finding suggested that MPR may not be indicated for routine assessment of central airway collapse [54].

Based on the data obtained from dynamic CT studies, radiology literature suggests the need for more rigorous criteria for diagnosing clinically relevant EDAC, with potentially separate diagnostic threshold levels for the trachea, right and left main stem bronchi [49, 6]. Clinical correlation of forced expiratory CT findings of EDAC with patient's symptoms and PFT is necessary in the decision-making process. In fact, it is the increasing use of dynamic CT that led to recognition of several morphologic types of ECAC [55, 56]. In one study, at inspiration, 94% of subjects demonstrated a normal tracheal configuration (round, oval, horseshoe, or inverted-pear shape), and 6% of subjects demonstrated an abnormal "lunate" tracheal configuration in which the coronal/sagittal diameter ratio is greater than 1. At expiration, 53% of subjects demonstrated a crescent-type, or "frown" shape; 6% of subjects demonstrated complete collapse; and 41% of subjects demonstrated other morphologies. Inspiratory tracheal morphology is almost always normal in patients with EDAC, with a lunate configuration only rarely observed. In contrast, an expiratory "frown sign" is observed in approximately 50% of patients with this condition.

Dynamic or Functional Bronchoscopy

Direct visualization of the airway with bronchoscopy remains the "gold standard" for the diagnosis of TBM [57]. Flexible bronchoscopy is the preferred modality for direct visualization and dynamic assessment of the central airways. Functional bronchoscopy consists of physiologic measurements during bronchoscopy and performance of dynamic bronchoscopy [4]. Dynamic flexible bronchoscopy allows for the assessment of airway collapsibility during tidal breathing or forced expiratory maneuvers. The patient follows commands and cooperates during the procedure with respiratory maneuvers and changes in body position during bronchoscopy. Patients are instructed to take a deep breath, hold it, and then blow it out. Airway dimension is estimated by dynamic flexible bronchoscopy as the anteroposterior distance between the midpoints of the posterior membrane and the anterior luminal aspects of the airway obtained during forced inspiration and expiration [58]. The presence of airway malacia is defined as greater than 50% expiratory reduction in the airway lumen on bronchoscopy. The severity of airway malacia is conventionally graded by the degree of airway collapse during forced expiration (intrathoracic malacia) or inspiration (extrathoracic malacia) [59]. Collapse less than 50% seems to be within normal limits, 50% to 75% is graded as mild, 75% to 90% as moderate, and 91% to 100% as severe malacia. Although most experts still agree that functional bronchoscopy is the gold standard for diagnosis, there are no standardized protocols guiding respiratory maneuvers and airway measurements during these procedures [59]. Recent survey based data show that 90% of clinicians diagnose TBM on dynamic bronchoscopy, but only 29% could identify TBM on bronchoscopy images [29]. For instance, a patient with malacia and orthopnea may not have the bronchoscopic findings of malacia unless the bronchoscopy is performed in a supine position [4]. Similarly, a patient with a history of tracheostomy and dyspnea when bending over or during neck flexion may have post tracheostomy stoma stricture with malacia, revealed only when the lesion becomes intrathoracic and increased pleural pressures during exhalation result in further narrowing of the airway lumen and cause flow limitation. Conversely, if the lesion is at the thoracic inlet, symptoms may occur only during inspiration if the lesion becomes extrathoracic, such as when the patient performs neck extension.

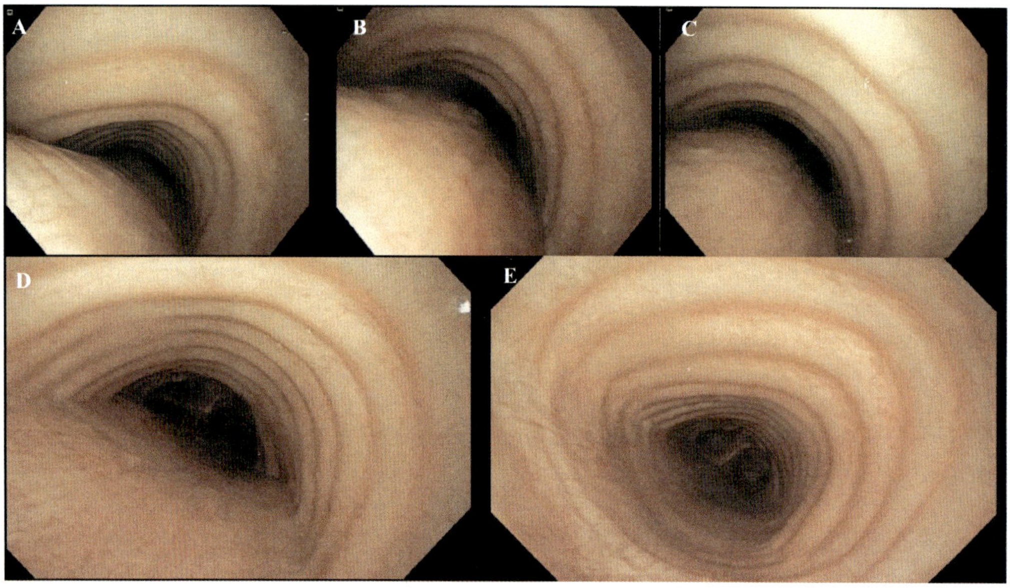

Fig. (3). Impact of respiratory maneuver and effort on degree of airway narrowing. Images (**A-E**) are obtained from the same patient undergonig flexible bronchoscopy. The tracheal cartilaginuous wall is intact during all respiratory maneuvers. Normal tracheal lumen during inspiration (**A**). TBM during coughing (**B**) and forced expiration (**C**). Physiologic, dynamic compression before CPAP with 10 cm H_20 (**D**). Normal tracheal lumen during CPAP with 10 cm H_20 (**E**).

Dynamic changes can be studied during quiet breathing, forced breathing maneuvers, coughing, and neck flexion/extension, and the impact on pressure change responsible for symptoms can be determined (Fig. **3**). Intraluminal catheter airway pressure measurements identified the choke point in the lower trachea in the ECAC [60]. Pressure catheter measurements in EDAC reveal no pressure drop along the collapsible central airway, in contrast to TBM. The measurements of central airway narrowing were derived from bronchoscopic videotapes and simultaneous pressure measurements in the trachea and esophagus in one study [30]. Airflow and transpulmonary pressure (PL) were measured to identify expiratory flow limitation during quiet breathing and to determine the critical PL required for maximum expiratory flow. In a prospective study, lateral airway pressure (Plat) during bronchoscopy using a double-lumen catheter was measured in 15 healthy subjects and 30 patients with tracheal obstruction located at the site of maximal obstruction and to estimate the outcome of intervention [26]. Pressure difference was used to evaluate the site of maximal obstruction. The direct measurement of pressure difference and the angle of the pressure–pressure curve represented a new assessment modality for the success of interventional bronchoscopy and could estimate the need for additional procedures better than bronchoscopy alone.

Assessment of the degree of airway narrowing in patients suspected with TBM is based on a semi-quantitative approximation made by the bronchoscopist during visual inspection. Accurate measurements of airway dimensions during bronchoscopy are relevant and objective measurement techniques (*i.e.* color histogram mode technique, CHMT) have been described [61].

Bronchoscopy allows direct visualization of the airway mucosa, can be performed in critically ill patients at the bedside, is not associated with ionizing radiation, and allows assessment of response to noninvasive positive pressure ventilation (NIPPV) when this is considered as a treatment alternative [4].

Dynamic Magnetic Resonance Imaging (MRI)

Although dynamic bronchoscopy is the current gold standard in patients with suspected TBM [57], it is an invasive procedure and requires sedation especially in pediatric patients. So provocative maneuvers such as forced expiration and coughing cannot be performed during bronchoscopy if patients are over sedated. Bronchoscopy also cannot provide exact measurements of airway dimensions comparable to that provided by imaging techniques, unless morphometric techniques are being used.

Magnetic resonance imaging (MRI) is mostly used for the diagnosis of TBM in pediatric patients, because it can characterize tracheal narrowing without using ionizing radiation or intravenous contrast medium in pediatric patients [62]. Due to its ability to evaluate vascular structures without iodinated contrast material, and direct multiplanar imaging capabilities, MRI is the preferred method to evaluate extrinsic airway abnormalities, including vascular compression syndromes [27]. Cine MRI provides extremely rapid acquisition of images, relationships of mediastinal structures and provides functional imaging of tracheal patency during the respiratory cycle for the evaluation of focal TM due to focal innominate artery compression [63]. In a study, inspiratory and expiratory spiral CT, cine CT, bronchoscopy, cine MRI were compared for localization and determination of collapse in patients with TBM before surgical procedure [64]. Temporal resolution of cine CT and cine MRI was sufficient; however, spatial resolution of cine MRI was inferior when compared to the CT. Significantly improved evaluation of respiratory collapse and further information of localized tracheal instability were obtained by cine CT.

Contrary to CT scanning, MRI has the advantage of avoiding radiation and offering superior contrast resolution and better characterizes soft tissue masses. MRI can delineate tracheal and main bronchial patency and their close anatomic relationship with the adjacent vascular structures. Modern MRI allows central airway imaging with adequate resolution [65]. As in CT scan, contrast agents are still used, but in the case of MRI, intravenous gadolinium contrast based agents are generally recommended unless contraindications exist. Images can be affected by respiratory and cardiac motion artifact, which makes interpretation of intrathoracic MRI images more difficult. Main stem bronchi trajectories are oblique and bias the accuracy of CSA measurement. Increased acquisition times often require the patient to stay still for at least several minutes at a time, which may not be possible in dyspneic, uncooperative, or critically ill patients [66]. The MRI examination for TBM takes about 15 minutes. Three dynamic measurements can be performed in the coronal, oblique, and transverse orientation. Minimal and maximal cross-sectional luminal diameters and tracheal lumen area can be calculated.

Spirometer controlled 3D cine-MRI is a promising method to assess static and dynamic changes in central airway dimensions in patient is suspected with TBM. Cine-MRI may be a more sensitive, faster and safer alternative for the diagnosis of static and dynamic TBM in cooperative children than bronchoscopy or cine-CT [67]. The most important advantage of 3D cine-MRI is that airway dimensions could be studied during standardized static and dynamic breathing maneuvers, such as forced expiration and cough. By acquiring simultaneous functional and morphological data, the severity of the TBM can be established in a standardized fashion. The second advantage of cine-MRI is that it allows physicians to obtain objective airway dimensions using post processing image analysis tools. The third advantage of 3D cine-MRI is that the procedure is less invasive, relative to bronchoscopy, since it does not require sedation. However, the most important advantage of cine-MRI compared with cine-CT was that it does not expose the children to ionizing, which is a greater risk for children than adults.

Cine-MRI also has a number of limitations, the most important of which is the need for optimal cooperation by the patient. The other limitation of cine-MRI is the low spatial resolution. The high spatial (submillimeter) and temporal resolution (10 frames/s) of dynamic CT cannot yet be obtained by MRI techniques. The dynamic (cine) MRI has been particularly useful to define pediatric TBM and is established as the standard modality for imaging the pediatric mediastinal airway [57, 62].

Radial Endobronchial Ultrasonography (EBUS)

Endobronchial ultrasonography (EBUS) was first introduced in the early 1990s. EBUS frequencies range from 5 to 30 MHz. Higher frequencies (20 MHz) do not penetrate as deep as lower ones (7.5 MHz). Superficial structures are thus better visualized using higher frequencies, while deeper structures are better visualized using lower frequency transducers. There are two types of probes for EBUS; the radial probe and convex (linear) probe. The 20 MHz balloon based radial EBUS probes are used for imaging airway wall layers, while 7.5 MHz linear EBUS probes are used for deeper structures such as lymph nodes and blood vessels.

Balloon based radial EBUS has been used to evaluate subepithelial edema in the asthmatic airway [68], degree of tracheal invasion and guiding in planning therapeutic interventions in patients with lung cancer [69, 70]. Radial EBUS is also useful in visualization of the laminar structure of the tracheobronchial wall, which is impossible with other diagnostic imaging methods [71, 72]. Radial EBUS can identify differences in central airway wall structure in patients with various forms of expiratory central airway collapse [73]. Radial EBUS in patients with TBM due to relapsing polychondritis reveals that the cartilage is thick and irregular while the membranous portion is normal. Whereas, in malacia due to chronic inflammation after tracheotomy, the cartilage is noted to be thick and irregular and the membranous portion is also thick. However, in EDAC associated with COPD, on the contrary, the cartilage is normal and the posterior membrane is thin when compared to the normal airway wall [73].

Radial EBUS uses a 20 MHz radial probe that reveals expiratory collapse (horizontalization) of the hyper-echogenic layer corresponding to the weakened airway wall cartilage, which is suggestive of TBM [60]. It also identifies hypo- and hyper-echoic layers that correlate with the laminar histological structures of the central airways. EBUS can also be used to identify structural differences in the membranous and cartilaginous portions of the central airways in patients with expiratory central airway collapse [73]. In TBM, the cartilage is destroyed, while in EDAC, the elastic fibers undergo atrophy, which explains why the posterior membrane is thinner than normal but the cartilage is intact. Radial EBUS may potentially distinguish between TBM and EDAC.

Endobronchial ultrasonography may be a useful adjunctive tool for the identification of adults at risk of postoperative TM where tracheopexy or airway stenting can be performed concurrently or sequentially if surgery is contemplated by showing destruction of the cartilaginous layer [74]. There is a need for future studies, to evaluate the role for Radial EBUS in the management of TBM and EDAC and also if it can to be used as a surrogate of histology.

Optical Coherence Tomography (OCT)

Optical coherence tomography (OCT) is a non-radiating imaging modality that uses infrared light to generate images at near microscopic resolution and with good correlation with histology specimens. OCT is able to generate images of the epithelial and sub-epithelial layers of the airway wall during bronchoscopy. OCT imaging enables characterization of the multilayered microstructural anatomy of the airways, with a maximum penetration depth up to 2 to 3 mm and 10-Am spatial resolution. The physical properties of OCT imaging are similar to those of ultrasonography, except that it uses light instead of ultrasound waves [75]. OCT enables the study of the in-vivo structure of lung tissue at a scale of tens of micrometers. It has been used to assess the layered structure of airway walls, quantify both airway lumen caliber and compliance, and image individual alveoli [76].

Image resolution of OCT is superior compared to ultrasound, CT, auto-fluorescence bronchoscopy and MRI. OCT, unlike ultrasound, does not require direct tissue contact or a coupling medium (such as a saline filled balloon) to produce an image. OCT is also an exceptionally safe technique as the broadband light is quite harmless to tissues and, unlike other imaging techniques, emits no ionizing radiation [77]. OCT has also a potential in the evaluation and treatment of patients with obstructive sleep apnea, tracheal stenosis, airway remodeling and inhalation injury [78].

Anatomical optical coherence tomography (aOCT) provides real-time measurements of obstructing central airway lesions that can assist therapeutic interventions such as selection of endobronchial stents and airway dilatation procedures [79]. aOCT has the capacity to measure the diameter and lumen area of the central airways accurately during bronchoscopy. The clinical use of aOCT imaging in the lower airways has been described in case series of three patients who has endobronchial pathologies [80]. aOCT could also be proved useful in the management of ECAC, where quantitative assessment of AC is desirable. This may be particularly useful in the setting of pediatric bronchoscopy, where longitudinal assessment of TBM is required, ideally without ionizing radiation [81].

The diagnosis of absent cartilage rings, suspected on bronchoscopy, can be confirmed by OCT [82]. OPT may be used for the diagnosis of TBM and also potentially differentiate TBM from EDAC, however further studies confirming these findings are needed.

Treatment Strategies

Identification of Symptoms and Impact on Functional Status and Quality of Life

Treatment decisions are based on the effects of patient`s symptoms, quality of life which are correlated with the findings of diagnostic studies. Tools like 6 Minute Walk Test (6MWT), Karnofsky performance status, modified Medical Research dyspnea score and St. George's Respiratory Questionnaire are used by the clinician for this purpose. Incidental diagnosis made during bronchoscopy or imaging studies are not treated [83].

Treatment of Associated Co-morbid Conditions

Common co-morbid conditions associated with EDAC are COPD, asthma, gastroesophageal reflux disease, obesity and recurrent aspiration. These conditions need to be identified and appropriately managed. TBM in relapsing polychondritis is common [84, 85], necessitating appropriate treatment with non-steroidal anti-inflammatory drugs or immunosuppressive agents [86]. Chronic irritation of the airway caused by smoking and chronic inflammation as seen in COPD and asthma are identified as risk factors for EDAC and hence optimal medical management should be initiated [87]. Airway clearance techniques (breathing out against a positive expiratory pressure resistance) in stable COPD patients improve health-related quality of life [88] and should be offered to patients who had difficulty clearing secretions.

Non-invasive Positive Pressure Ventilation (NIPPV)

In TBM, there is a reduction in the CSA of the airways that causes an increase in turbulence and airway resistance thus resulting in an increase in breathing and dyspnea. NIPPV increases the intraluminal pressure at the flow-limiting site and thereby maintains the patency of the airways, hence acting as a "pneumatic stent" [89] (Fig. **3**). NIPPV also decreases the airway resistance [90] and improves maximal expiratory flow at functional residual capacity [91] in patients with expiratory airflow obstruction. NIPPV is non-invasive, relatively simple to use and has been used in adult TBM patients [90, 92, 93]. It is difficult to recommend optimal NIPPV settings for TBM patients as there are no controlled studies evaluating the use of NIPPV in adult patients with TBM. However, physicians can consider NIPPV- Assisted Bronchoscopy to evaluate the changes and the degree of airway collapse and assess patient's symptoms and to possibly prescribe settings for NIPPV. Currently, there is no standardization of this technique [94]. Also, studies that compare continuous positive airway pressure (CPAP) *vs.* Bi-level positive airway pressure for TBM or use of facemask *vs.* nose mask are lacking.

The following protocol for NIPPV-Assisted Bronchoscopy is recommended. After informed consent, the airway dynamics should be evaluated without CPAP to access for the degree of airway narrowing (in upright and supine positions). Thereafter, after applying the facemask, the bronchoscope should be advanced to the nares through the swivel adapter and the facemask. The initial pressure setting is 0 cm H_2O that is gradually titrated upward in the increments of 3 cm H_2O until airway lumen during exhalation is at least 50% of that noted during inspiration (Fig. **3**).

Bronchoscopic Management

If respiratory symptoms persist even after optimal medical management of associated conditions and use of NIPPV, a short-term (10-14 days) stent trial for airway stabilization may be considered, especially for the true TBM patients. The stent trial serves to differentiate whether symptoms are from underlying TBM or related to associated disease and to evaluate the contribution of ECAC to the patient's symptoms. It also acts as a surrogate for the effects of airway stabilization from surgery. A prospective observational study [95], and case series [95 - 97] have shown stent insertion to improve respiratory symptoms, quality of life, and functional status, as it makes airflow less turbulent, however, this is not associated with improvement in FEV_1 or 6MWT.

Before stent insertion, baseline functional status should be determined. Also, dynamic bronchoscopy is performed to identify the location FLS, and stent insertion is considered only if the FLS is located in the trachea or the main stem bronchi. Dynamic bronchoscopy will also help to identify if there are any associated strictures or endobronchial lesions that will require dilation or removal before stent placement. Ideally, FLS should be identified by intraluminal airway pressure monitoring, not just by imaging.

Silicone stents are preferred over metallic stents for the management of TBM due to the ease of customization, repositioning, and its removal (Fig. **4**); however, their major drawbacks are stent migration, stent obstruction and mucus plugging. Their placement requires rigid bronchoscopy under general anesthesia. Though there are few case reports of use of the metallic stent in the TBM [98 - 102], their use in the TBM is not recommended [103]. Metallic stents are relatively easy to place, have low inner-to-outer diameter ratio, but they are also difficult to reposition or remove once it has been seated completely within the airway and they have the propensity to cause granulation tissue formation at the end of the stent [104]. However, in a few cases, covered metallic stents have been successfully removed even after 12-24 months post placement [102], but these procedures require expertise [105, 106]. Hence, the Food and Drug Administration recommends caution in their use in benign airway conditions [107].

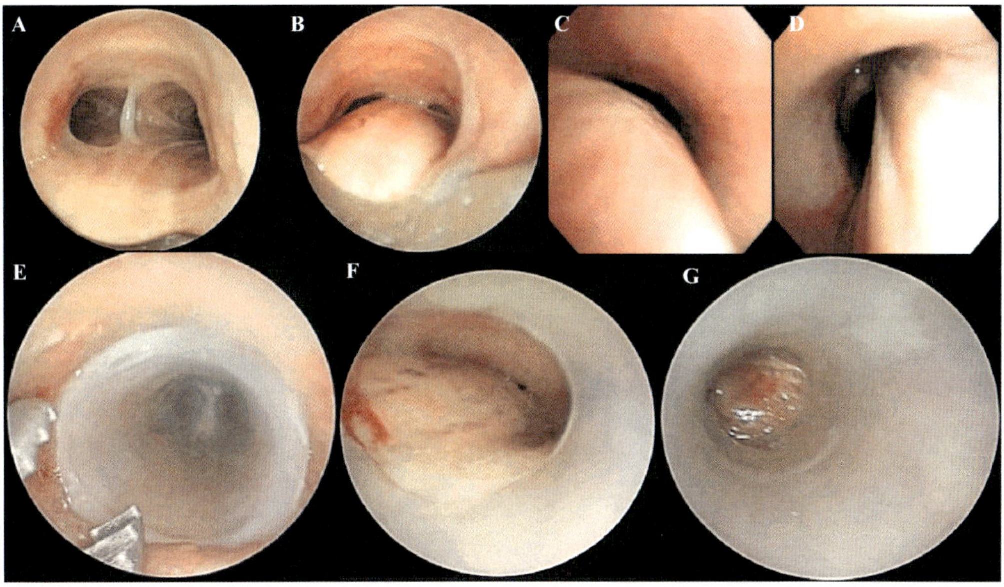

Fig. (4). Normal tracheal lumen during inspiration (**A**). EDAC during expiration (**B, C, D**). Rigid bronchoscopic image after stent insertion during inspiration (**E**). Follow-up bronchoscopy shows airway collpase distal to the left and right bronchial arms of Y silicone stent, consistent with the migration of choke points (**F, G**).

The type, length and diameter of airway stents are determined based on the location and severity of ECAC. If associated bronchomalacia is noted, an L-shaped or Y-shaped stent is recommended. Diffused or multifocal or larger affected areas require more than one stent, and tracheobronchomegaly necessitates larger stents (with a diameter greater than 16mm) that pose a technical challenge in their placements. Airway stents commonly used are - studded Dumon (Bryan Corp), ringed (Hood, Woburn, Massachusetts), or Y silicone stents (Bryan Corp). Stent-related complications in ECAC include granulation tissue formation, mucous plugging, stent migration, post-obstructive pneumonia and stent fracture [108]. It is hypothesized that this is due to dynamic features of ECAC (which causes continuous friction between the stent and the airway walls) and inflamed mucosa that is responsible for high risk for stent-related events [97].

Patients with indwelling airway stents require follow-up bronchoscopy in weeks following the insertion procedure, mainly to evaluate the possible stent-related complications and migration of choke points. The absence of distal migration of choke point and improvement in patient's symptoms on follow-up necessitate the removal of the stent if patients are considered for open surgical airway splinting. In selected patients with improvement in symptoms but who are not surgical candidates, stents could be considered as a long-term treatment, but they require carefully monitoring [109].

Open Surgical Procedures

The type of surgical procedures depends on the location of ECAC - focal or diffuse. For focal TBM, tracheal resection [110] with end-to-end anastomosis is considered to remove the abnormal airway segment for the focal disease. When resection is not possible, Montgomery T-tubes, silicone stents and tracheostomy placement are considered as alternatives. With Montgomery T-tubes, complications like stent dislocation, endoluminal granulomas, subglottic edema and sputum retention are encountered [111]. Silicone stents (Dumon TD Tracheal silicone stent) can be used but have a high risk of migration and require external fixation with nonabsorbable sutures [112] Endo Close suturing device and an external silicone button [109], or percutaneous endoscopic gastrostomy tube fastener [113].

For diffuse ECAC, stabilization of the airway is achieved by suturing a knitted polypropylene mesh (Marlex) to the extraluminal posterior membranous wall of the intrathoracic trachea and both main stem bronchi. This narrows the membranous wall of the airways so that the cartilage of the airways is brought into a more normal "C shape" and permanently relieves ECAC. Right posterolateral thoracotomy is required for this intervention [83, 114, 115]. So far, only two cases of tracheobronchoplasty by a video-assisted thoracoscopic surgical approach with combined with nitinol Ultraflex Microvasive non-covered stent placement [116] have been reported.

In a retrospective review study [117] which included 63 patients who underwent tracheobronchoplasty after successful stent trial, clinical and statistically significant improvements were noted in their quality of life, dyspnea, functional status and mean exercise capacity but there were no significant changes in FEV_1. In a similar prospective observational study [115] of 14 patients who underwent tracheobronchoplasty (without prior stent trial) reported improvement in dyspnea and cough. Though the study reported a significant improvement in FEV_1, only five out of 14 had improvement of 200 cc in their FEV_1. The average length of hospital stay in both studies was eight days. 3.2% mortality reported in the former study while no mortality was reported in the later study. Other complications included postoperative respiratory infection, prolonged mechanical ventilation, tracheostomy, atrial fibrillation and hemothorax. Late complications like severe symptomatic cervical TM which occurs superior to the uppermost extent of the mesh splint and which requires repeat operative intervention like cervical tracheoplasty have been reported [118].

Miscellaneous Treatments and Future Directions

Laser Therapy

Laser therapy in the treatment of TBM is an intriguing therapeutic approach. In a case report, the Neodymium-Yttrium aluminum perovskite (Nd:YAP) laser was used to treat TBM in Mounier-Kuhn syndrome. This laser emits light at 1340nm and is absorbed by water approximately 20 times more avidly than the Nd:YAG laser and may theoretically provide better photocoagulation and devascularization of the target lesion [119, 120]. It induces fibrosis of the posterior membranous wall and this results in less movement of the posterior wall during expiration and hence reduces the degree of airway collapse [121]. However, concerns remain over its use as the posterior membranous wall is about 3-5 mm thick.

Laser therapy was also used for the treatment of dynamic "A-shape" tracheal stenosis (DATS) that results in a dynamic stenosis with anterior fracture of tracheal cartilage and frequently associated posterior malacia [122]. Posterior TM was successfully treated in selected cases, avoiding stent placement. The study suggests that laser therapy is promising and should be considered for these selected patients.

Sclerosing Agents

Injection of the sclerosing agent like sodium morrhuate in the pericartilaginous tissue to produce fibrosis (either blindly or after skin incision) has been reported in pediatric patients [123]. This is based on the rationale that the peritracheal fibrosis provides external support to the airways. However, so far the use of sclerosing agents in adults TBM has not been reported.

Intraoperative, Real Time Airway Pressure Monitoring

The direct measurement of pressure difference and the angle of the pressure-pressure curve represent a new assessment modality for the success of interventional bronchoscopy and measuring airway pressure can estimate the need for additional procedures better than bronchoscopy alone [124]. Intraluminal airway pressure can provide valuable physiological information during bronchoscopy. That is because flow limiting segments will result in a pressure drop; if not then the collapsing airway is not flow limiting and does not warrant treatment for the purpose of improving airflow [60].

Biodegradable Stents

These stents were used first for tracheobronchial stenosis in an experimental animal study in 1998 [125]. Various biodegradable materials have been used, but the polydioxanone airway stents are more commonly studied and used [126 - 128]. The animal airway model has demonstrated acceptable safety and biocompatibility of this novel biodegradable polydioxanone stent [126]. The polydioxanone stents are reported to be potential alternatives to metallic or silicone stents for airway collapse or external compression of the trachea in children [127]. Biodegradable airway stents seemed to be safe, effective, and caused fewer complications than other types of stents for severe tracheal stenosis or malacia in small children [129]. Biodegradable polydioxanone stents can also be relevant for the treatment of adult patients with tracheal narrowing, but more experience and further research are needed in order to establish and assess this treatment in patients with TBM.

ABBREVIATIONS

CSA	Cross-sectional area
DAC	Dynamic airway collapse
ECAC	Excessive central airway collapse
TBM	Tracheobronchomalacia
EDAC	Excessive Dynamic Airway Collapse
MDCT	Multi-detector computed tomography
TM	Tracheomalacia
COPD	Chronic Obstructive Pulmonary Disease
CT	Computed tomography
EPP	Equal pressure point
FLS	Flow-limiting segment
PFT	Pulmonary function test
TLC	Total lung capacity
FEV1	Forced expiratory volume in 1 s
IOS	Impulse oscillometry
FVL	Flow-volume loop
AC	Airway collapse
MPR	Multiplanar reformatted

PL	Transpulmonary pressure
Plat	Lateral airway pressure
NIPPV	Non-invasive positive pressure ventilation
MRI	Magnetic resonance imaging
EBUS	Endobronchial ultrasonography
OCT	Optical coherence tomography
aCOT	Anatomical optical coherence tomography
6MWT	6 Minute Walk Test
CPAP	Continuous positive airway pressure

CONFLICT OF INTEREST

The authors declare no conflict of interest, financial or otherwise.

ACKNOWLEDGEMENTS

Declared none.

REFERENCES

[1] Leong P, Bardin PG, Lau KK. What's in a name? Expiratory tracheal narrowing in adults explained. Clin Radiol 2013; 68(12): 1268-75. [http://dx.doi.org/10.1016/j.crad.2013.06.017] [PMID: 23953005]

[2] Ridge CA, O'donnell CR, Lee EY, Majid A, Boiselle PM. Tracheobronchomalacia: current concepts and controversies. J Thorac Imaging 2011; 26(4): 278-89. [http://dx.doi.org/10.1097/RTI.0b013e3182203342] [PMID: 22009081]

[3] Fraser RG. Measurements of the calibre of human bronchi in three phases of respiration by cinebronchography. J Can Assoc Radiol 1961; 12: 102-12. [PMID: 13894769]

[4] Murgu S, Colt H. Tracheobronchomalacia and excessive dynamic airway collapse. Clin Chest Med 2013; 34(3): 527-55. [http://dx.doi.org/10.1016/j.ccm.2013.05.003] [PMID: 23993822]

[5] Murgu SD, Colt HG. Tracheobronchomalacia: untangling the Gordian knot. J Bronchology Interv Pulmonol 2005; 12(4): 239-44.

[6] Boiselle PM, O'Donnell CR, Bankier AA, *et al.* Tracheal collapsibility in healthy volunteers during forced expiration: assessment with multidetector CT. Radiology 2009; 252(1): 255-62. [http://dx.doi.org/10.1148/radiol.2521081958] [PMID: 19420322]

[7] Litmanovich D, O'Donnell CR, Bankier AA, *et al.* Bronchial collapsibility at forced expiration in healthy volunteers: assessment with multidetector CT. Radiology 2010; 257(2): 560-7. [http://dx.doi.org/10.1148/radiol.10100219] [PMID: 20829540]

[8] Boiselle PM, Michaud G, Roberts DH, *et al.* Dynamic expiratory tracheal collapse in COPD: correlation with clinical and physiologic parameters. Chest 2012; 142(6): 1539-44. [http://dx.doi.org/10.1378/chest.12-0299] [PMID: 22722230]

[9] Dal Negro RW, Tognella S, Guerriero M, Micheletto C. Prevalence of tracheobronchomalacia and excessive dynamic airway collapse in bronchial asthma of different severity. Multidiscip Respir Med

2013; 8(1): 32.
[http://dx.doi.org/10.1186/2049-6958-8-32] [PMID: 23673082]

[10] Kalra A, Abouzgheib W, Gajera M, Palaniswamy C, Puri N, Dellinger RP. Excessive dynamic airway collapse for the internist: new nomenclature or different entity? Postgrad Med J 2011; 87(1029): 482-6.
[http://dx.doi.org/10.1136/pgmj.2010.111948] [PMID: 21565878]

[11] Baram D, Smaldone G. Tracheal collapse *versus* tracheobronchomalacia: normal function *versus* disease. Am J Respir Crit Care Med 2006; 174(6): 724.
[http://dx.doi.org/10.1164/ajrccm.174.6.724] [PMID: 16959923]

[12] Park JG, Edell ES. Dynamic airway collapse: distinct from tracheomalacia. Bronchology Interv Pulmonol 2005; 12(3): 143-6.

[13] Jokinen K, Palva T, Sutinen S, Nuutinen J. Acquired tracheobronchomalacia. Ann Clin Res 1977; 9(2): 52-7.
[PMID: 883758]

[14] Rayl JE. Tracheobronchial collapse during cough. Radiology 1965; 85: 87-92.
[http://dx.doi.org/10.1148/85.1.87] [PMID: 14303075]

[15] Murgu SD, Colt HG. Description of a multidimensional classification system for patients with expiratory central airway collapse. Respirology 2007; 12(4): 543-50.
[http://dx.doi.org/10.1111/j.1440-1843.2007.01094.x] [PMID: 17587421]

[16] Murgu SD, Colt HG. Expiratory central airway collapse: a concise review. Egypt J Bronchol 2007; 1(1): 87-99.

[17] Choo EM, Seaman JC, Musani AI. Tracheomalacia/Tracheobronchomalacia and hyperdynamic airway collapse. Immunol Allergy Clin North Am 2013; 33(1): 23-34.
[http://dx.doi.org/10.1016/j.iac.2012.10.005] [PMID: 23337062]

[18] Kano Y, Sakurai H, Shidara J, Toida S, Yasuda H. Histopathological and immunohistochemical studies of acquired tracheobronchomalacia: an autopsy case report. ORL J Otorhinolaryngol Relat Spec 1996; 58(5): 288-94.
[http://dx.doi.org/10.1159/000276855] [PMID: 8936481]

[19] Adliff M, Ngato D, Keshavjee S, Brenaman S, Granton JT. Treatment of diffuse tracheomalacia secondary to relapsing polychondritis with continuous positive airway pressure. Chest 1997; 112(6): 1701-4.
[http://dx.doi.org/10.1378/chest.112.6.1701] [PMID: 9404780]

[20] West JB. Respiratory physiology: the essentials. Lippincott Williams & Wilkins 2012.

[21] Dawson SV, Elliott EA. Wave-speed limitation on expiratory flow-a unifying concept. J Appl Physiol 1977; 43(3): 498-515.
[PMID: 914721]

[22] Aliverti A, Pelosi P, Zin WA, Eds. Respiratory system and artificial ventilation. Springer 2008; p. 31.

[23] Elliott EA, Dawson SV. Test of wave-speed theory of flow limitation in elastic tubes. J Appl Physiol 1977; 43(3): 516-22.
[PMID: 914722]

[24] Hammer J, Eber E, Eds. Paediatric pulmonary function testing. Karger Medical and Scientific Publishers 2005; p. 35.
[http://dx.doi.org/10.1159/isbn.978-3-318-01087-9]

[25] Smaldone GC, Smith PL. Location of flow-limiting segments *via* airway catheters near residual volume in humans. J Appl Physiol 1985; 59(2): 502-8.
[PMID: 4030602]

[26] Nishine H, Hiramoto T, Kida H, *et al.* Assessing the site of maximal obstruction in the trachea using

lateral pressure measurement during bronchoscopy. Am J Respir Crit Care Med 2012; 185(1): 24-33. [http://dx.doi.org/10.1164/rccm.201104-0701OC] [PMID: 21997334]

[27] Carden KA, Boiselle PM, Waltz DA, Ernst A. Tracheomalacia and tracheobronchomalacia in children and adults: an in-depth review. Chest 2005; 127(3): 984-1005. [http://dx.doi.org/10.1378/chest.127.3.984] [PMID: 15764786]

[28] Majid A, Sosa AF, Ernst A, *et al.* Pulmonary function and flow-volume loop patterns in patients with tracheobronchomalacia. Respir Care 2013; 58(9): 1521-6. [http://dx.doi.org/10.4187/respcare.02277] [PMID: 23481440]

[29] Matus I, Richter W, Mani SB. Awareness, Competencies, and Practice Patterns in Tracheobronchomalacia: A Survey of Pulmonologists. J Bronchology Interv Pulmonol 2016; 23(2): 131-7. [http://dx.doi.org/10.1097/LBR.0000000000000281] [PMID: 27058715]

[30] Loring SH, O'donnell CR, Feller-Kopman DJ, Ernst A. Central airway mechanics and flow limitation in acquired tracheobronchomalacia. Chest 2007; 131(4): 1118-24. [http://dx.doi.org/10.1378/chest.06-2556] [PMID: 17426218]

[31] O'Donnell CR, Bankier AA, O'Donnell DH, Loring SH, Boiselle PM. Static end-expiratory and dynamic forced expiratory tracheal collapse in COPD. Clin Radiol 2014; 69(4): 357-62. [http://dx.doi.org/10.1016/j.crad.2013.11.003] [PMID: 24361144]

[32] Ernst A, Odell DD, Michaud G, Majid A, Herth FF, Gangadharan SP. Central airway stabilization for tracheobronchomalacia improves quality of life in patients with COPD. Chest 2011; 140(5): 1162-8. [http://dx.doi.org/10.1378/chest.10-3051] [PMID: 21868463]

[33] Weinstein DJ, Hull JE, Ritchie BL, Hayes JA, Morris MJ. Exercise-associated Excessive Dynamic Airway Collapse in Military Personnel. Ann Am Thorac Soc 2016; 13(9): 1476-82. [http://dx.doi.org/10.1513/AnnalsATS.201512-790OC] [PMID: 27332956]

[34] Murgu SD, Colt HG. Tracheobronchomalacia and excessive dynamic airway collapse. Respirology 2006; 11(4): 388-406. [http://dx.doi.org/10.1111/j.1440-1843.2006.00862.x] [PMID: 16771908]

[35] Ellingsen I, Holmedahl NH. Does excessive dynamic airway collapse have any impact on dynamic pulmonary function tests? J Bronchology Interv Pulmonol 2014; 21(1): 40-6. [http://dx.doi.org/10.1097/LBR.0000000000000040] [PMID: 24419185]

[36] Baroni RH, Feller-Kopman D, Nishino M, *et al.* Tracheobronchomalacia: comparison between end-expiratory and dynamic expiratory CT for evaluation of central airway collapse. Radiology 2005; 235(2): 635-41. [http://dx.doi.org/10.1148/radiol.2352040309] [PMID: 15798155]

[37] Ferretti GR, Jankowski A, Perrin MA, *et al.* Multi-detector CT evaluation in patients suspected of tracheobronchomalacia: comparison of end-expiratory with dynamic expiratory volumetric acquisitions. Eur J Radiol 2008; 68(2): 340-6. [http://dx.doi.org/10.1016/j.ejrad.2007.08.029] [PMID: 17913426]

[38] Lee EY, Litmanovich D, Boiselle PM. Multidetector CT evaluation of tracheobronchomalacia. Radiol Clin North Am 2009; 47(2): 261-9. [http://dx.doi.org/10.1016/j.rcl.2008.11.007] [PMID: 19249455]

[39] Lee EY, Mason KP, Zurakowski D, *et al.* MDCT assessment of tracheomalacia in symptomatic infants with mediastinal aortic vascular anomalies: preliminary technical experience. Pediatr Radiol 2008; 38(1): 82-8. [http://dx.doi.org/10.1007/s00247-007-0672-1] [PMID: 18038169]

[40] Lee EY, Strauss KJ, Tracy DA, Bastos Md, Zurakowski D, Boiselle PM. Comparison of standard-dose and reduced-dose expiratory MDCT techniques for assessment of tracheomalacia in children. Acad Radiol 2010; 17(4): 504-10.

[http://dx.doi.org/10.1016/j.acra.2009.11.014] [PMID: 20207318]

[41] Lee KS, Boiselle PM. Update on multidetector computed tomography imaging of the airways. J Thorac Imaging 2010; 25(2): 112-24.
[http://dx.doi.org/10.1097/RTI.0b013e3181d7e721] [PMID: 20463531]

[42] Boiselle PM, Feller-Kopman D, Ashiku S, Weeks D, Ernst A. Tracheobronchomalacia: evolving role of dynamic multislice helical CT. Radiol Clin North Am 2003; 41(3): 627-36.
[http://dx.doi.org/10.1016/S0033-8389(03)00023-X] [PMID: 12797610]

[43] Gilkeson RC, Ciancibello LM, Hejal RB, Montenegro HD, Lange P. Tracheobronchomalacia: dynamic airway evaluation with multidetector CT. AJR Am J Roentgenol 2001; 176(1): 205-10. [http://dx.doi.org/10.2214/ajr.176.1.1760205] [PMID: 11133567]

[44] Lee KS, Sun MR, Ernst A, Feller-Kopman D, Majid A, Boiselle PM. Comparison of Dynamic Expiratory CT With Bronchoscopy for Diagnosing Airway Malacia: A Pilot Evaluation. Chest 2007; 131(3): 758-64.
[http://dx.doi.org/10.1378/chest.06-2164] [PMID: 17356090]

[45] Baroni RH, Ashiku S, Boiselle PM. Dynamic CT evaluation of the central airways in patients undergoing tracheoplasty for tracheobronchomalacia. AJR Am J Roentgenol 2005; 184(5): 1444-9.
[http://dx.doi.org/10.2214/ajr.184.5.01841444] [PMID: 15855094]

[46] Lee KS, Lunn W, Feller-Kopman D, Ernst A, Hatabu H, Boiselle PM. Multislice CT evaluation of airway stents. J Thorac Imaging 2005; 20(2): 81-8.
[http://dx.doi.org/10.1097/01.rti.0000149789.28967.03] [PMID: 15818206]

[47] Lee KS, Ashiku SK, Ernst A, *et al.* Comparison of expiratory CT airway abnormalities before and after tracheoplasty surgery for tracheobronchomalacia. J Thorac Imaging 2008; 23(2): 121-6.
[http://dx.doi.org/10.1097/RTI.0b013e3181653c41] [PMID: 18520570]

[48] McDermott S, Barry SC, Judge EP, *et al.* Tracheomalacia in adults with cystic fibrosis: determination of prevalence and severity with dynamic cine CT. Radiology 2009; 252(2): 577-86.
[http://dx.doi.org/10.1148/radiol.2522081956] [PMID: 19508990]

[49] Litmanovich D, O'Donnell CR, Bankier AA, *et al.* Bronchial collapsibility at forced expiration in healthy volunteers: assessment with multidetector CT. Radiology 2010; 257(2): 560-7.
[http://dx.doi.org/10.1148/radiol.10100219] [PMID: 20829540]

[50] Majid A, Guerrero J, Gangadharan S, *et al.* Tracheobronchoplasty for severe tracheobronchomalacia: a prospective outcome analysis. Chest 2008; 134(4): 801-7.
[http://dx.doi.org/10.1378/chest.08-0728] [PMID: 18842912]

[51] Yamashiro T, San José Estépar R, Matsuoka S, *et al.* Intrathoracic tracheal volume and collapsibility on inspiratory and end-expiratory ct scans correlations with lung volume and pulmonary function in 85 smokers. Acad Radiol 2011; 18(3): 299-305.
[http://dx.doi.org/10.1016/j.acra.2010.11.005] [PMID: 21215660]

[52] Boiselle PM, Lee KS, Lin S, Raptopoulos V. Cine CT during coughing for assessment of tracheomalacia: preliminary experience with 64-MDCT. AJR Am J Roentgenol 2006; 187(2): W175-7.
[http://dx.doi.org/10.2214/AJR.05.1456] [PMID: 16861507]

[53] Wagnetz U, Roberts HC, Chung T, Patsios D, Chapman KR, Paul NS. Dynamic airway evaluation with volume CT: initial experience. Can Assoc Radiol J 2010; 61(2): 90-7.
[http://dx.doi.org/10.1016/j.carj.2009.11.007] [PMID: 20060258]

[54] Ciet P, Boiselle PM, Michaud G, O'Donnell C, Litmanovich DE. Optimal imaging protocol for measuring dynamic expiratory collapse of the central airways. Clin Radiol 2016; 71(1): e49-55.
[http://dx.doi.org/10.1016/j.crad.2015.10.014] [PMID: 26611199]

[55] Heidinger BH, Occhipinti M, Eisenberg RL, Bankier AA. Imaging of Large Airways Disorders. AJR Am J Roentgenol 2015; 205(1): 41-56.

[http://dx.doi.org/10.2214/AJR.14.13857] [PMID: 26102379]

[56] Boiselle PM, Ernst A. Tracheal morphology in patients with tracheomalacia: prevalence of inspiratory lunate and expiratory "frown" shapes. J Thorac Imaging 2006; 21(3): 190-6. [http://dx.doi.org/10.1097/01.rti.0000213647.42041.d0] [PMID: 16915063]

[57] Hysinger EB, Panitch HB. Paediatric Tracheomalacia. Paediatr Respir Rev 2016; 17: 9-15. [PMID: 25962857]

[58] Majid A, Gaurav K, Sanchez JM, *et al.* Evaluation of tracheobronchomalacia by dynamic flexible bronchoscopy. A pilot study. Ann Am Thorac Soc 2014; 11(6): 951-5. [http://dx.doi.org/10.1513/AnnalsATS.201312-435BC] [PMID: 24960030]

[59] Kugler C, Stanzel F. Tracheomalacia. Thorac Surg Clin 2014; 24(1): 51-8. [http://dx.doi.org/10.1016/j.thorsurg.2013.09.003] [PMID: 24295659]

[60] Handa H, Miyazawa T, Murgu SD, *et al.* Novel multimodality imaging and physiologic assessments clarify choke-point physiology and airway wall structure in expiratory central airway collapse. Respir Care 2012; 57(4): 634-41. [PMID: 22005343]

[61] Masters IB, Eastburn MM, Wootton R, *et al.* A new method for objective identification and measurement of airway lumen in paediatric flexible videobronchoscopy. Thorax 2005; 60(8): 652-8. [http://dx.doi.org/10.1136/thx.2004.034421] [PMID: 16061706]

[62] Vogl T, Wilimzig C, Bilaniuk LT, *et al.* MR imaging in pediatric airway obstruction. J Comput Assist Tomogr 1990; 14(2): 182-6. [http://dx.doi.org/10.1097/00004728-199003000-00004] [PMID: 2312844]

[63] Faust RA, Rimell FL, Remley KB. Cine magnetic resonance imaging for evaluation of focal tracheomalacia: innominate artery compression syndrome. Int J Pediatr Otorhinolaryngol 2002; 65(1): 27-33. [http://dx.doi.org/10.1016/S0165-5876(02)00123-4] [PMID: 12127219]

[64] Heussel CP, Hafner B, Lill J, Schreiber W, Thelen M, Kauczor HU. Paired inspiratory/expiratory spiral CT and continuous respiration cine CT in the diagnosis of tracheal instability. Eur Radiol 2001; 11(6): 982-9. [http://dx.doi.org/10.1007/s003300100818] [PMID: 11419175]

[65] Ley-Zaporozhan J, Ley S, Kauczor HU. Morphological and functional imaging in COPD with CT and MRI: present and future. Eur Radiol 2008; 18(3): 510-21. [http://dx.doi.org/10.1007/s00330-007-0772-1] [PMID: 17899100]

[66] Kuo GP, Torok CM, Aygun N, Zinreich SJ. Diagnostic imaging of the upper airway. Proc Am Thorac Soc 2011; 8(1): 40-5. [http://dx.doi.org/10.1513/pats.201004-032RN] [PMID: 21364220]

[67] Ciet P, Wielopolski P, Manniesing R, *et al.* Spirometer-controlled cine magnetic resonance imaging used to diagnose tracheobronchomalacia in paediatric patients. Eur Respir J 2014; 43(1): 115-24. [http://dx.doi.org/10.1183/09031936.00104512] [PMID: 23598953]

[68] Yamasaki A, Tomita K, Sano H, *et al.* Measuring subepithelial thickness using endobronchial ultrasonography in a patient with asthma: a case report. Lung 2003; 181(3): 115-20. [http://dx.doi.org/10.1007/s00408-003-1012-3] [PMID: 14565685]

[69] Ernst A, Feller-Kopman D, Becker HD, Mehta AC. Central airway obstruction. Am J Respir Crit Care Med 2004; 169(12): 1278-97. [http://dx.doi.org/10.1164/rccm.200210-1181SO] [PMID: 15187010]

[70] Miyazu Y, Miyazawa T, Kurimoto N, Iwamoto Y, Kanoh K, Kohno N. Endobronchial ultrasonography in the assessment of centrally located early-stage lung cancer before photodynamic therapy. Am J Respir Crit Care Med 2002; 165(6): 832-7. [http://dx.doi.org/10.1164/ajrccm.165.6.2108092] [PMID: 11897652]

[71] Kurimoto N, Murayama M, Yoshioka S, Nishisaka T, Inai K, Dohi K. Assessment of usefulness of endobronchial ultrasonography in determination of depth of tracheobronchial tumor invasion. Chest 1999; 115(6): 1500-6.
[http://dx.doi.org/10.1378/chest.115.6.1500] [PMID: 10378540]

[72] Baba M, Sekine Y, Suzuki M, *et al.* Correlation between endobronchial ultrasonography (EBUS) images and histologic findings in normal and tumor-invaded bronchial wall. Lung Cancer 2002; 35(1): 65-71.
[http://dx.doi.org/10.1016/S0169-5002(01)00284-7] [PMID: 11750715]

[73] Murgu S, Kurimoto N, Colt H. Endobronchial ultrasound morphology of expiratory central airway collapse. Respirology 2008; 13(2): 315-9.
[http://dx.doi.org/10.1111/j.1440-1843.2007.01216.x] [PMID: 18339038]

[74] Lee P, Low SY, Liew HL, Tan D, Eng P. Endobronchial ultrasound for detection of tracheomalacia from chronic compression by vascular ring. Respirology 2007; 12(2): 299-301.
[http://dx.doi.org/10.1111/j.1440-1843.2006.01021.x] [PMID: 17298468]

[75] Murgu SD. Optical coherence tomography of the airways. Curr Respir Care Med 2014; 3: 13-8.
[http://dx.doi.org/10.1007/s13665-013-0069-6]

[76] McLaughlin RA, Noble PB, Sampson DD. Optical coherence tomography in respiratory science and medicine: from airways to alveoli. Physiology (Bethesda) 2014; 29(5): 369-80.
[http://dx.doi.org/10.1152/physiol.00002.2014] [PMID: 25180266]

[77] Coxson HO, Eastwood PR, Williamson JP, Sin DD. Phenotyping airway disease with optical coherence tomography. Respirology 2011; 16(1): 34-43.
[http://dx.doi.org/10.1111/j.1440-1843.2010.01888.x] [PMID: 21044229]

[78] Hou R, Le T, Murgu SD, Chen Z, Brenner M. Recent advances in optical coherence tomography for the diagnoses of lung disorders. Expert Rev Respir Med 2011; 5(5): 711-24.
[http://dx.doi.org/10.1586/ers.11.59] [PMID: 21955240]

[79] Williamson JP, McLaughlin RA, Phillips MJ, *et al.* Feasibility of Applying Real-time Optical Imaging During Bronchoscopic Interventions for Central Airway Obstruction. J Bronchology Interv Pulmonol 2010; 17(4): 307-16.
[http://dx.doi.org/10.1097/LBR.0b013e3181f9eaae] [PMID: 23168951]

[80] Williamson JP, McLaughlin RA, Phillips MJ, *et al.* Using optical coherence tomography to improve diagnostic and therapeutic bronchoscopy. Chest 2009; 136(1): 272-6.
[http://dx.doi.org/10.1378/chest.08-2800] [PMID: 19225058]

[81] Williamson JP, Armstrong JJ, McLaughlin RA, *et al.* Measuring airway dimensions during bronchoscopy using anatomical optical coherence tomography. Eur Respir J 2010; 35(1): 34-41.
[http://dx.doi.org/10.1183/09031936.00041809] [PMID: 19541718]

[82] Torre M, Speggiorin S, Roebuck DJ, McLaren CA, Elliott MJ. Congenital absence of cartilaginous tracheal rings associated with esophageal atresia and trifurcated carina: a novel anomaly? J Pediatr Surg 2012; 47(5): 1008-11.
[http://dx.doi.org/10.1016/j.jpedsurg.2012.01.077] [PMID: 22595591]

[83] Gangadharan SP. Tracheobronchomalacia in adults. Semin Thorac Cardiovasc Surg 2010; 22(2): 165-73.
[http://dx.doi.org/10.1053/j.semtcvs.2010.07.001] [PMID: 21092895]

[84] McAdam LP, O'Hanlan MA, Bluestone R, Pearson CM. Relapsing polychondritis: prospective study of 23 patients and a review of the literature. Medicine (Baltimore) 1976; 55(3): 193-215.
[http://dx.doi.org/10.1097/00005792-197605000-00001] [PMID: 775252]

[85] Ernst A, Rafeq S, Boiselle P, *et al.* Relapsing polychondritis and airway involvement. Chest 2009; 135(4): 1024-30.
[http://dx.doi.org/10.1378/chest.08-1180] [PMID: 19017885]

[86] Longo L, Greco A, Rea A, Lo Vasco VR, De Virgilio A, De Vincentiis M. Relapsing polychondritis: A clinical update. Autoimmun Rev 2016; 15(6): 539-43. [http://dx.doi.org/10.1016/j.autrev.2016.02.013] [PMID: 26876384]

[87] Murgu SD, Colt HG. Treatment of adult tracheobronchomalacia and excessive dynamic airway collapse : an update. Treat Respir Med 2006; 5(2): 103-15. [http://dx.doi.org/10.2165/00151829-200605020-00004] [PMID: 16512691]

[88] Osadnik CR, McDonald CF, Jones AP, Holland AE. Airway clearance techniques for chronic obstructive pulmonary disease. Cochrane Database Syst Rev 2012; (3): CD008328. [PMID: 22419331]

[89] Panitch HB, Allen JL, Alpert BE, Schidlow DV. Effects of CPAP on lung mechanics in infants with acquired tracheobronchomalacia. Am J Respir Crit Care Med 1994; 150(5 Pt 1): 1341-6. [http://dx.doi.org/10.1164/ajrccm.150.5.7952562] [PMID: 7952562]

[90] Ferguson GT, Benoist J. Nasal continuous positive airway pressure in the treatment of tracheobronchomalacia. Am Rev Respir Dis 1993; 147(2): 457-61. [http://dx.doi.org/10.1164/ajrccm/147.2.457] [PMID: 8430971]

[91] Davis S, Jones M, Kisling J, Angelicchio C, Tepper RS. Effect of continuous positive airway pressure on forced expiratory flows in infants with tracheomalacia. Am J Respir Crit Care Med 1998; 158(1): 148-52. [http://dx.doi.org/10.1164/ajrccm.158.1.9711034] [PMID: 9655721]

[92] Jiang AG, Gao XY, Lu HY. Diagnosis and management of an elderly patient with severe tracheomalacia: A case report and review of the literature. Exp Ther Med 2013; 6(3): 765-8. [http://dx.doi.org/10.3892/etm.2013.1195] [PMID: 24137262]

[93] Adliff M, Ngato D, Keshavjee S, Brenaman S, Granton JT. Treatment of diffuse tracheomalacia secondary to relapsing polychondritis with continuous positive airway pressure. Chest 1997; 112(6): 1701-4. [http://dx.doi.org/10.1378/chest.112.6.1701] [PMID: 9404780]

[94] Murgu SD. Pneumatic stenting for tracheobronchomalacia. J Bronchology Interv Pulmonol 2014; 21(2): 109-12. [http://dx.doi.org/10.1097/LBR.0000000000000053] [PMID: 24739682]

[95] Ernst A, Majid A, Feller-Kopman D, *et al.* Airway stabilization with silicone stents for treating adult tracheobronchomalacia: a prospective observational study. Chest 2007; 132(2): 609-16. [http://dx.doi.org/10.1378/chest.06-2708] [PMID: 17699133]

[96] Odell DD, Shah A, Gangadharan SP, *et al.* Airway stenting and tracheobronchoplasty improve respiratory symptoms in Mounier-Kuhn syndrome. Chest 2011; 140(4): 867-73. [http://dx.doi.org/10.1378/chest.10-2010] [PMID: 21493699]

[97] Murgu SD, Colt HG. Complications of silicone stent insertion in patients with expiratory central airway collapse. Ann Thorac Surg 2007; 84(6): 1870-7. [http://dx.doi.org/10.1016/j.athoracsur.2007.07.026] [PMID: 18036901]

[98] Furman RH, Backer CL, Dunham ME, Donaldson J, Mavroudis C, Holinger LD. The use of balloon-expandable metallic stents in the treatment of pediatric tracheomalacia and bronchomalacia. Arch Otolaryngol Head Neck Surg 1999; 125(2): 203-7. [http://dx.doi.org/10.1001/archotol.125.2.203] [PMID: 10037287]

[99] Ochoa S, Cheng GZ, Folch E, Majid A. Use of self-expanding metallic airway stents in tracheobronchomalacia. J Bronchology Interv Pulmonol 2015; 22(3): e9-e11. [http://dx.doi.org/10.1097/LBR.0000000000000179] [PMID: 26165905]

[100] Chan AL, Juarez MM, Allen RP, Albertson TE. Do airway metallic stents for benign lesions confer too costly a benefit? BMC Pulm Med 2008; 8(1): 7. [http://dx.doi.org/10.1186/1471-2466-8-7] [PMID: 18423035]

[101] Saad CP, Murthy S, Krizmanich G, Mehta AC. Self-expandable metallic airway stents and flexible bronchoscopy: long-term outcomes analysis. Chest 2003; 124(5): 1993-9.
[http://dx.doi.org/10.1378/chest.124.5.1993] [PMID: 14605078]

[102] Noppen M, Stratakos G, D'Haese J, Meysman M, Vinken W. Removal of covered self-expandable metallic airway stents in benign disorders: indications, technique, and outcomes. Chest 2005; 127(2): 482-7.
[http://dx.doi.org/10.1378/chest.127.2.482] [PMID: 15705985]

[103] Lund ME, Force S. Airway stenting for patients with benign airway disease and the Food and Drug Administration advisory: a call for restraint. Chest 2007; 132(4): 1107-8.
[http://dx.doi.org/10.1378/chest.07-0242] [PMID: 17934107]

[104] Wood DE. Airway stenting. Chest Surg Clin N Am 2001; 11(4): 841-60.
[PMID: 11780299]

[105] Murthy SC, Gildea TR, Mehta AC. Removal of self-expandable metallic stents: is it possible? Semin Respir Crit Care Med 2004; 25(4): 381-5.
[http://dx.doi.org/10.1055/s-2004-832711] [PMID: 16088481]

[106] Lunn W, Feller-Kopman D, Wahidi M, Ashiku S, Thurer R, Ernst A. Endoscopic removal of metallic airway stents. Chest 2005; 127(6): 2106-12.
[http://dx.doi.org/10.1378/chest.127.6.2106] [PMID: 15947327]

[107] FDA public health notification. Complications from metallic tracheal stents in patients with benign airway disorders. US FDA 2005. Available at: http://www.fda.gov/MedicalDevices/Safety/AlertsandNotices/PublicHealthNotifications/ucm062115.htm

[108] Popilevsky F, Al-Ajam MR, Ly V, Sanchez LD, Cutaia M, Dynamic Y. Dynamic Y stent fractures in crescentic tracheobronchomalacia. J Bronchology Interv Pulmonol 2012; 19(3): 206-10.
[http://dx.doi.org/10.1097/LBR.0b013e31825c6f57] [PMID: 23207463]

[109] Majid A, Fernandez-Bussy S, Kent M, *et al.* External fixation of proximal tracheal airway stents: a modified technique. Ann Thorac Surg 2012; 93(6): e167-9.
[http://dx.doi.org/10.1016/j.athoracsur.2012.01.094] [PMID: 22632539]

[110] Grillo HC. Surgical treatment of postintubation tracheal injuries. J Thorac Cardiovasc Surg 1979; 78(6): 860-75.
[PMID: 502569]

[111] Liu HC, Lee KS, Huang CJ, Cheng CR, Hsu WH, Huang MH. Silicone T-tube for complex laryngotracheal problems. Eur J Cardiothorac Surg 2002; 21(2): 326-30.
[http://dx.doi.org/10.1016/S1010-7940(01)01098-3] [PMID: 11825744]

[112] Colt HG, Harrell J, Neuman TR, Robbins T. External fixation of subglottic tracheal stents. Chest 1994; 105(6): 1653-7.
[http://dx.doi.org/10.1378/chest.105.6.1653] [PMID: 8205856]

[113] Musani AI, Jensen K, Mitchell JD, Weyant M, Garces K, Hsia D. Novel use of a percutaneous endoscopic gastrostomy tube fastener for securing silicone tracheal stents in patients with benign proximal airway obstruction. J Bronchology Interv Pulmonol 2012; 19(2): 121-5.
[http://dx.doi.org/10.1097/LBR.0b013e318251e238] [PMID: 23207354]

[114] Lagisetty KH, Gangadharan SP. Tracheobronchoplasty for the treatment of tracheobronchomalacia. J Thorac Cardiovasc Surg 2012; 144(3): S58-9.
[http://dx.doi.org/10.1016/j.jtcvs.2012.05.025] [PMID: 22676978]

[115] Wright CD, Grillo HC, Hammoud ZT, *et al.* Tracheoplasty for expiratory collapse of central airways. Ann Thorac Surg 2005; 80(1): 259-66.
[http://dx.doi.org/10.1016/j.athoracsur.2005.01.032] [PMID: 15975378]

[116] Tse DG, Han SM, Charuworn B, Kaufer ES. Video-assisted thoracoscopic surgical

tracheobronchoplasty for tracheobronchomalacia. J Thorac Cardiovasc Surg 2011; 142(3): 714-6. [http://dx.doi.org/10.1016/j.jtcvs.2010.11.037] [PMID: 21277600]

[117] Gangadharan SP, Bakhos CT, Majid A, *et al.* Technical aspects and outcomes of tracheobronchoplasty for severe tracheobronchomalacia. Ann Thorac Surg 2011; 91(5): 1574-80. [http://dx.doi.org/10.1016/j.athoracsur.2011.01.009] [PMID: 21377650]

[118] Wilson JL, Folch E, Kent MS, Majid A, Gangadharan SP. Posterior mesh tracheoplasty for cervical tracheomalacia: A novel trachea-preserving technique. Ann Thorac Surg 2016; 101(1): 372-4. [http://dx.doi.org/10.1016/j.athoracsur.2015.05.112] [PMID: 26694287]

[119] Dutau H, Breen DP. Endobronchial laser treatment: an essential tool in therapeutic bronchoscopy. Eur Respir J 2010; 48: 149-60.

[120] Lee HJ, Malhotra R, Grossman C, Wesley Shepherd R. Initial report of neodymium: Yttrium-aluminum-perovskite (Nd:YAP) laser use during bronchoscopy. J Bronchology Interv Pulmonol 2011; 18(3): 229-32. [http://dx.doi.org/10.1097/LBR.0b013e3182296615] [PMID: 23208565]

[121] Dutau H, Maldonado F, Breen DP, Colchen A. Endoscopic successful management of tracheobronchomalacia with laser: apropos of a Mounier-Kuhn syndrome. Eur J Cardiothorac Surg 2011; 39(6): e186-8. [http://dx.doi.org/10.1016/j.ejcts.2011.01.074] [PMID: 21382725]

[122] Plojoux J, Laroumagne S, Vandemoortele T, Astoul PJ, Thomas PA, Dutau H. Management of benign dynamic "A-shape" tracheal stenosis: a retrospective study of 60 patients. Ann Thorac Surg 2015; 99(2): 447-53. [http://dx.doi.org/10.1016/j.athoracsur.2014.08.037] [PMID: 25497072]

[123] Abu-Dalu K, Faught P, Grosfeld JL. Peritracheal fibrosis induced by sclerosing agents: a putative treatment for tracheomalacia. J Invest Surg 1996; 9(6): 433-7. [http://dx.doi.org/10.3109/08941939609025860] [PMID: 8981216]

[124] Nishine H, Hiramoto T, Kida H, *et al.* Assessing the site of maximal obstruction in the trachea using lateral pressure measurement during bronchoscopy. Am J Respir Crit Care Med 2012; 185(1): 24-33. [http://dx.doi.org/10.1164/rccm.201104-0701OC] [PMID: 21997334]

[125] Korpela A, Aarnio P, Sariola H, Törmälä P, Harjula A. Comparison of tissue reactions in the tracheal mucosa surrounding a bioabsorbable and silicone airway stents. Ann Thorac Surg 1998; 66(5): 1772-6. [http://dx.doi.org/10.1016/S0003-4975(98)00763-2] [PMID: 9875787]

[126] Novotny L, Crha M, Rauser P, *et al.* Novel biodegradable polydioxanone stents in a rabbit airway model. J Thorac Cardiovasc Surg 2012; 143(2): 437-44. [http://dx.doi.org/10.1016/j.jtcvs.2011.08.002] [PMID: 21885070]

[127] Vondrys D, Elliott MJ, McLaren CA, Noctor C, Roebuck DJ. First experience with biodegradable airway stents in children. Ann Thorac Surg 2011; 92(5): 1870-4. [http://dx.doi.org/10.1016/j.athoracsur.2011.07.042] [PMID: 22051281]

[128] Stehlik L, Hytych V, Letackova J, Kubena P, Vasakova M. Biodegradable polydioxanone stents in the treatment of adult patients with tracheal narrowing. BMC Pulm Med 2015; 15: 164. [http://dx.doi.org/10.1186/s12890-015-0160-6] [PMID: 26690793]

[129] Antón-Pacheco JL, Luna C, García E, *et al.* Initial experience with a new biodegradable airway stent in children: Is this the stent we were waiting for? Pediatr Pulmonol 2016; 51(6): 607-12. [http://dx.doi.org/10.1002/ppul.23340] [PMID: 26584412]

CHAPTER 11

Tracheal And Bronchial Stenosis: Etiologies, Bronchoscopic Interventions and Outcomes

Benjamin Young, Sonali Sethi, Thomas R. Gildea and **Michael Machuzak***

Department of Pulmonary Medicine, Respiratory Institute, Cleveland Clinic, Cleveland, OH, USA

Abstract: Central airway obstruction can arise from a variety of disease processes, both benign and malignant in etiology, and result in significant morbidity and mortality to the patient. Both surgical and endoscopic techniques can be used to successfully manage central airway obstruction. The decision regarding how to approach each patient should be based on their own unique anatomic and physiologic considerations. In this chapter, we will discuss the etiologies of tracheal and bronchial stenosis, the physiologic effects of central airway stenosis, and the various bronchoscopic techniques that can be applied to manage central airway obstruction.

Keywords: Airway stent, Balloon dilation, Bronchial stenosis, Central airway obstruction, Electrocautery, Laser, Post-intubation tracheal stenosis (PITS), Tracheal anatomy, Tracheal stenosis.

INTRODUCTION

Obstruction of the central airways causes significant morbidity and mortality, and can arise from a variety of different disease processes [1]. Although definitions vary in the literature, central airway obstruction (CAO) is generally defined as occlusion of >50% of the lumen of the trachea, mainstem bronchi, bronchus intermedius, or a lobar bronchus [2]. While the exact incidence of central airway obstruction is unknown, the increasing incidence of lung cancer would suggest that the overall incidence of CAO is increasing. An estimated 30% of lung cancer patients develop complications due to airway obstruction, and up to 40% of lung cancer deaths can be attributable to locoregional disease. In addition to malignant disease, the increased use of endotracheal intubation in a growing, aging population would suggest that the number of benign CAO is also increasing [1].

A combination of surgical and endoscopic techniques can be employed to manage central airway obstruction. In emergent central airway obstruction, endoscopic

* **Corresponding author Michael Machuzak:** Department of Pulmonary Medicine, Respiratory Institute, Cleveland Clinic, Cleveland, OH, USA; Tel: (216) 444-2718; E-mail: machuzm@ccf.org

Ali I. Musani (Ed.)

techniques to stabilize the airway are the procedure of choice. In non-emergent cases, surgical resection is the treatment of choice in selected patients if curative resection is possible. Endoscopic techniques can be employed to evaluate and stabilize the airway while surgical management is planned. However, care should be taken such that the endoscopic treatment does not interfere with the future potential surgical intervention. A multi-disciplinary approach is advocated, as the decision for a specific intervention is dictated by the individual needs of each patient and demands a high degree of expertise and collaboration between otolaryngologists, interventional pulmonologists, and thoracic surgeons [1, 3].

AIRWAY ANATOMY AND PHYSIOLOGY

Advanced knowledge of the anatomy of the central airways is critical in managing central airway obstruction and planning any airway procedure. The trachea originates at the inferior aspect of the cricoid cartilage, at approximately the level of the sixth or seventh thoracic vertebrae, and terminates at the main carina [4]. The suprasternal notch divides the trachea into the extrathoracic portion, which makes up approximately one third of its length, and the intrathoracic trachea, which makes up the remaining two thirds of its length. The normal adult trachea is 10-14 cm in total length [3]. The normal coronal diameter of the trachea is 13-25 mm in men, and is 10-21 mm in women. The normal tracheal sagittal diameter is 13-27 mm in men, and is 10-23 mm in women. On CT, the normal tracheal wall is 1-3 mm thick [4].

Histologically, the trachea consists of four layers, as seen in Fig. (**1**). There is an inner mucosal layer, a submucosal layer, cartilage and muscle (trachealis muscle), and an outer adventitial layer. The adventitial layer includes the lymphatics and connective tissue. The anterior trachea has between 16-24 C-shaped cartilaginous rings, which are 4-5 mm in height and linked together by annular ligaments of fibroconnective tissue, whose purpose is to support the trachea during expiration. The posterior tracheal wall, also referred to as the membranous portion of the trachea, is only supported by the trachealis muscle, a thin band of smooth muscle, with an inner transverse layer and an outer longitudinal layer [4, 5]. The blood supply of the trachea, which is shared with the esophagus, comes from a series of longitudinal arcades located on each side of the trachea. The arcades are supplied by multiple small arteries originating from the supreme intercostal, the inferior thyroid, the internal thoracic, the phrenic, and the bronchial arteries. The blood supply is segmental, with the arteries supplying a submucosal plexus that is the only source of blood to the tracheal cartilages [6].

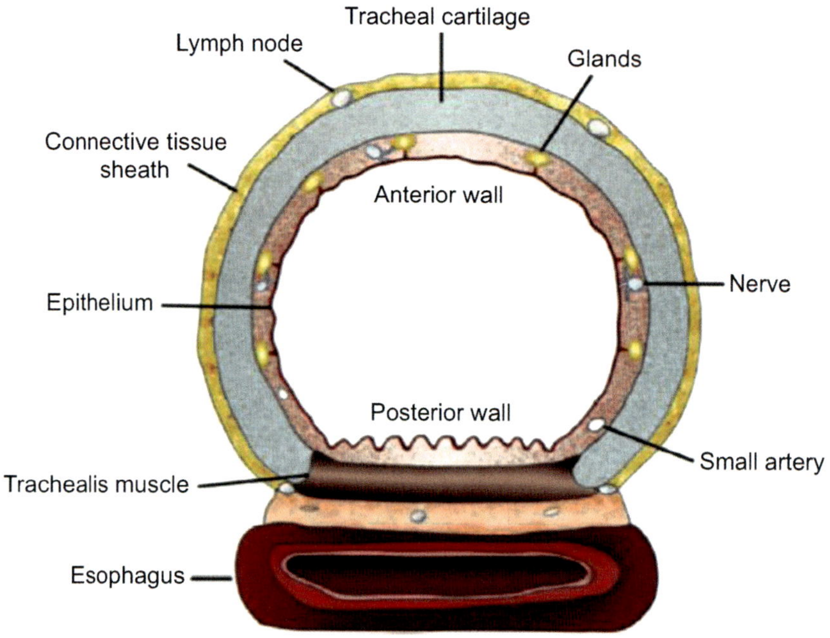

Fig. (1). Tracheal wall anatomy. Note the horseshoe-shaped cartilaginous ring extending along the anterior and lateral walls of the trachea. The mucosa and submucosa are difficult to delineate on computed tomography in a normal trachea. (Reprinted with permission [4]).

The main carina marks the distal end of the trachea, and bifurcates the trachea into the right and left mainstem bronchi. The main carina is located at the left of the fifth to sixth thoracic vertebrae, or the manubriosternal junction [3]. The left mainstem bronchus extends from the main carina to the secondary carina, dividing the left upper and lower lobes. The left mainstem bronchus is approximately 4 cm in length, with a diameter of approximately 13 mm. The left mainstem bronchus diverges from the trachea at approximately a 45° angle [3] and courses laterally and inferiorly to the left pulmonary artery [4]. The right mainstem bronchus extends from the main carina to the right upper lobe orifice, and is approximately 2 cm in length, with an approximate diameter of 15 mm. It diverges from the trachea at an angle of 25-30° from midline [3] and courses posteriorly and superiorly to the right pulmonary artery [4]. The bronchus intermedius is a continuation of the right mainstem bronchus distal to the right upper lobe orifice, and extends to the right middle and lower lobe bifurcation. The bronchus intermedius is approximately 2 cm in length [3]. The configuration of the proximal tracheobronchial tree can be seen in Fig. (**2**).

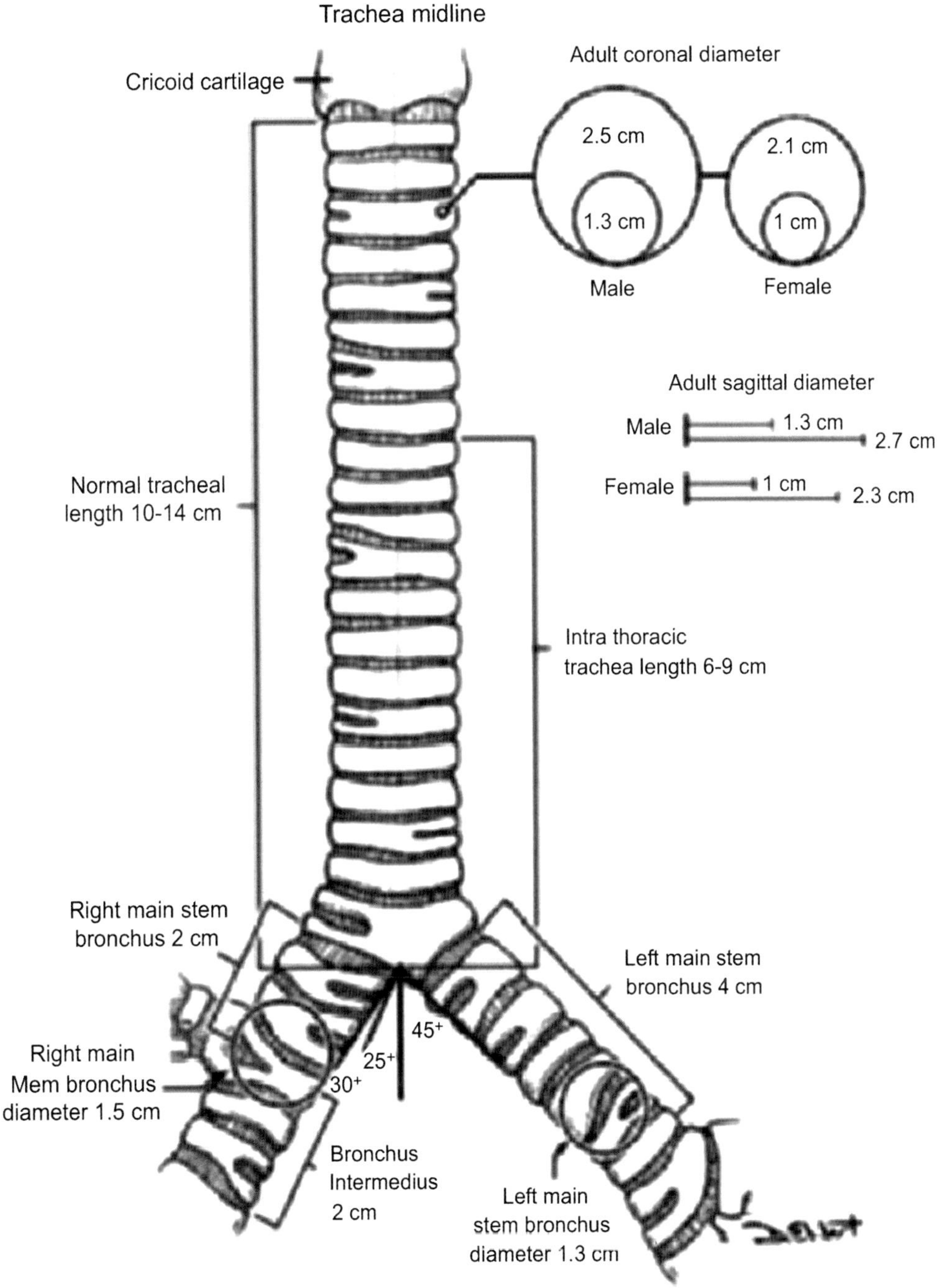

Fig. (2). Anatomy of the proximal tracheobronchial tree (Reprinted with permission [7]).

The intrathoracic tracheal diameter is dynamic. It expands during inspiration and recoils with expiration [3]. CT imaging can demonstrate the physiologic anterior bowing of the posterior membranous portion of the trachea during expiration, with little change in the cartilaginous anterolateral tracheal wall [4], as shown in Fig. (**3**).

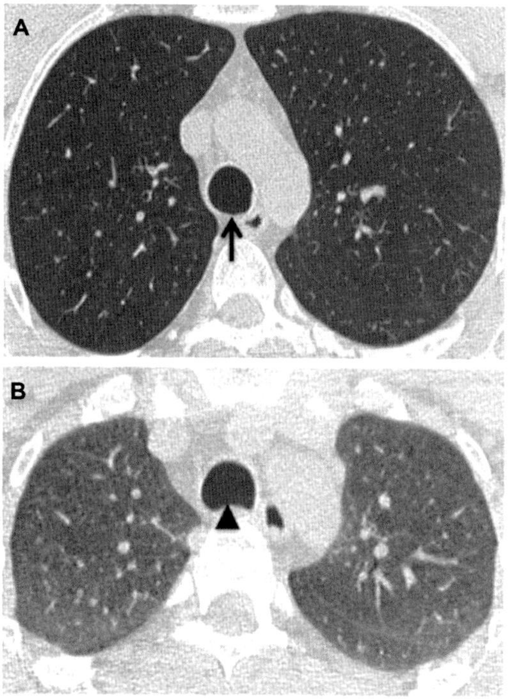

Fig. (3). Normal inspiratory and expiratory computed tomography images. On inspiration (A), note that the membranous wall of the trachea bows posteriorly (arrow). On expiration (B), the membranous wall bows anteriorly (arrowhead). Note that the anterolateral walls change little in their morphologic appearance, due to the cartilaginous support. (Reprinted with permission [4]).

Alvin Barach, in 1935, hypothesized that the sensation of air hunger in patients with central airway obstruction was caused by "the increased effort required to obtain the normal velocity of air delivered to and from the lungs." In cases of mild airflow obstruction, there may be little effect on airflow, and as such patients may remain asymptomatic [1]. The work of breathing depends on the change in pressure along the stenotic airway, and is influenced mainly by the degree of obstruction and the airflow velocity. Computer modeling of tracheal stenosis show a relationship to the squared ratio of bulk flow to stenosis lumen cross section, predicting a dramatic and relatively sudden increase in respiratory impairment once a relatively severe degree of stenosis is reached that correlates to what is observed in clinical practice [8], as shown in Fig. (**4**).

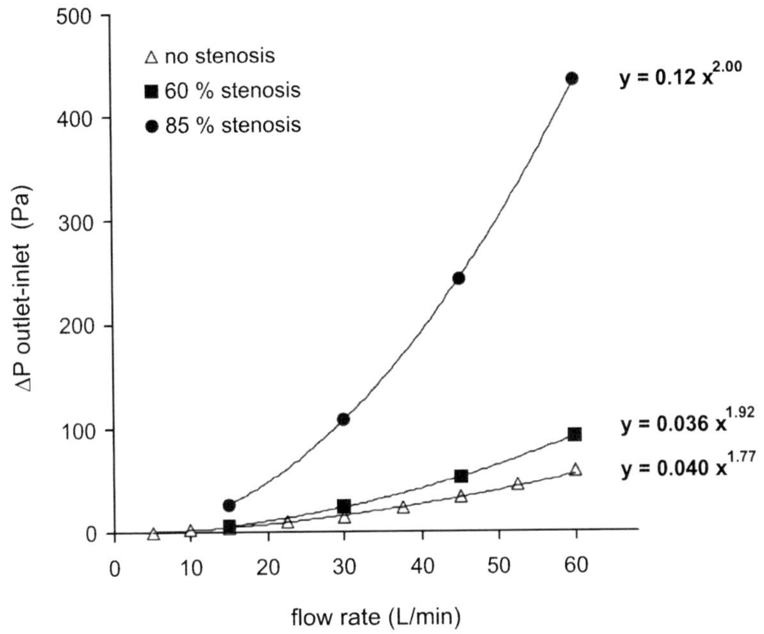

Fig. (4). CFD-simulated pressure drops between model inlet and outlet for different flows up to 60 l/min in the case of no stenosis (Δ), of 60% constriction (▪) and 85% constriction(●). The line plots are the corresponding best-fit power laws, leading to power values of 1.77 (no stenosis), 1.92 (60% stenosis), and 2.00 (85% stenosis). (Reprinted with permission [8]).

In mild tracheal narrowing, with a reduction of ≤50% of the tracheal lumen, the changes in cross-sectional area and pressure drop is similar to that which occurs normally through the glottis, and is unlikely to cause symptoms. With increased stenosis of the trachea, 51-70% reduction of the cross-sectional area, significant pressure drops can occur at higher flow rates, such as those that occur during exertion. As such, patients are likely to report variable symptoms that occur with activity [2]. The trachea is usually narrowed to less than 8 mm in diameter before exertional symptoms are present [1]. More severe stenosis, with cross-sectional area reduced >71%, results in significant pressure drop even at low flow rates. Patients with this degree of stenosis generally report symptoms at rest [2]. The tracheal lumen is usually less than 5 mm in diameter at this point [1].

Pulmonary function testing, specifically spirometry and flow volume loops, can be used to evaluate patients before and after interventions. The typical blunting of the flow volume loop on inspiration and expiration commonly seen in central airway obstruction is typically seen before spirometry yields abnormal expiratory flows, however the tracheal lumen needs to be narrowed to 6-8mm in diameter [2].

MORPHOLOGY & CLASSIFICATION

Tracheal stenosis may be classified according to the morphological aspects of simple or complex stenosis. Simple stenosis is comprised of short segments (<1 cm) which are web-like, concentric, membranous lesions without cartilage damage. Complex stenosis is characterized by extensive endoluminal occlusion (>1 cm), circumferential contraction scarring and/or associated with malacia or loss of cartilaginous support.

Laryngotracheal stenosis was first classified by *Cotton* in 1984, then revised by *Myer et al* in 1994. The Myer-Cotton classification system determines the degree of tracheal stenosis using standard endotracheal tubes as guides and observing how they pass through the narrowest point. Together, the Myer-Cotton system is based on circumferential stenosis with four staging degrees based on the percentage of reduction in cross-sectional area, using cutoff values of 50% and 70% narrowing to define grades, as shown in Fig. (**5**). Location and length are noted, but do not affect the grade of stenosis [9].

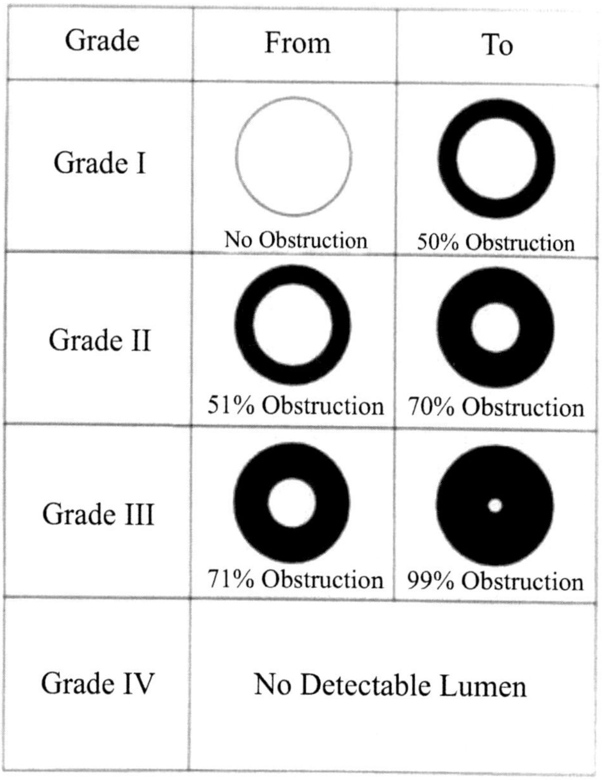

Fig. (5). Proposed stenosis classification system (Reprinted with permission [9]).

In general, stage I lesions have the highest success rate while stage IV lesions have the lowest. In addition, complex stenosis has a lower endoscopic treatment success rate compared to simple stenosis.

Tracheal stenosis includes various morphologic descriptions such as A-shaped, circumferential, web-like, complex, eccentric, pseudo-stenosis, and mixed, with certain morphologies being characteristic of etiology. For example, post-tracheostomy stenosis are typically A-shaped or triangular; idiopathic subglottic stenosis is typically a circumferential (concentric) simple lesion; and post-intubation tracheal stenosis can be hourglass or complex. Morphology can affect flow dynamics, symptoms, and response to certain therapeutic interventions. For example, in post-tracheostomy stenosis, the stricture is often anterior, sparing the posterior membranous portion of the airway. Because the injury is anterior and the mobile posterior membrane remains unaffected, dilation alone is often ineffective. In addition, completely circumferential strictures are shown to have poorer outcomes requiring more interventions than eccentric localized hypertrophic tissue [10].

ETIOLOGY

Throughout the past century, the etiologies of central airway obstruction have evolved. In the early 20th century, central airway obstruction was primarily caused by aspiration or infections, such as syphilis, diphtheria, typhoid fever, and tuberculosis [11]. In 1897, Dr. Gustav Killian performed rigid bronchoscopy to remove a pork bone from a farmer's airway, ushering in the era of modern bronchoscopy [12 - 14]. In 1917, Chevalier Jackson first described high tracheostomy as a risk factor in the development of laryngotracheal stenosis. After World War II, blunt trauma, primarily from motor vehicle accidents, became the major etiology of laryngotracheal stenosis. Trauma as the primary etiology of laryngotracheal stenosis began to decline in the 1970's as motor vehicle safety features improved, as well as the institution of a national speed limit [11]. As traumatic airway injury was on the decline, there was an increase in the use of endotracheal intubation and positive pressure mechanical ventilation. The incidence of tracheostomy, used for patients requiring mechanical ventilator for more than 5-7 days, increased by 15-fold from 1947 to 1959 [15]. Prolonged intubation was believed to be responsible for >90% of cases of laryngotracheal stenosis [11]. At the time, post-intubation tracheal stenosis was thought to be rare, but a prospective study of patients after intubation or tracheostomy revealed a 20% incidence of tracheal stenosis. Through a series of cadaver and animal studies, Dr. Hermes Grillo confirmed the role of pressure necrosis in the development of post-intubation tracheal stenosis, and was instrumental in demonstrating the benefits of a high-volume, low-pressure cuff in minimizing the risk for post-intubation tracheal stenosis [15]. Currently, etiologies resulting in tracheal stenosis are idiopathic, congenital, post-intubation tracheal stenosis, tracheostomy, neoplasms, radiation therapy, previous airway surgeries, infection, and inflammatory conditions.

Congential Tracheal Stenosis (CTS)

Congenital tracheal stenosis describes a wide range of tracheal abnormalities which may be the result of an abnormality inherent to the trachea itself or may be the effect of external forces compressing the airway. In the majority of cases, it consists of a funnel-shaped part of the trachea characterized by complete circular cartilaginous tracheal rings and is often associated with other congenital malformations. Although this type of stenosis is uncommon, it is the third most frequent congenital airway problem. In 1964, *Cantrell and Guild* classified 3 morphological types of CTS as generalized hypoplasia, funnel-shaped stenosis and segmental stenosis. CTS is rarely managed successfully with endoscopic techniques [16].

Post-Intubation / Post-Tracheostomy Tracheal Stenosis

Currently, the leading cause of tracheal stenosis is endotracheal intubation. Post-intubation tracheal stenosis (PITS) was first recognized as an entity in 1880, after MacEwen instituted prolonged endotracheal intubation in four patients with upper airway obstruction [17]. Since then, several risk factors have been identified which include prolonged intubation, traumatic intubation, a large-caliber endotracheal tube, history of a previous intubation or tracheostomy, need for reintubation, high tracheostomy site, frequent displacement of the endotracheal tube, local infection while intubated, steroid usage, obesity, and the concomitant existence of a nasogastric tube [11, 18].

Among all intubated patients, the reported incidence of PITS and post-tracheostomy tracheal stenosis (PTTS) ranges from 10-22%, but only 1-2% of patients have severe stenosis or are symptomatic [18]. Severe PITS and PTTS have an estimated incidence of 4.9 cases per million per year in the general population [19].

The most widely accepted theory is that PITS and PTTS is caused either by cuff-induced ischemic damage to the trachea, stomal injury from a tracheostomy, or a combination of the two. Cuff-induced damage occurs when high pressure from a tube or cuff exceeds the capillary pressure of the airway wall with loss of regional blood flow to the tracheal wall. This leads to local ischemia, and possibly necrosis. Stenosis subsequently develops during the phase of healing of an area of transmural injury to the airway wall. Local inflammation and ischemia result in upregulation of the fibrinolytic pathways, including C and S proteins locally, which leads to proliferation and airway remodeling with the creation of a membranous web-like stenosis [20]. Prolonged intubation can result in tracheal stenosis at various levels within the trachea. Stenosis can occur anywhere from the level of the endotracheal tube tip, up to the glottic and subglottic area. However, the most common sites are where the endotracheal cuff has been in contact with the tracheal wall and at the tracheal stoma site after a tracheostomy procedure. This ischemic injury begins within the first few hours of intubation, and healing of the damaged region can result in web-like fibrosis within 3-6 weeks [15, 21].

Tracheal stenosis following tracheostomy can occur as a complication of a previous tracheostomy, percutaneous tracheostomy, cricothyroidotomy, or surgical treatment for airway neoplasms. Stenosis may be above the stoma, at the same level of the stoma, at the cuff site, or at the tip of the cannula. PTTS most commonly results from abnormal would healing with excess granulation tissue formation around the tracheal stoma site or over fractured cartilage which can occur during the tracheostomy procedure [22, 23].

Idiopathic Tracheal Stenosis (ITS)

Idiopathic tracheal stenosis is a rare inflammatory process of unknown cause and is an exclusion diagnosis based on the absence of recent intubation or trauma, or other rare disease that can affect the trachea.

Some reports advocate a hormonal etiology since most patients are females in the 20-50 year age range. Estrogen and progesterone receptor studies in resected surgical specimens have revealed positive staining of fibroblasts, suggesting a hormonal role [24]. It has been postulated that estrogen increases levels of transforming growth factor B1 and fibronectin, both of which affect the wound healing response. Transforming growth factor B1 promotes early extracellular matrix production, fibrosis, and deposition of type I and III collagens. Fibronectin is thought to enhance collagen deposition and wound contraction, all possibly causing ITS [25].

Others have advocated that laryngopharyngeal reflux resulting in severe coughing and mechanical trauma is a possible etiological factor. Up to 70% of tracheal stenosis, whether or not an underlying cause has been identified, have abnormal laryngeal acid exposure and may benefit from anti-reflux therapy [11]. Gastroesophageal reflux has been proposed as a medical condition that may exacerbate the pathogenesis of tracheal stenosis, be a single cause for stenosis, or cause restenosis after repair. The recognition of, routine screening for, and widespread use of effective medication for the treatment of GERD has significantly reduced a major source of chronic airway inflammation and has improved patency following surgery.

Inflammatory Conditions

Granulomatosis with Polyangiitis (GPA)

Granulomatosis with polyangiitis (GPA) is a multi-systemic disease characterized by necrotizing vasculitis and granuloma formation. Airway involvement is uncommon, but if present may occur either as a presenting feature or a late-stage manifestation of the disease and will occur in approximately 10-20% of cases [26]. Tracheobronchial manifestations of GPA may take place after remission has been achieved with appropriate immunosuppressive therapy. However, the development of airway stenosis does not necessarily indicate failure of immuno-suppressive therapy. The stenosis often occurs or progresses independently of other features of active disease. Only 20-26% with GPA-related tracheal strictures respond to glucocorticoids alone or in combination with another immuno-suppressant. The remaining 74-80% of patients usually require interventional therapies.

The subglottis and upper trachea are most commonly involved, with the most common finding being circumferential scarring and critical narrowing of the airway. Evidence suggests that this may be because airway obstruction is caused by fibrotic scarring rather than active inflammation. The evaluation and diagnosis of a patient with suspected tracheobronchial GPA disease requires a combination of clinical assessment, serologic testing, sinus and chest imaging, pulmonary function tests, bronchoscopy, and tissue biopsy. The diagnosis is established when serologic and histopathologic evidence of vasculitis and granulomatous inflammation are present in a patient with a compatible clinical presentation. For those patients who remain symptomatic despite appropriate medical management, endoscopic management is an option with topical corticosteroids, laser incisions or resection, serial dilatations, and local mitomycin-C application. Patients often require multiple mechanical dilations and other therapy to restore airway patency. Overall 10 year survival is 75%.

Relapsing Polychondritis (RP)

Relapsing polychondritis is a multi-system immune-mediated disease characterized by recurrent episodes of inflammation of cartilaginous structures. One-third of cases develop in association with another connective tissue disease, and generally occurs between the ages of 40-60 years. In the active stage, the disease may involve the laryngotracheobronchial tree and cause red, painful swelling of the cartilage. After the inflammatory stage, significant destruction may occur with diffuse, smooth thickening of the larynx, trachea, and proximal bronchi. This can lead to tracheal wall nodularity, diffuse narrowing of the tracheobronchial tree, thickened, densely calcified cartilaginous rings with spared posterior tracheal membrane, or major airway collapse secondary to destruction of cartilaginous rings. Medical management of RP focuses on suppression the acute inflammatory process. However, it is feasible to palliate or stabilize the airway with endoscopic procedures such as stenting, and dilatation [4, 27].

Amyloidosis

Amyloidosis is a disorder characterized by extracellular tissue deposition of fibrillar proteins and can involve the respiratory tract. Sites in the larynx that shows a predilection for nodular or polypoid amyloidosis include the ventricles, false vocal cords, aryepiglottic folds, subglottis, and there may be diffuse narrowing and wall thickening with circumferential airway involvement. Bronchoscopy reveals multiple plaques or localized tumor-like masses. Tissue biopsy stained with Congo red and examined under polarized light shows the characteristic submucosal extracellular deposits of amyloid protein. Endoscopic procedures have been suggested as a possible method for dealing with airway stenosis, however surgery, when possible, remains the treatment of choice in localized stenosis [4, 27].

Infection

Airway stenosis secondary to chronic infection is rare, except in certain endemic geographic areas. It has been described in patients with tuberculosis, syphilis, typhoid fever, scarlet fever, diphtheria, leprosy, and laryngeal scleroma secondary to Klebsiella rhinoscleromatis. Endotracheal tuberculosis may result in significant airway obstruction related to the initial lesion or subsequent stricture formation, despite appropriate anti-tuberculosis therapy. Although infrequent in western countries, this is one of the most common etiologies where TB is endemic [4] [27].

Airway Complications After Lung Transplant

Initial attempts at lung transplantation were limited by anastomotic failure, thought to be due to bronchial ischemia, in up to 80% of cases. Some complications, such as granulation tissue and anastomotic dehiscence, occur at the anastomotic site, while other complications, such as infection, mucosal slough, fibrotic stricture, and bronchomalacia, can occur anywhere in the transplanted airway. By the early to mid-1990s, due to improvements in surgical technique and immune suppression, airway complications requiring intervention occurred in only approximately 10% of lung transplants. Risk factors for airway complications included single lung transplantation, the use of simple interrupted suturing, telescoping the anastomosis, size discrepancy and longer duration of postoperative mechanical ventilation [1].

Malignant Airway Obstruction

Malignancy can affect any part of the airway. The most common cause of malignant airway obstruction is direct extension from an adjacent tumor, most commonly a bronchogenic carcinoma. Other tumors that frequently invade the airway are esophageal and thyroid carcinoma. Primary tumors of the airway are rare, with an estimated incidence of 600-700 cases per year. Primary tracheal tumors are due to either squamous cell carcinoma or adenoid cystic carcinoma in 70-80% of cases. Carcinoid tumors account for the majority of primary airway tumors distal to the trachea. Metastases to the airway are not uncommon, with the most frequent primary sites being renal cell, colorectal, breast, thyroid carcinoma and melanoma [1, 27].

MANAGEMENT

No definitive medical therapies have been found to treat the disease process of all forms of airway stenosis. Surgical resection with end-to-end anastomosis is considered the definitive treatment for airway stenosis in appropriate patients. However, mortality rates have been reported up to 5% for tracheal resection [28], and more distal airways may not be amenable to surgical treatment. Interventional bronchoscopy procedures can serve as a bridge to surgical treatment and most importantly, can constitute definitive therapy for many patients, including those that are surgical candidates [29].

When endoscopically managing benign disease in the airway, it is important to be cognizant of an overall therapeutic plan that requires a combination of modalities, and the potential need for future therapies. In patients with strictures less than 1 cm in length, good results are often achieved with endoscopic therapy, although open surgical laryngotracheal resection is viewed as preferable in patients who are operable. However, surgical treatment of strictures 4 cm and longer are often associated with anastomotic complications consisting of granulation, dehiscence, or stenosis. Therefore, although tracheal resection often provides curative treatment in patients, the surgical resection may not be feasible for lengths greater than 4-6 cm in adults [30]. Morphologically, web-like stenosis can be managed by endoscopic dilation repeatedly, however complex stenosis may be best treated by stent implantation in experienced hands with close follow-up required.

Instrumentation

The basic instrumentation for endoscopic management of airway stenosis includes rigid laryngoscopes and bronchoscopes with dilators, and flexible fiberoptic bronchoscopes. The rigid bronchoscope is a stainless-steel tube that ranges in diameter from 8-14 mm and in length from 27-40 cm. It allows for the simultaneous delivery of oxygen and anesthetic agents, as well as the passage of large instruments, while maintaining a generous view of the trachea. The distal end of the rigid bronchoscope is beveled and can be used as a coring device resulting in a blunt dilation to stenotic areas and furthermore stent the airway open. Various sized dilators can be passed through a larger size rigid scope, allowing for a more gentle dilation of the stricture without damage to normal mucosa [3].

Balloon Dilation

Focal circumferential strictures are endoscopically managed best by balloon dilation of the airway. Balloon bronchoplasty of the stenotic airway is safe, rapid, and effective. Balloon dilation has been successful alone when a fibrotic process caused the stenosis without cartilage destruction. Airway balloons can be inserted through the working channel of the flexible bronchoscope or through a rigid bronchoscope or over a guide-wire. The stricture should be seated in the middle of the expanding balloon. As the balloon expands, the energy is transmitted to the area of least resistance. The balloon should be inflated in increments with frequent deflation to observe progress and any potential airway injury. Apnea is required during the periods of balloon inflation in the trachea and some desaturation may occur, limiting the inflation time. Potential complications include perforation, airway wall injury or rupture, bleeding, pneumothorax, bronchospasm, mediastinitis, chest pain, and recurrent stenosis [1, 3, 27].

LASER

Endoscopic laser techniques rely on laser-tissue interactions based on biologic, chemical, or thermal reactions. It has sufficient power to vaporize tissue and produces an excellent coagulation effect. Knowledge of tissue effects in specific settings is important since inappropriate laser settings or resection techniques can enhance laser-related adverse effects and alter local anatomy. Factors found to be associated with poor results or failure include circumferential strictures longer than 1 cm in vertical dimension, trachcomalacia, posterior laryngeal inlet scarring with arytenoids fixation, and a previous history of severe bacterial infection associated with tracheostomy. It should be recognized that some experts believe that tissue damage caused by laser therapy, secondary to deep coagulation damages to blood flow, promotes fibrosis, scarring, and granulation tissue which consequently leads to re-stenosis [1, 27, 31].

CO_2 Laser

Based on laser-tissue interactions, the CO_2 laser is the preferred laser for treating benign stenosis. There is no scatter and no deep penetration therefore the risk for collateral mucosal damage or airway perforation is lower. It is an excellent cutting tool with an almost scalpel-like precision.

Nd:YAG Laser

This laser is best used in conjunction with dilation to release the tension of the stricture by performing radial incision in the stenotic tissues. Nd:YAG has greater depth of penetration compared to CO_2 and hence, should at all times be directed parallel to the tracheal wall, skimming the surface of the target tissue to avoid damage to the underlying cartilage rings. There are experts who believe that this should not be used as primary treatment since it could cause more scarring and complicate further options for open surgical interventions.

Electrocautery

In an attempt to reduce local injury cause by laser therapy, and to favor re-epithelialization after resection, electrocautery knife can be used in the endoscopic management of web-like benign airway stenosis [32]. It works by contact and can easily cut through the tracheal wall and cartilage with radial incisions typically performed at 4-, 8-, and 12-o'clock positions. Macroscopically, a clean cut is observed in the tissue. Use of electrocautery knife instead of laser results in several advantages; cost of equipment for electrocautery is less expensive, it offers more precise and limited tissue vaporization, and may be safer to use.

Cryotherapy

Cryotherapy utilizes extreme cold (below -40°C) in repeated freeze-thaw cycles to destroy tissue. The physical effects result from freezing and recrystallization of cellular water on thawing, as well as cellular rehydration. The vascular effects result in tissue ischemia from vasoconstriction, platelet aggregation, and increased blood viscosity. The overall tissue effect is determined by the rapidity of freezing and thawing, the lowest temperature achieved, the number of freeze-thaw cycles, and the water content of tissues. Nitrous oxide is a commonly used cryogen which can result in temperatures of -89°C at the tip of the cryoprobe within several seconds. One of the primary advantages of cryotherapy is its relative safety. Fibrous tissue and cartilage have low water content, and as such are cryoresistant, leading to a markedly reduced incidence of airway perforation. Bleeding is also uncommon due to the hemostatic effects of cryotherapy. These advantages have led some to recommend cryotherapy as first-line treatment for patients with post-transplant anastomotic strictures and granulation tissue [1].

Cryodebridement is a technique that takes advantage of the extreme cold to form a tissue block that can be extracted from the airway by removal of the cryoprobe. It is an excellent technique for removing more gelatinous airway obstructions for which mechanical debulking is ineffective [3]. A recent study of the use of cryodebridement, in combination with other modalities, on 156 patients showed the procedure to be effective (95% of patients achieved either partial or complete airway patency) and safe (overall complication rate of 11%, with all the complications being relatively minor and self-limited) [33].

Stents

In the last two decades, progress has been made in the management of tracheal stenosis using silicone, metal, and hybrid stents to support and maintain the airway lumen, restore integrity of a disrupted airway, support an airway wall from a compressing extraluminal mass, and preoperatively to restore airway patency prior to surgical treatment. Silicone stents are helpful for splinting extensive post-intubation stenosis, and are appropriate for palliating airway narrowing in nonsurgical candidates. Long-term stenting trials with silicone stents has been reported as an effective means of treating PITS/PTTS in 50% of patients. *Brichet et al* endoscopically dilated and stented patients with post-intubation stenosis and stent removal at about one year. Roughly half of the patients did not require follow-up intervention and operable patients who recurred were able to undergo surgery without deleterious stent effects [29]. Metal stent insertion should never be used in patients who are potential candidates for resection, as they are associated with significant complications including granulation tissue, extension of stenosis, perforation, and hemoptysis. Metal stents in patients with benign airway disorders should only be considered after all other treatment options have been exhausted. Metal stents, especially covered metal stents, are useful in restoring patency in airways compromised by extraluminal compression from tumors [1].

Montgomery T-Tube

A Montgomery T-tube is warranted for patients with a critical stenosis who are not candidates for surgery or indwelling airway stent insertions, and develop recurrence after dilation techniques. T-tubes are a silicone stent which should be inserted through the area of stenosis and additionally conserve airway not involved by the stenotic lesion. For most patients who do not require mechanical ventilatory support, a silicone T-tube provides functional capability. In a large case series consisting of 53 patients with complex tracheal stenoses, silicone T-tube insertion was effective in 70% of patients with limited complications. Concurrent cardiopulmonary disease and intractable infection were the two major causes of failure after T-tube placement [34]. Granulation tissue formation at the proximal and distal end of the T-tube can occur as well, as chronic airway irritation inciting infection. Frequent bronchoscopies may be necessary to remove thick mucus plaques and maintain stent patency.

OUTCOMES

In a study of a mixed population of 53 patients with malignant (45%) and non-malignant (55%) central airway obstruction at Duke University from 2010 to 2013, spirometry and quality of life date were collected pre- and post-intervention. Patients in the benign non-malignant central airway obstruction were more likely to undergo balloon dilation and stent placement, whereas patients with malignant airway obstruction were more likely to have heat therapy and debridement. FEV_1 increased by an average of 0.4 L and FVC increased by an average of 0.5 L after intervention in both groups. There was a strong correlation between improvement in FEV_1 and symptoms and quality of life. There was no difference in the improvement in spirometry or quality of life measures between the two groups. Location of intervention was not associated with change in lung function or quality of life [35].

The American College of Chest Physicians Quality Improvement Registry, Evaluation, and Education (AQuIRE) collected data from multiple participating centers performing therapeutic bronchoscopy from 2009 to 2013. A total of 1,115 procedures were performed on 947 patients with malignant airway obstruction at 15 different centers. The technical success rate (reopening of the airway to >50% of normal diameter) was 93%, with endobronchial obstruction and stent placement being associated with the highest technical success rates. Of the 187 patients who had pre- and post-intervention Borg scores measured, there was an overall decrease in dyspnea (mean ΔBorg, 0.9 ±2.2), with patients with higher baseline Borg scores receiving the most benefit. Pre- and post-intervention quality of life scores were measured in 183 patients showed overall improvement, with the most improvement seen in patients with higher baseline dyspnea and without lobar obstruction. The overall complication rate in the registry was 3.9%, with a procedural related mortality rate of 0.5% [36].

CONCLUSION

Central airway obstruction can occur from a variety of disease processes, resulting in the potential for significant morbidity and mortality. A combination of endoscopic tools and techniques can be applied to successfully manage central airway obstruction, and the decision on which modalities to use should be driven by each patient's underlying disease process and unique anatomic and physiologic considerations. When endoscopic therapy is used to treat central airway obstruction, it should be without significant sequelae and not interfere with the potential for future surgical management. Therefore, the therapeutic process involves a selection between conservative, endoscopic, and surgical procedures, and a multidisciplinary approach is usually recommended, as the decision for a specific intervention demands a high degree of expertise and collaboration between otolaryngologists, interventional pulmonologists, and thoracic surgeons.

CONFLICT OF INTEREST

The authors declare no conflict of interest, financial or otherwise.

ACKNOWLEDGEMENTS

Declared none.

REFERENCES

[1] Ernst A, Feller-Kopman D, Becker HD, Mehta AC. Central airway obstruction. Am J Respir Crit Care Med 2004; 169(12): 1278-97. [http://dx.doi.org/10.1164/rccm.200210-1181SO] [PMID: 15187010]

[2] Murgu SD, Egressy K, Laxmanan B, Doblare G, Ortiz-Comino R, Hogarth DK. Central Airway Obstruction: Benign Strictures, Tracheobronchomalacia, and Malignancy-related Obstruction. Chest 2016; 150(2): 426-41. [http://dx.doi.org/10.1016/j.chest.2016.02.001] [PMID: 26874192]

[3] Gorden JA, Ernst A. Endoscopic management of central airway obstruction. Semin Thorac Cardiovasc Surg 2009; 21(3): 263-73. [http://dx.doi.org/10.1053/j.semtcvs.2009.08.002] [PMID: 19942126]

[4] Lawrence DA, Branson B, Oliva I, Rubinowitz A. The wonderful world of the windpipe: a review of central airway anatomy and pathology. Can Assoc Radiol J 2015; 66(1): 30-43. [http://dx.doi.org/10.1016/j.carj.2014.08.003] [PMID: 25623009]

[5] Lunn W. Obstruction of the central airways: evaluation and management.Thoracic Endoscopy: Advances in Interventional Pulmonology. Malden, Massachusetts: Blackwell Publishing 2006; pp. 323-9. [http://dx.doi.org/10.1002/9780470755969.ch22]

[6] Gaissert HA, Burns J. The compromised airway: tumors, strictures, and tracheomalacia. Surg Clin North Am 2010; 90(5): 1065-89. [http://dx.doi.org/10.1016/j.suc.2010.06.004] [PMID: 20955884]

[7] Gorden JA, Wood DE. Rigid Bronchoscopy.Thoracic Endoscopy: Advances in Interventional Pulmonology. Malden, Massachusetts: Blackwell Publishing 2006; pp. 121-33.

[8] Brouns M, Jayaraju ST, Lacor C, *et al.* Tracheal stenosis: a flow dynamics study. J Appl Physiol 1985; 102(3): 1178-84.

[9] Myer CM III, O'Connor DM, Cotton RT. Proposed grading system for subglottic stenosis based on endotracheal tube sizes. Ann Otol Rhinol Laryngol 1994; 103(4 Pt 1): 319-23. [http://dx.doi.org/10.1177/000348949410300410] [PMID: 8154776]

[10] Simpson GT, Strong MS, Healy GB, Shapshay SM, Vaughan CW. Predictive factors of success or failure in the endoscopic management of laryngeal and tracheal stenosis. Ann Otol Rhinol Laryngol 1982; 91(4 Pt 1): 384-8.
[http://dx.doi.org/10.1177/000348948209100412] [PMID: 7114718]

[11] Koshkareva Y, Gaughan JP, Soliman AM. Risk factors for adult laryngotracheal stenosis: a review of 74 cases. Ann Otol Rhinol Laryngol 2007; 116(3): 206-10.
[http://dx.doi.org/10.1177/000348940711600308] [PMID: 17419525]

[12] Kollorath O. Entfernung eines Knochenstucks aus dem rechten Bronchus auf naturlichem Wege und unter Anwendung der directen Laryngoscopie. Munch Med Wochenschr 1897; 1038-9.

[13] Semaan R, Yarmus L. Rigid bronchoscopy and silicone stents in the management of central airway obstruction. J Thorac Dis 2015; 7 (Suppl. 4): S352-62.
[PMID: 26807283]

[14] Panchabhai TS, Mehta AC. Historical perspectives of bronchoscopy. Connecting the dots. Ann Am Thorac Soc 2015; 12(5): 631-41.
[http://dx.doi.org/10.1513/AnnalsATS.201502-089PS] [PMID: 25965540]

[15] Wain JC. Postintubation tracheal stenosis. Chest Surg Clin N Am 2003; 13(2): 231-46.
[http://dx.doi.org/10.1016/S1052-3359(03)00034-6] [PMID: 12755310]

[16] Herrera P, Caldarone C, Forte V, *et al.* The current state of congenital tracheal stenosis. Pediatr Surg Int 2007; 23(11): 1033-44.
[http://dx.doi.org/10.1007/s00383-007-1945-3] [PMID: 17712567]

[17] Macewen W. General Observations on the Introduction of Tracheal Tubes by the Mouth, Instead of Performing Tracheotomy or Laryngotomy. BMJ 1880; 2(1021): 122-4.
[http://dx.doi.org/10.1136/bmj.2.1021.122] [PMID: 20749630]

[18] Kastanos N, Estopá Miró R, Marín Perez A, Xaubet Mir A, Agustí-Vidal A. Laryngotracheal injury due to endotracheal intubation: incidence, evolution, and predisposing factors. A prospective long-term study. Crit Care Med 1983; 11(5): 362-7.
[http://dx.doi.org/10.1097/00003246-198305000-00009] [PMID: 6839788]

[19] Nouraei SA, Ma E, Patel A, Howard DJ, Sandhu GS. Estimating the population incidence of adult post-intubation laryngotracheal stenosis. Clin Otolaryngol 2007; 32(5): 411-2.
[http://dx.doi.org/10.1111/j.1749-4486.2007.01484.x] [PMID: 17883582]

[20] Spittle N, McCluskey A. Lesson of the week: tracheal stenosis after intubation. BMJ 2000; 321(7267): 1000-2.
[http://dx.doi.org/10.1136/bmj.321.7267.1000] [PMID: 11039970]

[21] Weymuller EA Jr. Laryngeal injury from prolonged endotracheal intubation. Laryngoscope 1988; 98(8 Pt 2) (Suppl. 45): 1-15.
[http://dx.doi.org/10.1288/00005537-198808001-00001] [PMID: 3398673]

[22] Anand VK, Alemar G, Warren ET. Surgical considerations in tracheal stenosis. Laryngoscope 1992; 102(3): 237-43.
[http://dx.doi.org/10.1288/00005537-199203000-00002] [PMID: 1545649]

[23] Grillo HC, Donahue DM, Mathisen DJ, Wain JC, Wright CD. Postintubation tracheal stenosis. Treatment and results. J Thorac Cardiovasc Surg 1995; 109(3): 486-92.
[http://dx.doi.org/10.1016/S0022-5223(95)70279-2] [PMID: 7877309]

[24] Mark EJ, Meng F, Kradin RL, Mathisen DJ, Matsubara O. Idiopathic tracheal stenosis: a clinicopathologic study of 63 cases and comparison of the pathology with chondromalacia. Am J Surg Pathol 2008; 32(8): 1138-43.
[http://dx.doi.org/10.1097/PAS.0b013e3181648d4a] [PMID: 18545144]

[25] Park SS, Streitz JM Jr, Rebeiz EE, Shapshay SM. Idiopathic subglottic stenosis. Arch Otolaryngol

Head Neck Surg 1995; 121(8): 894-7.
[http://dx.doi.org/10.1001/archotol.1995.01890080062012] [PMID: 7619417]

[26] Waxman J, Bose WJ. Laryngeal manifestations of Wegener's granulomatosis: case reports and review of the literature. J Rheumatol 1986; 13(2): 408-11.
[PMID: 3723501]

[27] Puchalski J, Musani AI. Tracheobronchial stenosis: causes and advances in management. Clin Chest Med 2013; 34(3): 557-67.
[http://dx.doi.org/10.1016/j.ccm.2013.05.002] [PMID: 23993823]

[28] Maassen W, Greschuchna D, Vogt-Moykopf I, Toomes H, Lüllig H. Tracheal resection--state of the art. Thorac Cardiovasc Surg 1985; 33(1): 2-7.
[http://dx.doi.org/10.1055/s-2007-1014071] [PMID: 2579455]

[29] Brichet A, Verkindre C, Dupont J, *et al.* Multidisciplinary approach to management of postintubation tracheal stenoses. Eur Respir J 1999; 13(4): 888-93.
[http://dx.doi.org/10.1034/j.1399-3003.1999.13d32.x] [PMID: 10362058]

[30] Wright CD, Grillo HC, Wain JC, *et al.* Anastomotic complications after tracheal resection: prognostic factors and management. J Thorac Cardiovasc Surg 2004; 128(5): 731-9.
[http://dx.doi.org/10.1016/j.jtcvs.2004.07.005] [PMID: 15514601]

[31] Khemasuwan D, Mehta AC, Wang KP. Past, present, and future of endobronchial laser photoresection. J Thorac Dis 2015; 7 (Suppl. 4): S380-8.
[PMID: 26807285]

[32] Tremblay A, Coulter T, Mehta AC. Modification of a Mucosal-Sparing Technique Using Electrocautery and Balloon Dilatation in the Endoscopic Management of Web-Like Benign Airway Stenosis. J Bronchol 2003; 10(4): 268-71.
[http://dx.doi.org/10.1097/00128594-200310000-00006]

[33] Inaty H, Folch E, Berger R, *et al.* Unimodality and Multimodality Cryodebridement for Airway Obstruction. A Single-Center Experience with Safety and Efficacy. Ann Am Thorac Soc 2016; 13(6): 856-61.
[http://dx.doi.org/10.1513/AnnalsATS.201508-486OC] [PMID: 26999041]

[34] Liu HC, Lee KS, Huang CJ, Cheng CR, Hsu WH, Huang MH. Silicone T-tube for complex laryngotracheal problems. Eur J Cardiothorac Surg 2002; 21(2): 326-30.
[http://dx.doi.org/10.1016/S1010-7940(01)01098-3] [PMID: 11825744]

[35] Mahmood K, Wahidi MM, Thomas S, *et al.* Therapeutic bronchoscopy improves spirometry, quality of life, and survival in central airway obstruction. Respiration 2015; 89(5): 404-13.
[http://dx.doi.org/10.1159/000381103] [PMID: 25925488]

[36] Ost DE, Ernst A, Grosu HB, *et al.* AQuIRE Bronchoscopy Registry. Therapeutic bronchoscopy for malignant central airway obstruction: success rates and impact on dyspnea and quality of life. Chest 2015; 147(5): 1282-98.
[http://dx.doi.org/10.1378/chest.14-1526] [PMID: 25358019]

CHAPTER 12

Airway Stenting in Benign and Malignant Diseases

David P. Breen* and **Mohammed Ahmed**

Department of Respiratory Medicine, Galway University Hospitals, Galway, Ireland

Abstract: Airway stenting is an important technique for the treatment of central airway obstruction and is a major component of an integrated Interventional Pulmonology service. Indications for this intervention can be broadly divided into malignant and benign conditions. Malignant airway obstruction is the commonest indication and can happen due to endobronchial tumors or external compression. Benign conditions include stenosis, fistula and airway malacia. An important consideration in benign conditions is patient longevity. Two groups of stents are available- silicon and metallic. Each is associated with advantages and disadvantages and the choice of stents depends on a number of factors including airway and disease related factors, physician choice and expertise and the available equipment within the endoscopy unit. Silicone stents require rigid bronchoscopy for placement while metallic stents can be deployed using flexible bronchoscopy. Irrespective of prosthesis type, stent related complications occur and include migration, stent obstruction from mucus, tumor ingrowth or granulation tissue and stent fracture. Finally, novel drug eluting and biodegradable stents are being studied with promising early results.

Keywords: airway, bronchoscopy, fistula, malacia, malignant, metallic, silicone, stents, stenosis.

INTRODUCTION

In mid-19th century, a widely respected French physician named Armand Trousseau was assigned by the French government to investigate epidemics that were ravaging across Europe. In 1851 he introduced the first double lumen tracheotomy tube that was life-saving in many cases of diphtheria, croup and typhus. Few years later on, the complications of such intervention were widely encountered by internists and surgeons in the form of tracheal stenosis. Some pioneers tried to surgically treat tracheal strictures by inserting what was later known as metallic airway stents (after a British dentist, Charles Stent) [1]. The first reports in the literature came from Trendelenburg (1872) and Bond (1891) [2]. It was not until the development of the Montgomery T tube in the sixties and

* **Corresponding author David P Breen:** Department of Respiratory Medicine, Galway University Hospitals, Galway, Ireland; Tel/Fax: 0035391524222; E-mail david.breen@hse.ie

Ali I. Musani (Ed.)

the Dumon stent in the mid-1980s that stenting became an integral part of the management of airway compromise from a number of benign and malignant conditions [3, 4]. Indications for airway stenting are shown in Table **1** and will be discussed in detail later. The primary indication for an airway stent is to reestablish patency of the airway [5]. It is important to emphasize that stenting, whether for benign or malignant disease, should be considered a palliative procedure and hence should be used only when all other treatment options are exhausted or contraindicated due to patient factors such as associated irreversible co-morbid conditions [6]. In rare situations stents may be used as a bridge to definitive therapy. Examples of this might include cases of benign tracheal stenosis and stent placement in the setting of fistula formation [7 - 9]. In highly selected cases airway stents can be used as first line definitive intervention as in the case of post lung transplantation bronchial stenosis.

Table 1. indications for the insertion of airway stents

Malignant Conditions	**Benign Conditions**
Endobronchial disease	Post Intubation Tracheal Stenosis
Extrinsic compression	Post Tracheostomy Tracheal Stenosis
Mixed intrinsic and extrinsic obstructions	Airway fistula (bronchopleural or trachea-esophageal)
	Post lung transplantation bronchial stenosis
	Airway malacia
	Miscellaneous

TYPES OF STENTS

Two major groups of stents are currently in use –silicone and metallic stents [10 - 12]. Inherently, both types of stents have limitations and a group of hybrid stents has been developed in order to overcome these. There is also ongoing research into the utility of biodegradable and drug eluting stents in the footsteps of the evolution of coronary stents. Silicone stents require rigid bronchoscopy for deployment while metallic stents can be placed with flexible bronchoscopy. To fit with the anatomic structure of the airways, stents have been designed in different shapes, straight, bifurcating (Y stents) and T tubes.

Self-Expandable Metallic Stents (SEMS)

SEMS are available as fully covered, partially covered or uncovered stents. While their primary advantage is that they can be placed with flexible bronchoscopy, the addition of rigid bronchoscopy allows greater airway manipulation and control. Another advantage is that they conform to the airway due to their self-expanding nature. The Food and Drug Administration of the USA (FDA) advised caution with the use of metallic stents in benign disease. Many of the concerns raised by the FDA have been discussed previously – stents should only be deployed as a last option after all other treatment options have been explored but also in the case of benign diseases metallic stents are difficult to remove and when this is tried complications like bleeding are common. Commercially available SEMS include the Silmet stent (Novatech, La Ciotat, France) (see Fig. **1**), Aero Tracheobronchial Stent (Merit Medical Systems, Inc. Utah, USA), and the Ultraflex stent (Boston Scientific, Natick, Massachusetts, USA). Finally, industry customized stents are available.

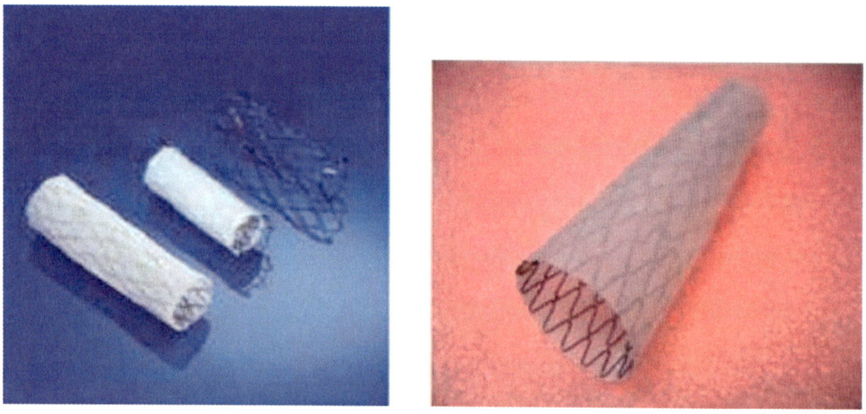

Fig. (1). Self Expandable Metallic Stents (SEMS). These are available in fully covered, partially cover, uncovered and custom made conical stents. Novatech, LaCiotat, France. [Courtesy Dr Hervé Dutau].

We previously described two such scenarios where customized stents were necessary, the conical SEMS for post pneumonectomy fistula and a 28mm customized metallic stent to manage severe malacia in a patient with Marfan's syndrome associated tracheomegaly [9, 13] (see Fig. **2**).

Silicone Stents

All silicone stents require rigid bronchoscopy for placement. They are available in all designs; straight, Y stent and T tube varieties. A major advantage of silicone stents is that they are easy to remove if needed but on the other hand their design means they have a higher rate of migration. Another significant advantage is that they are easily adjustable compared to metallic stents. The gold standard stent remains the Dumon stent (Tracheobronxane®, Novatech, La Ciotat, France). These prostheses are the most widely used stents worldwide. They have studs on the outside that minimize migration and reduce mucosal ischemia by limiting contact with the airway wall. The stents are available in a wide range of sizes and diameters (up to 18 mm in external diameter and 60 mm in length). This ensures

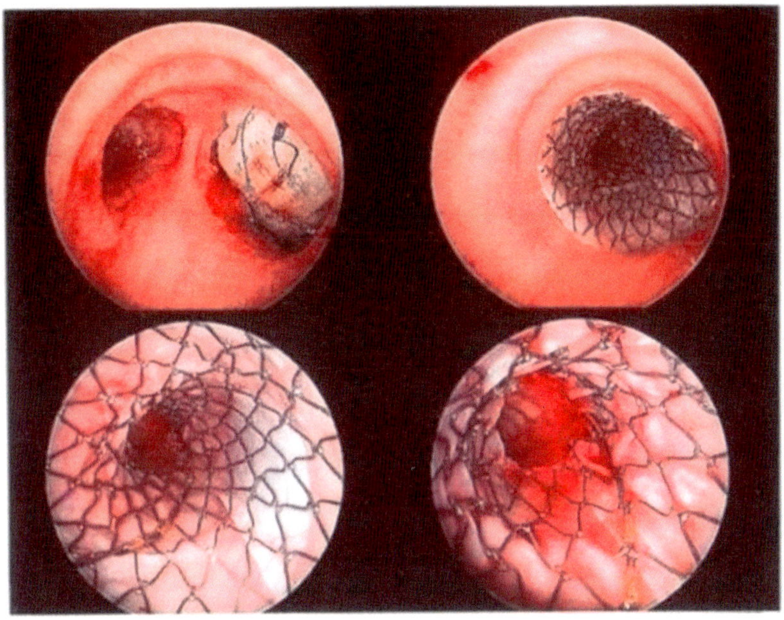

Fig. (2). The use of a custom made conical stent (Silmet, Novatech, LaCiotat, France to cover a large post pneumonectomy fistula. Courtesy Dr Hervé Dutau.

that the stent can be sized to the required length to encompass the stenosis and 0.5 cm of normal mucosa above and below the stenosis. This minimizes the length of the stent and assists clearance of secretions and patient tolerance. The rims of each stent are polished to reduce the risk of granuloma formation. The Marseille group has described a number of customizations to improve the functionality of the stent for an individual's airway. This includes cutting the stent to minimize its impact on the airway and the addition of windows in the stent using the Dutau Forceps (Novatech, La Ciotat, France) (see Fig. **3**). This improves ventilation of sub segmental bronchi, which would otherwise be covered [14]. In addition, recent advances include radiopaque studs–the Dumon Gold Studded Stent (Novatech, La Ciotat, France). which improves radiographic visualization. The Dumon silicone stent is also available in a Y design for disease at the level of the carina. Unlike the straight stent, the Y stent is more difficult to place correctly and requires a significant amount of time to position across the carina using rigid grasping forceps. Hour glass stents are available and these are particularly suitable for benign stenosis. Other silicone stents such as the Hood stent (Hood Laboratories, Pembroke, MA, USA), and the Noppen stent (MTW, Essen, Germany), are no longer commercially available. Finally, dynamic stents are also available. These have a flexible posterior wall, which mimics the posterior wall of the trachea. This improves secretion clearance.

Hybrid Stents

This group of stents was developed to remedy the deficiencies of the silicone and the SEMS. As the name implies, more than one material is included in the stent structure. The Polyflex stent (Boston Scientific, Natick, Massachusetts, USA) is made from polyethylene threads built into the silicone. The stent may adapt better to an hourglass stenosis when compared to the Dumon silicone stent; however, it has a higher migration rate, as it is more easily compressed than the Dumon stent [15]. The Aero (previously the Alveolus) stent (Merit Endotek) is another hybrid design. It is made of nitinol completely covered by polyurethane. Its length is modifiable and it can be introduced using a flexible scope. Despite what is in theory a good design, an increased rate of need for early removal has been reported mostly due to migration [16].

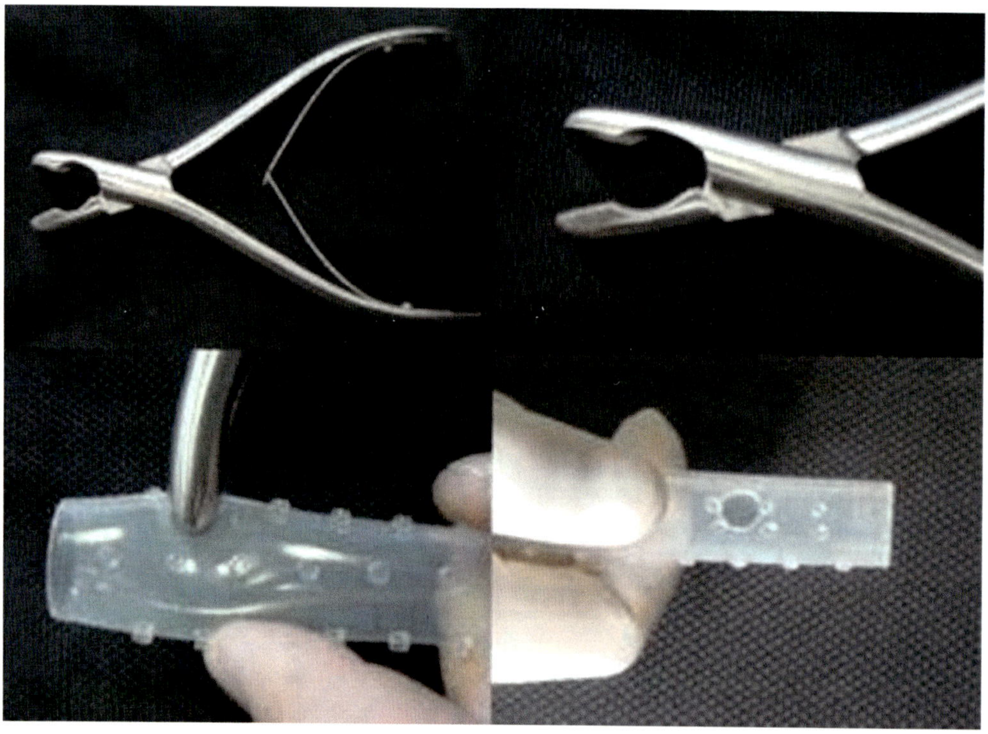

Fig. (3). The Dutau forceps (Novatech, LaCiotat, France). Courtesy Dr Hervé Dutau.

Drug Eluting and Biodegradable Stents

In the pursuit of a reduced incidence of restenosis and airway stent occlusion, an approach similar to the one utilized in coronary artery drug eluting stents was suggested. Stents releasing drugs like mitomycin and cisplatin has been used in animal experiments [17]. In the case of benign disease, the idea of a biodegradable stent that will safely disintegrate over time is appealing as it avoids a second rigid bronchoscopy procedure for removing a silicon stent and all the associated risks. Chao *et al* studied a cisplatin coated biodegradable stent first in vitro and it showed a strength comparable to the Ultraflex SEMS. Studies on rabbits then showed sustained cisplatin levels in the trachea for > 5 weeks and an intact ciliated epithelium in the stented area [18]. Results from another animal study suggested the use of bio-absorbable stents coated with mitomycin c were also promising [19]. There is only a limited body of evidence when it comes to human studies. One pilot study by Lischke *et al.* evaluated the safety and efficacy of polydioxanone stents (Ella-Cs Ltd., Hradec Králové, Czeck Republic) in post lung transplantation anastomotic bronchial stenosis. Six patients were included and 22 stents were successfully implanted. The median intervention free duration was 24 months (rang 7-44 months) [20]. No drug eluting airway stent is currently in use in clinical practice and further research is required in this promising area.

INDICATIONS

Benign Conditions

Benign Stenosis

Benign tracheal stenosis can occur from a number of etiologies. Despite technological improvements post intubation (PITS) and post tracheostomy (PTTS) tracheal stenosis remain the most commonly encountered [21, 22]. A number of conditions have been associated with this complication including the use of the inert materials, tube size, lateral wall pressure, movement, hypotension, local infection, use of steroids, and the duration of intubation. Although subglottic stenosis most commonly results from endotracheal tube damage, it may occur after damage of the 1st tracheal ring or cricoid cartilage during tracheostomy. In about half the cases the stenosis occurs at the cuff site. Other causes of benign tracheal stenosis are relatively rare. These include beam radiation and acid aspiration among others.

Post Intubation Tracheal Stenosis (PITS) and Post Tracheostomy Tracheal Stenosis (PTTS)

In the past the widespread use of high-pressure, low volume cuffs was associated with a high risk of PITS [23]. Although high volume low-pressure cuffs and/or early tracheotomy reduced the rate of stenosis at the cuff site they have not totally prevented this complication. The reported incidence of tracheal stenosis following tracheostomy and endotracheal intubation ranges from 0.6% to 21% and 6% to

21%, respectively. PITS is commonly seen in the form a web-like stenosis. The pathogenesis for this stenosis appears to be related to the compromise of the tracheal blood supply by excessive mucosal pressure from the inflated cuff. Previous studies have demonstrated that there is obstruction to mucosal blood flow with lateral wall pressures exceeding 22 mm Hg, with total occlusion of flow to the mucosa over the tracheal rings and posterior tracheal wall at a lateral wall pressure of 37 mm Hg. It has been hypothesized that large volume cuffs achieve a sparing effect on capillary blood flow over the cartilaginous rings by applying pressure to the arterioles in the intercartilaginous submucosa, thus raising the effective perfusion pressure.

In contrast, the most important reason for stenosis in PTTS is damaged cartilage. Risks for stenosis include a large stoma and excessive force whilst placing the tracheostomy tube through the stoma. Wound sepsis and previous cervical or tracheal trauma affect healing of the stoma. In one study, wound sepsis was a causative factor in approximately 42% of the cases of stomal stenosis following open tracheostomy. PITS tend to be longer in length than PTTS (mean 2.6 cm compared to 1.2 cm, respectively) [24]. In most cases, airway stenting is reserved for those considered to be not fit for surgery or as a bridge to definite intervention. In selected cases with simple stenosis (<10 mm in length and no airway malacia or damaged cartilage) airway stenting following incision using a rigid scope and/or other endoscopic therapies like balloon dilatation and Laser treatment can be used as first line [25]. Such cases have to be discussed at the multidisciplinary meeting.

Post Lung Transplantation

Stenosis can also occur at the anastomosis site in lung transplant recipients. The reported incidence of this complication ranges from 1.6% to 32% [26 - 29]. Two types of stenosis have been reported – directly at the anastomosis site and distant from the site; known as segmental non-anastomosis bronchial stenosis with a reported incidence of 2.5 to 3%. In one study silicon stent insertion was associated with improvement in FEV1 and symptoms and in most cases the stent was removed after a median of six months with stable lung function on follow up [30]. This represents an exceptional situation where airway stents can be used as definite treatment.

Idiopathic Tracheal Stenosis

It is increasingly recognized that tracheal stenosis can occur without a history of antecedent airway injury or a clear disease process [31, 32]. There is evidence that this might be an inflammatory condition with activation of the IL-23/IL-17A pathway [33]. Such cases of idiopathic tracheal stenosis have received attention of late with groups describing the clinicopathological features and the outcomes from a multidisciplinary airway intervention including mechanical or thermal dilatation (rigid, laser or electrocoagulation) and stent placement. In total, 18% of patients received a stent. All procedures were effective; however, recurrence occurred in the majority of patients over a prolonged follow up period (87% at 5 years).

Miscellaneous

Benign stenosis can also occur in a myriad of localized and systemic diseases that may affect the airways. This includes tuberculosis, sarcoidosis, papillomatosis and granulomatosis with polyangiitis (previously known as Wegener's).

Fistula

A fistula is a non-anatomical communication between the airway and an adjoining structure. Fistulas can occur between the airway and the oesophagus - (tracheo-oesophageal fistula, (TOF)), mediastinum or pleura (Bronchopleural fistula, (BPF)). The same principles of airway management apply as in airway stenosis; *i.e.* definitive treatment should be undertaken if possible prior to resorting to stent placement. However, stents may offer excellent palliation and rarely they may act as a bridge to definitive therapy.

Bronchopleural Fistula

Post resection fistula can be a devastating complication of thoracic surgery with an incidence of 4.5-20% post lobectomy and pneumectomy. The incidence is lower for benign conditions compared to patients with a known malignancy and it can also be classified as acute, subacute, or chronic. The acute form is usually related to dehiscence or technical complications and requires early reoperation. The subacute and chronic forms are related to infection in immunocompromised or debilitated patients with associated comorbidities. Postoperative radiotherapy is a risk factor for late bronchopleural fistulas. Complications of BPF include pyothorax, aspiration pneumonia, spillage of contaminated secretions into the contralateral lung and adult respiratory distress syndrome (ARDS). These complications are frequently resistant to non-surgical treatment and result in significant morbidity and prolonged hospital and intensive care stays. Irrespective of the incidence, this complication is associated with significant morbidity and mortality. Patients are frequently debilitated secondary to the underlying primary diagnosis, recent surgery and in some cases neoadjuvant therapy. The mortality rate amongst patients who develop a fistula post pneumonectomy ranges from 15% to 71%. Sirbu *et al.* reported their experience with 490 patients post lung resection for non-small cell lung cancer. The overall incidence was 4.4%

(22/490). Bronchopleural Fistula (BPF) after pneumonectomy occurred in 12 patients (54.6%) and post lobectomy in 9 (40.9%) [34, 35]. The wide variability in incidence is related to a number of factors including the extent of the resection, the resection technique used and the experience of the surgeon. In addition, a number of pre and post-operative risk factors have been identified. Pre-operative factors include fever, steroid use, H. influenzae in the sputum, elevated erythrocyte sedimentation rate, and anemia. Postoperative risk factors which have been implicated include fever, steroid use, leukocytosis, the presence of a tracheostomy and need for bronchoscopy with excessive suctioning. This is often performed for sputum impaction and/or mucus plugging. In addition, residual tumor at the resection margins, a long bronchial stump, excessive tightness of individual sutures, extensive peribronchial, and paratracheal dissection have been associated with an increased incidence of fistulization. All these factors increase the risk of ischemic necrosis and/or pooling of secretions with subsequent colonization and bacterial overgrowth.

Management of BPF depends on a number of factors including the underlying etiology, size, time of onset of the fistula postoperatively and health status of the patient [36]. Surgery is the treatment of choice of this condition but endoscopic techniques have been advocated as an option when surgery is not possible or has to be postponed. In patients with small fistulas, bronchoscopic options have included the use of silver nitrate, ethanol, cyanoacrylate glue, fibrin glue injection, polyethylene glycol, laser and, in cases with large fistulas, stent placement has been attempted - both silicone and metallic stents. Large dehiscences (> 8 mm) are generally considered not to be amenable to successful primary closure using bronchoscopic techniques. However, in this scenario, the role of endoscopic techniques is twofold, to act as a bridge until definitive surgical therapy, thus allowing an improvement in the patients' clinical status before surgery and, in cases that are not fit for further surgery, bronchoscopic intervention may provide adequate palliation of symptoms.

Tracheoesophageal Fistula

Acquired tracheoesophageal fistula again can be caused by benign or malignant disease. In the case of lung and esophageal cancer it is associated with significantly increased morbidity and deterioration in patient's quality of life. Airway stenting provides effective palliation of patient symptoms but the type of stent and location of insertion should be decided carefully in a multidisciplinary meeting setting. In a significant proportion of cases an esophageal stent is also required [37].

Airway Malacia

Tracheomalacia is defined as a weakness of the trachea due to atrophy of the longitudinal elastic fibers of the pars membranacea, or impaired cartilage integrity resulting in an airway that is softer and more susceptible to collapse [38]. Multiple interventions have been tried to improve ventilation in patients with severe obstruction secondary to malacia. Stents have also been used to try to stabilize the airway with mixed results. In addition, the placement of a stent may only serve to alter the choke point therefore extending the area of malacia. Stenting may be the only available treatment option in patients who are not candidates for surgical intervention. Alternatively, in surgical candidates, stents may be seen as a stabilizing tool prior to definitive treatment. Patients who obtain a good clinical response to a stent are likely to benefit from surgery. Both metallic and silicone stents have been used with most authors favoring the silicone prosthesis because they have a lower rate of complications in this particular population.

Malignant Disease

The most common indication for stenting is to recanalize an obstructed airway in the setting of malignant obstruction. This is most frequently secondary to primary lung malignancy. Indeed, it is estimated that 20–30% of all patients with a primary bronchogenic carcinoma will present with malignant central airway obstruction (CAO), which may result in haemorrhage, dyspnea, atelectasis, and pneumonia. In addition, after initial treatment, 30–50% of patients will present with local recurrences [39]. Other thoracic malignancies; thyroid, laryngeal and esophageal tumors, may directly invade the central airways causing compromise. Finally, nearly all extra-thoracic malignancies have been reported to metastasize to the airway.

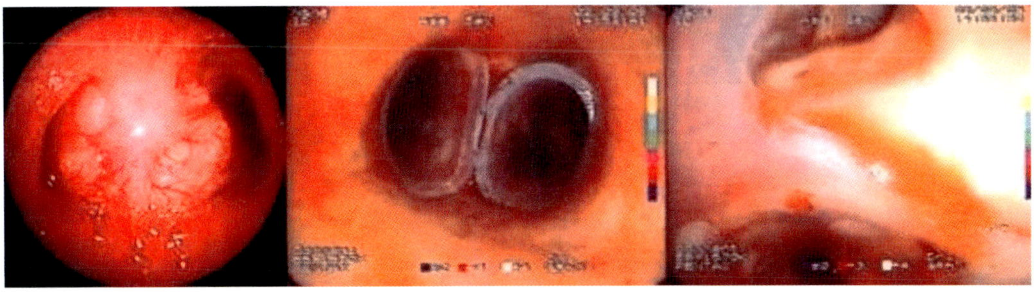

Fig. (4). A tumour at the level of the main carina. Post mechanical debulking, 2 silicone stents were placed. The right stent had a window cut to allow ventilation of the right upper lobe. [Courtesy Dr Hervé Dutau].

Malignant obstruction of the airway can occur through three mechanisms –extrinsic, intrinsic and a mixed pattern [40]. Treatment of malignant stenosis is dependent on the type and degree of obstruction. Any pathology, which results in a stenosis greater than 50% of the normal caliber may be an indication for stenting. In most centers, stenting is just one component of a comprehensive airway management programme which may include mechanical debulking (rigid bronchoscope), techniques for recanalization which includes immediate effect techniques – laser, argon plasma coagulation and electrocoagulation and delayed effect techniques – cryotherapy and photodymanic therapy [41, 42]. If, however the airway remains compromised after the use of debulking/dilatation with either mechanical debulking or accessory tools, then a stent may be indicated (Fig. **4**). Splinting with a stent is required more often in the setting of extrinsic compression from malignant nodal involvement or extraluminal tumor. However, in some situations, post debulking, the lumen remains stenosed greater that 50% and a stent may be required. In addition, in cases where an intrinsic tumor rapidly re-obstructs the lumen a decision may be made by the endoscopist to place a stent at the second intervention.

Stent Choice

The stent of choice will depend on a number of factors that include disease and patient characteristics, airway anatomy, physician/surgeon expertise and available equipment. The authors' preference is for a silicone stent. Metallic stents should not be used for the treatment of benign stenosis considering the issue of removability even in the case of uncovered stents. As stated in the British Thoracic Society (BTS) guideline the use of rigid bronchoscopy allows airway stability, adequate ventilation and rapid control of hemorrhage and clot removal. In addition, the silicone stent is easily customized and its position can be adjusted with ease after deployment. It can also be removed later on if the clinical situation dictates. In our unit, a SEMS is employed when there is a distorted airway with excessive tortuosity; in these situations, the silicone stent does not conform to the airway anatomy and, if placed, often results in kinking with ongoing airway stenosis and high risk of complications. The SEMS more easily conforms to this type of airway. In addition, conical SEMS are particularly useful in cases where the diameter of the airway varies from distal to the proximal extremity. However, unlike the recommendation of the BTS guideline, when placing a SEMS our department utilizes rigid bronchoscopy and intubation.

Once a decision is made to place a stent, the length of stenosis and required diameter needs to be measured. This can be performed with dedicated measuring forceps. The required stent size is estimated from the diameter of the rigid tube and the length can be measured using a flexible bronchoscope. The size of the stent should exceed the size of the stenosis by 1 cm therefore allowing 0.5cm clearance at the distal and proximal margin. The stent should oversize the stenosis so that there is adequate radial force to keep the prosthesis in position. Only experienced bronchoscopists who are capable to responding and managing the early and late complications of advanced airway disease should place stents. Therapeutic bronchoscopy should be available to all patients with central airway obstruction. The recent National Institute of Health and Clinical Excellence (NICE) guidance in the UK advises that all cancer networks should offer this service to their patients.

PROCEDURE PLANNING AND STENT PLACEMENT

A decision to stent the airway should be taken by a multidisciplinary team. As previously discussed, stenting should be viewed as a palliative procedure and in the majority of cases it should be the last therapeutic option. For example, in the setting of benign tracheal stenosis, surgical resection is the preferred treatment. However, this may not be possible and an airway stent should be assessed as a treatment choice. It is preferable that these procedures are planned and that the patient is reviewed in clinic prior to undertaking the intervention. This allows optimization of the medical condition and review of all available imaging. In addition, the anesthetist can assess the patient and optimize any reversible conditions. However, these cases are often emergencies and are therefore performed with minimal pre assessment. Rigid bronchoscopy is required for the placement of silicone stents while metal stents can be placed by either rigid or flexible bronchoscopy. The recent British Thoracic Society (BTS) guideline for advanced diagnostic and therapeutic flexible bronchoscopy in adults does not address silicone stent placement and therefore concentrates on the use of the SEMS [43]. Most respiratory physicians have obtained competency in the use of the flexible bronchoscope under local anesthesia. A small proportion will place expandable stents using the flexible scope. Although rigid bronchoscopy does require general anesthesia it has an advantage over flexible bronchoscopy in that it ensures safe and adequate ventilation and airway control – removal of large pieces of tumor and control of hemorrhage. However, the BTS guideline states that there is limited expertise with this technique amongst respiratory physicians and therefore the recommendation is to perform therapeutic procedures with a flexible scope through either a laryngeal mask or endotracheal tube. It is the opinion of the authors that all therapeutic airway procedures should be performed with a rigid scope passed into the airway to ensure patency with adequate ventilation but a flexible bronchoscope must also be available.

In addition, the rigid bronchoscope provides a wider spectrum of interventions; rapid airway recanalization through immediate mechanical debulking, use of accessory tools such as laser, APC or coagulation therapy and insertion of stent either silicone or metallic. The flexible scope can be passed through the barrel of the rigid scope thus allowing treatment of lesions located in the distal airway, toileting of the airway and management of disease in smaller sub segmental bronchi. If fiberoptic bronchoscopy is planned as the first intervention in critically ill patients it should be performed in the operating room and the endoscopists should be capable of proceeding to rigid bronchoscopy if the clinical and anatomical findings necessitate it.

Flexible bronchoscopy is performed using an adult bronchoscope with a large working channel (2.8 to 3.2 mm) to allow adequate suction and delivery of laser probes, balloon dilators, and stent delivery devices. Larger stent delivery catheters should be introduced under fluoroscopy after placing external radiopaque markers.

In the setting of a simple benign stenosis it should be radially incised in three locations before serial dilatation with the rigid bronchoscope and a tracheal stent deployed. Benign stenoses at the level of the main bronchi (after sleeve lobectomy, transplantation *etc.*) can be more difficult to dilate. The stenosis is often extremely tight and may require the use of a balloon or pediatric rigid scopes for the first dilatation.

When the tumor is located at the level of the carina it often straddles the main bronchi. In these situations, it is essential to rapidly obtain a viable airway for ventilation. Once ventilatory stability is obtained then further debulking can be performed and the airway can be maintained with a Y stent.

COMPLICATIONS

Stent related complications are listed in Table **2** [44, 45].

Table 2. Potential complications associated with the insertion of airway stents.

Complication	Comment
Stent migration	More likely with silicone stents, stent removal often necessary
Obstruction	Due to poor mucus clearance, granulation tissue or malignant disease progression
Stent fracture	Associated with metallic stents. In some cases can lead to wall erosion, bleeding or fistula formation
Infection	Commonly isolated organisms are *staph aureus* and *pseudomonas sp*

Migration

All stents can migrate. This risk is highest for a straight stent, however even Y stents can alter position and there have been a few reports of T tube dislodgement.

Stent migration can occur early and is usually due to incorrect stent size or as a late complication when there are changes in the stenotic caliber secondary to adjuvant treatments such as chemotherapy and radiotherapy. Migration has been reported in approximately 10% of malignant stenosis and is estimated to be double this rate for benign disease. Even if a stent migrates it is unlikely to cause life threatening complications as long as the lumen is patent. However, the patient's symptoms may deteriorate with increasing cough, dyspnea and/or stridor. When stent migration occurs it mandates repeat endoscopy and stent removal. If the airway remains stenosed then a further larger diameter stent may need to be placed. An exception is if migration occurred due to a clinical response to antineoplastic therapy then further stenting may not be required.

Obstruction

A stent can obstruct due to inspissated secretions, granulation tissue and tumor ingrowth. Mucoid impaction is estimated to occur in 3.6% of all stents. This can lead to airway obstruction in rare cases but is more likely to result in halitosis, superimposed infection and recurrence of symptoms due to airway narrowing. Some patients appear to be more prone to mucus impaction; these include current smokers and diabetics. In addition, the underlying disease process may result in muscle weakness and poor cough reflex thus increasing the difficulty to clear impacted secretions. Granulation tissue can obstruct a stent over time. This usually develops at the proximal or distal end of the stent due to the friction forces between the stent and the airway. When granulation tissue narrows the lumen to less than 50% of its normal caliber symptoms are likely to recur. Overall granulation tissue is found in 50% of all cases and becomes clinically significant in 25% of cases. This often requires further intervention including using mechanical or thermal tools to remove the granulation tissue. Occasionally the stent needs to be removed and replaced – often with a longer prosthesis. Tumor ingrowth will occur in all cases of malignant airway disease if no further antineoplastic therapy is administered and frequently even with treatment. The obstruction may occur early if a partially covered stent is used because the tumor can readily grow through the uncovered metal matrix. When disease progression occurs in the airway the case should be re-discussed at the multidisciplinary tumor team meeting prior to planning further endoscopic treatment. Frequently the airway can be salvaged by using a longer stent but on many occasions performing no further intervention can be more appropriate depending on the clinical situation. If a stent is replaced it usually requires a longer prosthesis and therefore a greater proportion of the airway is covered which comes at the expense of increased risk of mucus retention and impaction.

Infection

Noppen *et al.* prospectively assessed patients post airway stenting and reported a 78% rate of stent colonization in 3-4 weeks post insertion [46]. Staphylococcus and pseudomonas appear to be the most frequent organisms causing stent associated respiratory tract infections with fungi isolated in 22% of cases included in a systematic review [47]. From current data it is difficult to discern whether an etiological relationship exists between airway stents and respiratory tract infections. In rare case reports, removal of the stent was associated with clinical improvement.

Stent Fracture

This is an important complication that can occur with metallic stents. All metallic stents have been reported to fracture. The Gianturco stent had the highest rate of fracture, reported at 25% with an associated 12.5% rate of fistula formation. There was also a risk of wall and vascular erosion with resulting massive hemoptysis. Fracture can also lead to the stent becoming embedded in the wall of the airway in which case stent removal becomes very challenging and hazardous.

PATIENT MANAGEMENT POST STENT INSERTION

Various different protocols have been suggested from different groups to attempt to reduce stent related complications. It is universally agreed that all patients should be given a stent pack documenting the type and size of stent placed. This acts as an alert to other health care workers if an airway related emergency occurs. Airway clearance may be improved with normal saline nebulization. The exact nature of this has not been elucidated and indeed the requirements are likely to alter due to a number of patient and environmental factors. For example, mucoid impaction may occur with greater frequency in regions with a dry arid climate. Suggested protocols include mist inhalation, nebulized saline, nebulized hypertonic saline and acetylcysteine inhalation. In addition, some authors suggest humidification in the bedroom at night. The surveillance pattern is variable and may include radiological and endoscopic surveillance techniques. It is accepted that if new or worsening symptoms develop it is mandatory to reassess the stent for position and function. Some patients will have particular problems with mucus retention and halitosis which may be significantly relieved with direct stent toileting. Finally, even if a complication is seen at surveillance it may not necessitate stent removal. This decision must be made by the endoscopist taking into account the patients symptoms, possible future complications if the stent associated complication progresses and the continued need for a stent. For example, a single fracture may not require stent removal if the airway remains patent and the fracture is not in contact with the mucosa. However, the development of non-obstructing granulation tissue may require immediate intervention because progression may significantly compromise the airway in future.

CONCLUSION

Stents are an important tool in the palliation of airway related pathology. However, they are associated with a significant complication rate and therefore they should only be used if all other treatment options are exhausted or contraindicated. Stents are grouped into metal and silicone prostheses. It is the authors' practice to perform all stent deployments at the time of rigid bronchoscopy to ensure adequate ventilation and control of treatment complications such as tumor debris and hemorrhage. The role of interventional airway management has been strengthened recently by the publication of the NICE guideline, CG121 which states that all cancer networks should offer access to a team capable of providing interventional endobronchial treatments.

CONFLICT OF INTEREST

The authors declare no conflict of interest, financial or otherwise.

ACKNOWLEDGEMENTS

Declared none.

REFERENCES

[1] Ring ME. How a dentist's name became a synonym for a life-saving device: the story of Dr. Charles Stent. J Hist Dent 2001; 49(2): 77-80.
[PMID: 11484317]

[2] Bond CJ. Note on the treatment of tracheal stenosis by a new T-shaped tracheostomy tube. Lancet 1891; 137(3523): 539.
[http://dx.doi.org/10.1016/S0140-6736(02)16426-9]

[3] Montgomery WW. T-tube tracheal stent. Arch Otolaryngol Chic Ill 1960 1965; 82: 320-1.

[4] Dumon JF. A dedicated tracheobronchial stent. Chest 1990; 97(2): 328-32.
[http://dx.doi.org/10.1378/chest.97.2.328] [PMID: 1688757]

[5] Freitag L. Airway Stents. Eur Respir Mon 2010; (48): 190-217.
[http://dx.doi.org/10.1183/1025448x.00991409]

[6] Gompelmann D, Eberhardt R, Herth FJ. Advanced malignant lung disease: what the specialist can offer. Respiration 2011; 82(2): 111-23.
[http://dx.doi.org/10.1159/000329703] [PMID: 21778793]

[7] Foccoli P, Scappaticci E, Rea F, Revello F, Bezzi M, Cavaliere S. Management of post-intubation and/or tracheotomy tracheal stenoses. Monaldi Arch Chest Dis 2011; 75(1): 82-5.
[PMID: 21627001]

[8] Rahman NA, Fruchter O, Shitrit D, Fox BD, Kramer MR. Flexible bronchoscopic management of benign tracheal stenosis: long term follow-up of 115 patients. J Cardiothorac Surg 2010; 5: 2.

[http://dx.doi.org/10.1186/1749-8090-5-2] [PMID: 20078894]

[9] Dutau H, Breen DP, Gomez C, Thomas PA, Vergnon J-M. The integrated place of tracheobronchial stents in the multidisciplinary management of large post-pneumonectomy fistulas: our experience using a novel customised conical self-expandable metallic stent. Eur J Cardiothorac Surg 2011; 39(2): 185-9.
[http://dx.doi.org/10.1016/j.ejcts.2010.05.020] [PMID: 20591685]

[10] Casal RF. Update in airway stents. Curr Opin Pulm Med 2010; 16(4): 321-8.
[http://dx.doi.org/10.1097/MCP.0b013e32833a260] [PMID: 20531080]

[11] Lee P, Kupeli E, Mehta AC. Airway stents. Clin Chest Med 2010; 31(1): 141-50. [Table of Contents.].
[http://dx.doi.org/10.1016/j.ccm.2009.08.002] [PMID: 20172440]

[12] Ranu H, Madden BP. Endobronchial stenting in the management of large airway pathology. Postgrad Med J 2009; 85(1010): 682-7.
[http://dx.doi.org/10.1136/pgmj.2009.089011] [PMID: 20075408]

[13] Dutau H, Cavailles A, Fernandez-Navamuel I, Breen DP. Tracheal compression in a patient with Marfan's syndrome-associated tracheomegaly treated by an XXL stent: the largest diameter airway stent ever placed in a previously undescribed airway condition. Respiration 2009; 77(1): 97-101.
[http://dx.doi.org/10.1159/000108784] [PMID: 17890846]

[14] Breen DP, Dutau H. On-site customization of silicone stents: towards optimal palliation of complex airway conditions. Respiration 2009; 77(4): 447-53.
[http://dx.doi.org/10.1159/000205396] [PMID: 19246883]

[15] Gildea TR, Murthy SC, Sahoo D, Mason DP, Mehta AC. Performance of a self-expanding silicone stent in palliation of benign airway conditions. Chest 2006; 130(5): 1419-23.
[http://dx.doi.org/10.1378/chest.130.5.1419] [PMID: 17099019]

[16] Dooms C, De Keukeleire T, Janssens A, Carron K. Performance of fully covered self-expanding metallic stents in benign airway strictures. Respiration 2009; 77(4): 420-6.
[http://dx.doi.org/10.1159/000203364] [PMID: 19223681]

[17] Dutau H, Musani AI, Laroumagne S, Darwiche K, Freitag L, Astoul P. Biodegradable Airway Stents - Bench to Bedside: A Comprehensive Review. Respiration 2015; 90(6): 512-21.
[http://dx.doi.org/10.1159/000442054] [PMID: 26613524]

[18] Chao Y-K, Liu K-S, Wang Y-C, Huang Y-L, Liu S-J. Biodegradable cisplatin-eluting tracheal stent for malignant airway obstruction: in vivo and in vitro studies. Chest 2013; 144(1): 193-9.
[http://dx.doi.org/10.1378/chest.12-2282] [PMID: 23349039]

[19] Zhu GH, Ng AH, Venkatraman SS, *et al.* A novel bioabsorbable drug-eluting tracheal stent. Laryngoscope 2011; 121(10): 2234-9.
[http://dx.doi.org/10.1002/lary.22175] [PMID: 21823127]

[20] Lischke R, Pozniak J, Vondrys D, Elliott MJ. Novel biodegradable stents in the treatment of bronchial stenosis after lung transplantation. Eur J Cardiothorac Surg 2011; 40(3): 619-24.
[PMID: 21334911]

[21] Gaissert HA, Burns J. The compromised airway: tumors, strictures, and tracheomalacia. Surg Clin North Am 2010; 90(5): 1065-89.
[http://dx.doi.org/10.1016/j.suc.2010.06.004] [PMID: 20955884]

[22] Grillo HC, Donahue DM, Mathisen DJ, Wain JC, Wright CD. Postintubation tracheal stenosis. J Thorac Cardiovasc Surg 1995; 109(3): 486-93.
[http://dx.doi.org/10.1016/S0022-5223(95)70279-2]

[23] Seegobin RD, van Hasselt GL. Endotracheal cuff pressure and tracheal mucosal blood flow: endoscopic study of effects of four large volume cuffs. Br Med J (Clin Res Ed) 1984; 288(6422): 965-8.
[http://dx.doi.org/10.1136/bmj.288.6422.965] [PMID: 6423162]

[24] McCaffrey TV. Classification of laryngotracheal stenosis. Laryngoscope 1992; 102(12 Pt 1): 1335-40. [http://dx.doi.org/10.1288/00005537-199212000-00004] [PMID: 1453837]

[25] Galluccio G, Lucantoni G, Battistoni P, *et al.* Interventional endoscopy in the management of benign tracheal stenoses: definitive treatment at long-term follow-up. Eur J Cardio-Thorac Surg Off J Eur Assoc Cardio-Thorac Surg 2009; 35(3): 429-934. [http://dx.doi.org/10.1016/j.ejcts.2008.10.041]

[26] Schmid RA, Boehler A, Speich R, Frey HR, Russi EW, Weder W. Bronchial anastomotic complications following lung transplantation: still a major cause of morbidity? Eur Respir J 1997; 10(12): 2872-5. [http://dx.doi.org/10.1183/09031936.97.10122872] [PMID: 9493676]

[27] Van De Wauwer C, Van Raemdonck D, Verleden GM, *et al.* Risk factors for airway complications within the first year after lung transplantation. Eur J Cardiothorac Surg 2007; 31(4): 703-10. [http://dx.doi.org/10.1016/j.ejcts.2007.01.025] [PMID: 17306556]

[28] Kapoor BS, May B, Panu N, Kowalik K, Hunter DW. Endobronchial stent placement for the management of airway complications after lung transplantation. J Vasc Interv Radiol 2007; 18(5): 629-32. [http://dx.doi.org/10.1016/j.jvir.2007.02.021] [PMID: 17494844]

[29] Mulligan MS. Endoscopic management of airway complications after lung transplantation. Chest Surg Clin N Am 2001; 11(4): 907-15. [PMID: 11780302]

[30] Sundset A, Lund MB, Hansen G, Bjørtuft Ø, Kongerud J, Geiran OR. Airway complications after lung transplantation: long-term outcome of silicone stenting. Respiration 2012; 83(3): 245-52. [http://dx.doi.org/10.1159/000334905] [PMID: 22343478]

[31] Mark EJ, Meng F, Kradin RL, Mathisen DJ, Matsubara O. Idiopathic tracheal stenosis: a clinicopathologic study of 63 cases and comparison of the pathology with chondromalacia. Am J Surg Pathol 2008; 32(8): 1138-43. [http://dx.doi.org/10.1097/PAS.0b013e3181648d4a] [PMID: 18545144]

[32] Perotin J-M, Jeanfaivre T, Thibout Y, *et al.* Endoscopic management of idiopathic tracheal stenosis. Ann Thorac Surg 2011; 92(1): 297-301. [http://dx.doi.org/10.1016/j.athoracsur.2011.03.129] [PMID: 21718860]

[33] Gelbard A, Katsantonis N-G, Mizuta M, *et al.* Idiopathic subglottic stenosis is associated with activation of the inflammatory IL-17A/IL-23 axis. Laryngoscope 2016; 126(11): E356-61. [http://dx.doi.org/10.1002/lary.26098] [PMID: 27296163]

[34] Sirbu H, Busch T, Aleksic I, Schreiner W, Oster O, Dalichau H. Bronchopleural fistula in the surgery of non-small cell lung cancer: incidence, risk factors, and management. Ann Thorac Cardiovasc Surg 2001; 7(6): 330-6. [PMID: 11888471]

[35] Lois M, Noppen M. Bronchopleural fistulas: an overview of the problem with special focus on endoscopic management. Chest 2005; 128(6): 3955-65. [http://dx.doi.org/10.1378/chest.128.6.3955] [PMID: 16354867]

[36] West D, Togo A, Kirk AJ. Are bronchoscopic approaches to post-pneumonectomy bronchopleural fistula an effective alternative to repeat thoracotomy? Interact Cardiovasc Thorac Surg 2007; 6(4): 547-50. [http://dx.doi.org/10.1510/icvts.2007.159319] [PMID: 17669932]

[37] Wang H, Tao M, Zhang N, *et al.* Airway Covered Metallic Stent Based on Different Fistula Location and Size in Malignant Tracheoesophageal Fistula. Am J Med Sci 2015; 350(5): 364-8. [http://dx.doi.org/10.1097/MAJ.0000000000000565] [PMID: 26422803]

[38] Carden KA, Boiselle PM, Waltz DA, Ernst A. Tracheomalacia and tracheobronchomalacia in children

and adults: an in-depth review. Chest 2005; 127(3): 984-1005.
[http://dx.doi.org/10.1378/chest.127.3.984] [PMID: 15764786]

[39] Noppen N. Interventional palliative treatment options for lung cancer. Ann Oncol 2002; 13 (Suppl. 4): 247-50.
[http://dx.doi.org/10.1093/annonc/mdf666] [PMID: 12401697]

[40] Gorden JA, Ernst A. Endoscopic management of central airway obstruction. Semin Thorac Cardiovasc Surg 2009; 21(3): 263-73.
[http://dx.doi.org/10.1053/j.semtcvs.2009.08.002] [PMID: 19942126]

[41] Williamson JP, Phillips MJ, Hillman DR, Eastwood PR. Managing obstruction of the central airways. Intern Med J 2010; 40(6): 399-410.
[http://dx.doi.org/10.1111/j.1445-5994.2009.02113.x] [PMID: 19849741]

[42] Zarić B, Canak V, Sarcev T, Marković M, Jovanović S, Budisin E. Interventional pulmonology techniques for immediate desobstruction of malignant central airway obstruction. J BUON 2007; 12(1): 11-22.
[PMID: 17436396]

[43] Du Rand IA, Barber PV, Goldring J, *et al.* BTS Interventional Bronchoscopy Guideline Group. Summary of the British Thoracic Society guidelines for advanced diagnostic and therapeutic flexible bronchoscopy in adults. Thorax 2011; 66(11): 1014-5.
[http://dx.doi.org/10.1136/thoraxjnl-2011-201052] [PMID: 22003155]

[44] Kunst P, Burgers S, Onderwater S, vd Heuvel M. Stenting of airways: beware of the complications. Ann Thorac Surg 2011; 92(2): 774.
[http://dx.doi.org/10.1016/j.athoracsur.2011.01.086] [PMID: 21801946]

[45] Davis N, Madden BP, Sheth A, Crerar-Gilbert AJ. Airway management of patients with tracheobronchial stents. Br J Anaesth 2006; 96(1): 132-5.
[http://dx.doi.org/10.1093/bja/aei267] [PMID: 16257995]

[46] Noppen M, Piérard D, Meysman M, Claes I, Vincken W. Bacterial colonization of central airways after stenting. Am J Respir Crit Care Med 1999; 160(2): 672-7.
[http://dx.doi.org/10.1164/ajrccm.160.2.9812081] [PMID: 10430745]

[47] Agrafiotis M, Siempos II, Falagas ME. Infections related to airway stenting: a systematic review. Respiration 2009; 78(1): 69-74.
[http://dx.doi.org/10.1159/000213244] [PMID: 19365108]

CHAPTER 13

Point of Care Ultrasonography for Interventional Pulmonologist

Amit Taneja*

Division of Pulmonary & Critical Care Medicine, Department of Medicine, Medical College of Wisconsin, Milwaukee WI , USA

Abstract: Point of Care Ultrasound use is becoming an extension of physical examination in a variety of situations and particularly in the Emergency Departments and Intensive care units. Ultrasound is an important tool in the arsenal of Interventional Pulmonologist. Thoracic ultrasound is easily available bedside tool that is more sensitive than conventional x-ray in rapid diagnosis of pleural effusion and pneumothorax. Ultrasound use has become the standard of care for pleural procedures as it minimizes complications. Understanding and recognition of basic pleuro-pulmonary ultrasound patterns are keys to proper usage and incorporation of this technology in the daily practice of Interventional Pulmonary. Ultrasound is also being increasingly used for percutaneous tracheostomy for optimizing patient selection and minimizing inadvertent vascular injury.

Keywords: Interventional Pulmonary, Thoracic ultrasound, tracheostomy, Ultrasound guided pleural procedures.

INTRODUCTION

Thoracic Ultrasound is a readily available and easy to use bedside tool that can be used to make rapid bedside diagnoses (*e.g.* pleural effusion, consolidation, pulmonary edema); and also to exclude certain diagnoses (*e.g.* pneumothorax). With adequate training, ultrasound can be easily learned by those in training and practice of interventional pulmonology and thus used to perform bedside ultrasound guided pleural procedures (*e.g.* chest tube insertion, thoracentesis, needle biopsy of pleural-based mass) and to also exclude pneumothorax as a complication after pleural or bronchoscopic procedures. Ultrasound has been shown to be more sensitive than a chest x-ray in detecting the presence of an effusion; and also more sensitive and a lot quicker than a chest x-ray in ruling out

* **Corresponding author Amit Taneja:** Division of Pulmonary & Critical Care Medicine, Department of Medicine, Medical College of Wisconsin, Milwaukee WI, USA; Tel: 414-955-7040; Fax: 414-955-6211; E-mail: ataneja@mcw.edu

Ali I. Musani (Ed.)

pneumothorax. Furthermore, ultrasound with a high-frequency probe (vascular probe) can be of invaluable help in percutaneous dilatational tracheostomy. We use it prior to starting the procedure to rule out any aberrant vasculature in the neck. It has also been used to guide the entire procedure without any bronchoscopic visualization.

This article summarizes the current evidence for the use of point of care ultrasound as it applies to the field of Interventional Pulmonology. Pleural and chest ultrasonography will be discussed; however the ultrasonography of the heart, assessment of volume responsiveness, assessment of DVT *etc.* are beyond the scope of this review.

EQUIPMENT

The phased array transducer used for cardiac imaging is also optimal for pleural and thoracic ultrasonography. Some machines have a lung preset which optimizes the settings; otherwise abdominal preset can also be used. Indeed, per Dr. Lichtenstein-one of the pioneers in the field-"any machine and any probe can work more or less" [1]. High frequency or vascular probes provide greater detail of the pleural surface and peripheral pathology; however are not suitable for deeper structures and at times in morbidly obese patients.

PERFORMING THORACIC ULTRASOUND

Ultrasound can be done in upright or supine positions. For pleural procedures, we prefer that patient be in the most comfortable posture/position and yet most compatible with the safest access to the intended area in the pleural space. We scan the chest with the ultrasound prior to starting the procedure and clean and drape only after doing ultrasound exam and selecting not only the correct area but also most ergonomic (for the physician) and most comfortable patient position. Basic knowledge of "knobology" is essential to use the ultrasound machine with a reasonable understanding of depth (*i.e.* how deep is the ultrasound looking); gain (this is very similar to brightness control) and orientation. (*e.g.* cephalad to caudad). Depth and gain, for example, can be controlled with respective knobs on most machines. Often times the auto-gain feature is a good starting point. The transducer is held longitudinally with the marker facing cephalad. It is moved between intercostal spaces while holding it firmly and perpendicular to the chest wall. Ideally, multiple areas on the chest wall should be scanned with ultrasound - both in front and back. Ultrasound produces characteristic lines and artifacts-the recognition of which is essential in interpreting the ultrasound picture. These are discussed briefly in the next section.

NORMAL ULTRASOUND EXAM

In a normally aerated lung, in between the rib shadows, one can see a bright shimmering horizontal line. This is the pleural line (Figs. **1** & **2**). On further observation, this shimmering line moves with respiration and this represents the sliding of the visceral pleura in relation to the parietal pleura. This is the so-called lung sliding sign (Fig. **2**) and as should be obvious, it indicates a lung that is expanding with ventilation; and where the visceral and parietal pleura are in close approximation to each other. As such, therefore, this rules out a pneumothorax. It should be noted however that absence of lung sliding simply means that the lung is not expanding or the visceral and parietal pleura are separated. This does not rule in a pneumothorax as for example areas with bullous emphysema may have an absence of lung sliding. Once the pleural line is identified, one can identify an artifact called the A-line. (Artifact, as this is simply a result of reverberation, akin to multiple back and forth echoes- causing repetition of the same sound). A-lines are equidistant bright lines parallel to the pleural line (Fig. **1**). The distance between consecutive A-lines is the same as the distance between the skin surface and the pleural line; as the A-lines are simply repeated reverberation artifacts of this. Lung sliding and A-lines are the hallmarks of normal lung ultrasound exam [2].

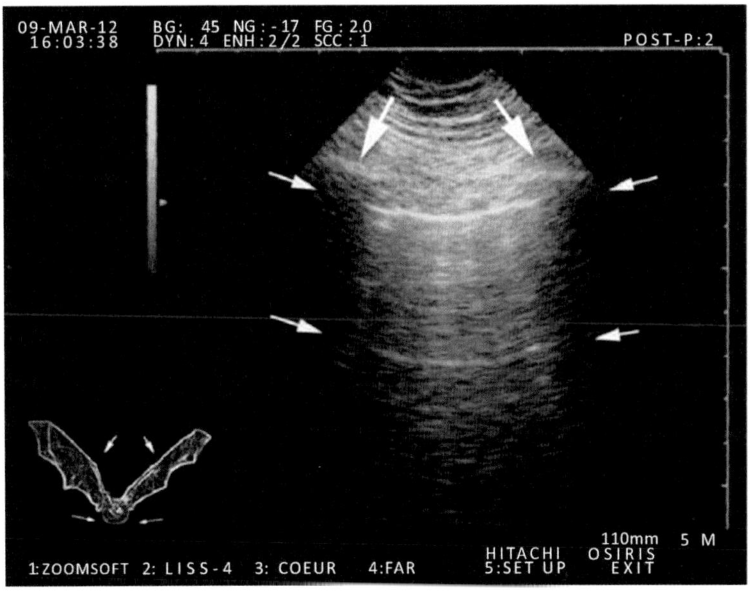

Fig. (1). Pleural line and A-lines. Note the ribs marked by vertical arrows. The upper horizontal arrows show the pleural line. The lower horizontal arrows show the A-lines [2].

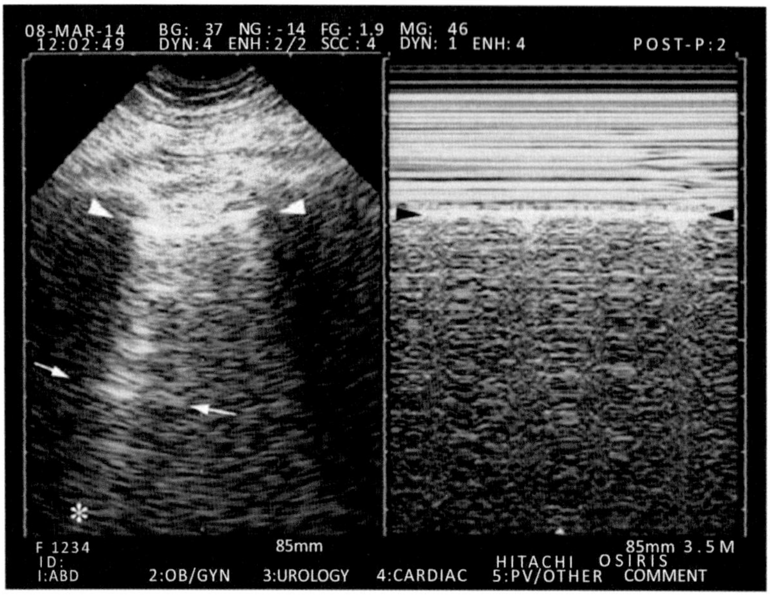

Fig. (2). Once again notice the A lines. A real-time ultrasound would show that pleural line shimmers and moves with breathing. This is the lung sliding. The right-hand panel shows M-mode ultrasound. The black arrowheads indicate the pleural line. There is a clear cut difference between top half due to motionless skin/soft tissue and the bottom half of the M mode picture creating the sea shore pattern. This essentially rules out pneumothorax [2].

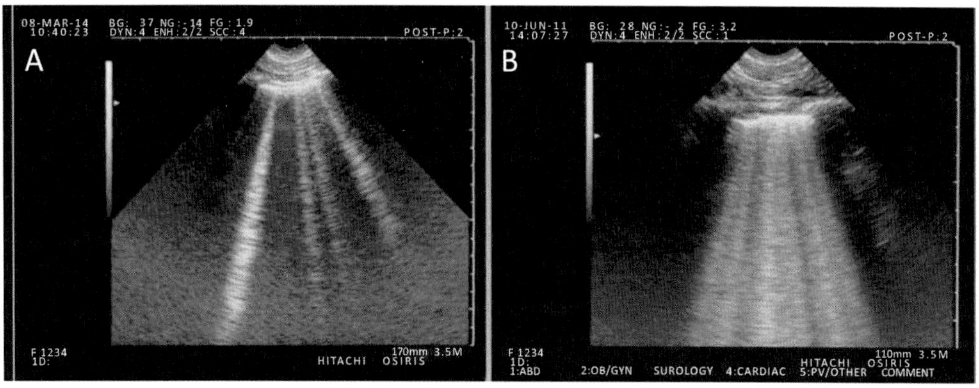

Fig. (3). Note the pleural line and the bright perpendicular artifacts arising from the pleural line. These are the B-lines. These are long and reach up to the edge of the screen and are as hyperechoic as the pleural line. B lines also rule out pneumothorax. A predominant B-line pattern is seen in alveolar-interstitial syndromes [2].

Another artifact that can be seen is called comet tail. These are vertical lines arising from the pleural line extending to variable depths into the lung parenchyma. B-lines are comet tail artifacts that always arise from the pleural line; move in concert with lung sliding; are long and extending deep into the ultrasound picture; obliterate the A-lines and are as hyperechoic as the pleural line (Fig. **3**). A few B-lines at the lung bases are of questionable significance. Sonographic exam of predominant B-lines suggests alveolar-interstitial syndrome-this can be from cardiogenic or non- cardiogenic edema or interstitial fibrosis. The presence of B-lines also rules out a pneumothorax. Notably, the presence of A-lines and absence of B-lines would strongly argue against cardiogenic pulmonary edema. This pattern has been shown to reliably predict wedge pressure of < 18 mm Hg [3].

ULTRASOUND PATTERNS IN PLEURO-PULMONARY PATHOLOGY

Pleural Effusion

Pleural fluid appears as anechoic or hypoechoic space within the thorax. Anechoic means that it appears dark as no or minimal ultrasound waves are reflected back to the transducer. This is in contrast to the appearance of the lung, diaphragm and caudally located liver or spleen. Thus the presence of fluid is easily detectable. It is useful to remember Dr. Lichtenstein's gravity rules (fluid to bottom and gas rises). Thus we start by scanning the most dependent part of the thorax, identify diaphragm and liver or spleen as the case may be and then scan somewhat cephalad to this to locate effusion. Of course, loculated effusions may not be strictly in the dependent portion. Identification of diaphragm is crucial to avoid any confusion of ascites with pleural fluid and inadvertent puncture of liver or spleen during attempted pleural procedure. Effusion causes compressive atelectasis of adjacent lung. This can often be seen floating and flapping in the pleural fluid. Ultrasound is much more sensitive than physical examination and chest X-ray for detection of small pleural effusions [2]. Further, ultrasound provides an easy and direct visualization of the nature of the fluid with the presence or absence of septations and debris floating in the fluid (See Figs. **4-6**). The presence of such septations and complexity in the pleural fluid suggest an exudative process.In pleural effusions with cellular debris, one can see "plankton" sign, in which the debris can be seen floating in the fluid when agitated by cardiac or respiratory motion. In loculated pleural effusions, thick strands can be seen oscillating within the pleural space, also due to the cardiac or respiratory motion. Echogenicity of the pleural effusion must be carefully evaluated, as it may give a clue to the underlying etiology. Understanding the terminology of echogenicity is also important. An anechoic effusion has no echogenicity within; a complex non-septated pattern has evidence of complexity within the fluid but no fibrin strands or septations; a complex septated pattern has fibrin strands and septations within, and the homogeneously echogenic pattern has evenly distributed hypoechoic density within the effusion [4]. Although initial studies demonstrated that all transudative effusions are anechoic, a subsequent study revealed that transudative

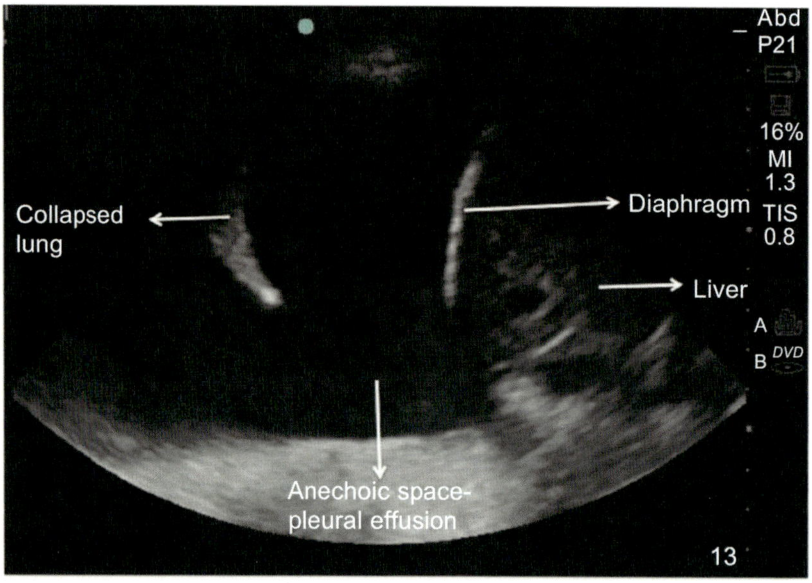

Fig. (4). typical anechoic, simple pleural effusion with usual anatomic boundaries [18].

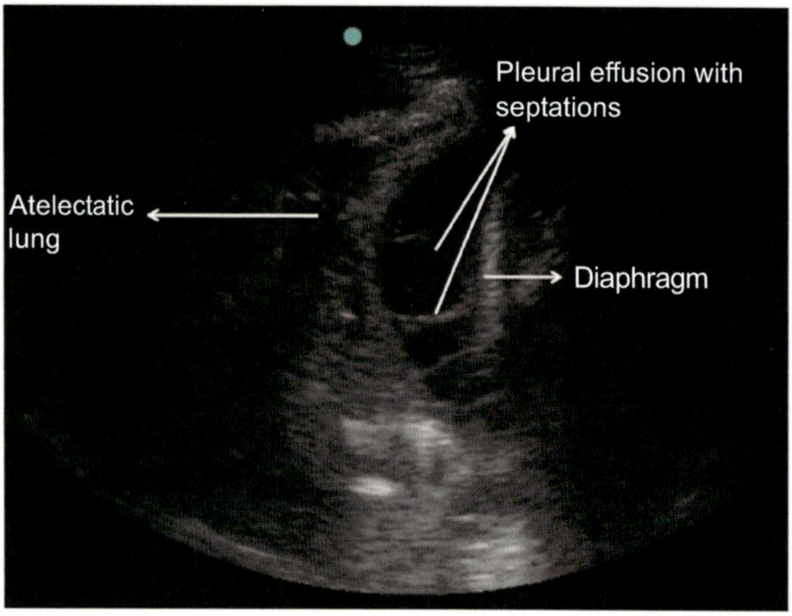

Fig. (5). Complex pleural effusion with septations [18].

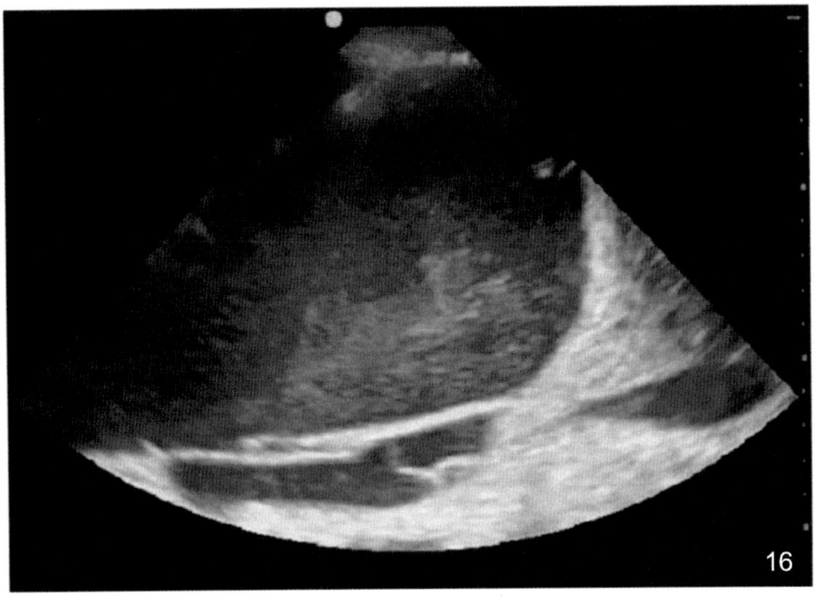

Fig. (6). Echogenic material in pleural fluid with layering. This suggests hemothorax [18].

effusions may be either anechoic or complex non-septated but never complex septated or homogeneously echogenic [5]. On the contrary, exudative effusions may have any of the four patterns described. Homogenously echogenic patterns are characteristic of hemothorax or empyema, while sonographic evidence of pleural nodules [6] associated parenchymal lesions, or pleural thickening is associated with exudative effusions. In patients with suspected malignant pleural effusion, findings consistent with malignancy include pleural thickening greater than 1 cm, pleural nodularity, and diaphragmatic thickening greater than 7 mm [7].

Consolidation

Consolidated lung looks like liver. Indeed one is reminded of the classic pathological description of bacterial pneumonia; wherein the affected lung goes through stages of gray and red *hepatization*. Not only does lung look and feel like liver to a gross pathologist; it also looks like liver on the ultrasound picture. There are no A-lines in the affected area. Obviously, this is cephalad to diaphragm. With experience, one can make out air-bronchograms in the consolidated lung (Fig. 7). These are the exact counterparts of air bronchograms seen on conventional radiographs or CT scans. Whereas air bronchograms appear as dark/radiolucent lines going through the lung parenchyma on the CT scan; on the ultrasound picture these appear bright (not black!), punctate and very echogenic foci. Often times, these bright echogenic foci are seen to move during the respiratory cycle. These are called dynamic air bronchograms and may help differentiate true consolidation from atelectasis. Early small consolidations appear as sub- pleural defects and gradually enlarge to assume a wedge- shaped appearance as more lung parenchyma is involved. The interface of the consolidation with the unaffected aerated lung creates an irregular hyperechoic border called the *shred* sign.

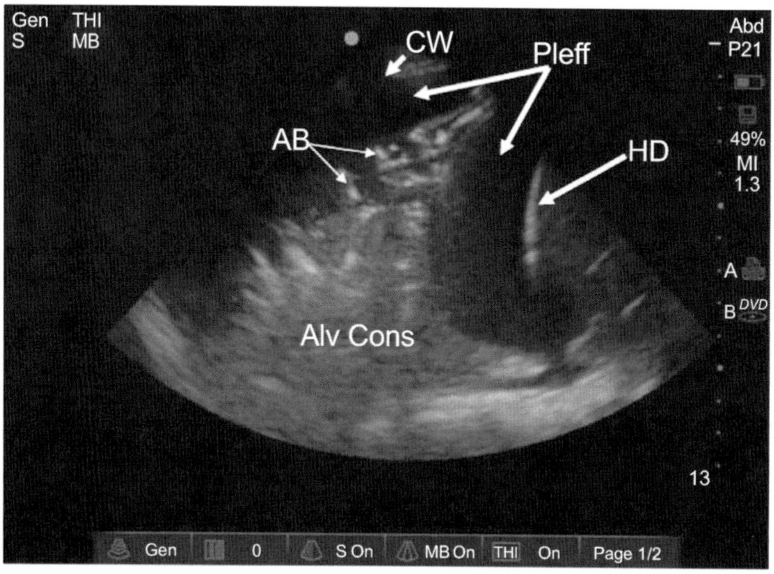

Fig. (7). Note liver like consolidated lung. AB – white punctate air bronchograms in consolidated lung. Pleff- pleural effusion. CW-chest wall, HD-hemidiaphragm [19].

Pneumothorax

One of the greatest uses of point of care ultrasound is in rapid and accurate ruling out of pneumothorax in an acutely unstable patient or after a thoracic procedure. The presence of lung sliding bilaterally and over multiple sites essentially rules out pneumothorax [8, 9]. As stated previously, lung sliding is detected as the shimmering movement of the pleural line along with phases of the respiratory cycle. This indicates that as the lung expands, that visceral and parietal pleura are in close approximation with each other. A similar finding is called lung pulse. As the name suggests, in concert with cardiac motion, sliding seen along the pleural surface is called lung pulse. Once again, this essentially rules out pneumothorax. Note that A-lines can still be seen even if pneumothorax is present. As mentioned previously, these are simply reverberation artifacts of the pleural line, so their presence doesn't help exclude pneumothorax. Of course, if A-lines are present with no lung sliding or lung pulse, pneumothorax should be considered. The presence of B-lines also excludes pneumothorax.

In addition, M-mode can be used. M stands for motion; and when scanning the area of interest, on selecting M mode, a distinct sonographic picture is created. If there is motion below the pleural line (due to lung expansion), a distinctive pattern is created. The picture above the pleural line consists of a stratified pattern due to motionless soft tissue; whereas the area below the pleural line appears sandy; hence the so-called seashore sign. The presence of motion on M mode thus helps to rule out pneumothorax (See Figs. **8** and **9**).

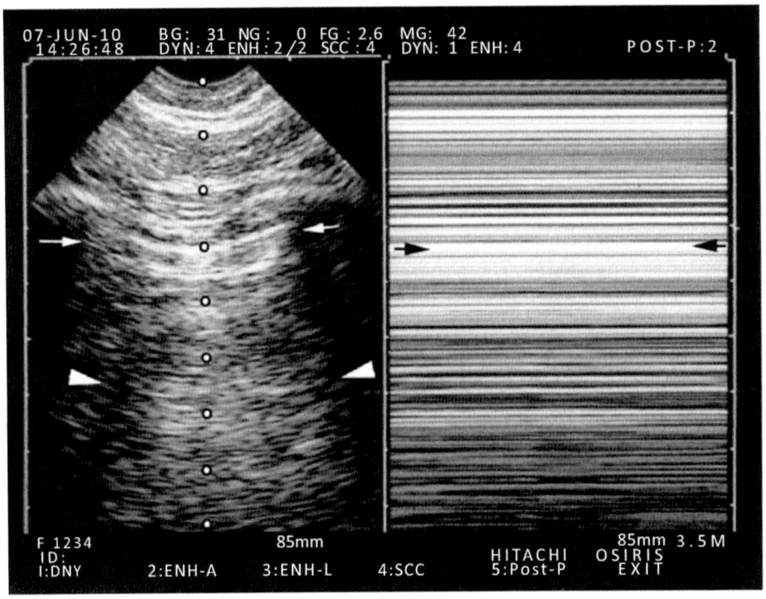

Fig. (8). On the left panel A-lines can be seen. In real time ultrasound, there is no shimmering movement of the pleural line with breathing or cardiac pulsation. That is, there is no lung sliding. On the right panel, when this area is interrogated on M mode, part above and below the pleural line (arrowhead) looks identical due to lack of motion. This picture is the so-called stratosphere sign [2]. Compare this to picture in Fig. (**2**).

Note that presence of lung sliding, lung pulse, B lines, and motion on M mode rule out pneumothorax. The converse is not true. Thus, these findings have a near 100% negative predictive value; but are not necessarily specific for the diagnosis of pneumothorax.

The most specific sign of pneumothorax is the presence of a lung point [10]. Once absence of lung sliding is found, one scans to more dependent or posterior location of the chest till interface with a more normal appearing sonographic pattern is encountered. Of course, if the pneumothorax is massive, there may be no interface with the normal pattern. However, if the interface with normal sonographic pattern can be found, this is called the lung point. This is the interface between normal lung sliding (or pathological B-lines) and pneumothorax pattern (absence of lung sliding with exclusive A-lines). This can be further confirmed with M-mode scanning, where the distinct patterns can be seen side by side; often these come in and out with different phases of respiration. The lung point thus marks the location of the pneumothorax. The finding of lung point is 100% specific for pneumothorax but is only 66% sensitive [10].

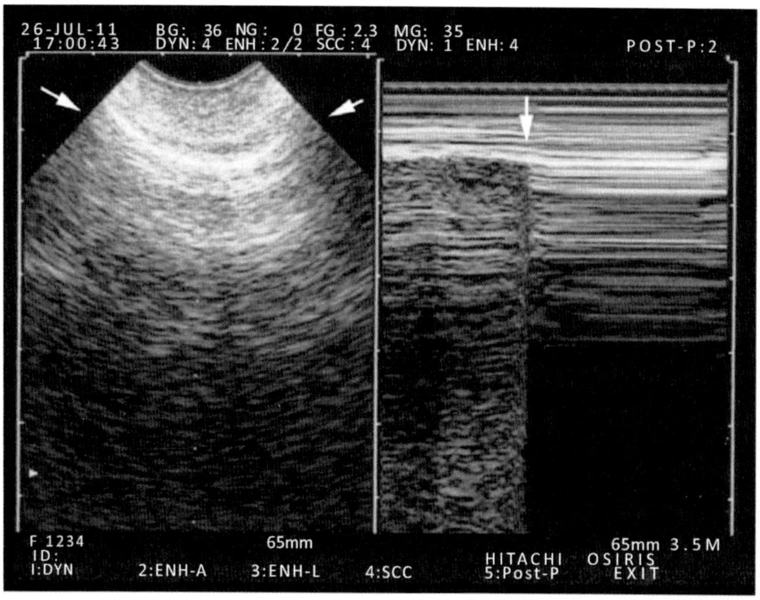

Fig. (9). Demonstration of lung point. On the left panel, A-lines are seen. There was no lung sliding on real-time ultrasound. Initial M mode exam showed a picture similar to Fig. (**8**). On further scanning of the chest, at a particular location, M mode picture changed such that normal lung motion came in and out of the picture with respiratory cycle. This is pathognomonic of pneumothorax [2].

The location of lung point correlates with the size of the pneumothorax and correlates with the need for chest tube insertion [10]. An anterior lung point correlates with a small pneumothorax and is usually of limited clinical significance. However, a lung point that is located more laterally or posteriorly is usually indicative of a larger and more symptomatic pneumothorax that frequently requires intervention.

Thus, ultrasound provides a rapid, easily repeatable bedside assessment to rule out pneumothorax. This is invaluable both before and after pleural or bronchoscopic procedures and in rapid assessment of a dyspneic patient. Indeed it is more effective and much more rapid way of ruling out pneumothorax than a portable chest x-ray.

Lung Abscess

Peripheral lung abscess abutting the pleura can be seen within the consolidated lung. These appear as masses with irregular borders of varying echogenicity. Ultrasound has been used to sample and drain peripheral lung abscess percutaneously [11].

The obvious concern is for soilage of pleural space resulting in empyema. It is suggested that if there is no lung sliding in the area, it may indicate spontaneous pleurodesis that may have happened already as a result of inflammation; and thus may minimize the risk of pleural cavity soilage.

Pleural-based Tumors

Pleural-based lung or pleural tumors can be easily visualized with ultrasound. These appear as hypoechoic rounded areas with relatively normal lung surrounding them. Lung ultrasound [12] has been shown to be more sensitive and specific than CT scan to show chest wall invasion; it has also been proposed that color flow signals can be used to help differentiate benign from malignant lesions.

POINT OF CARE ULTRASOUND FOR PLEURAL PROCEDURES

Thoracentesis and Chest Tube Insertion

Ultrasound is an invaluable tool for accessing pleural space- both for diagnostic tap; or a more therapeutic procedure. Indeed ultrasound guidance is now considered standard of care for bedside pleural procedures. Ultrasound guidance has been shown to reduce the incidence of pneumothorax to 3% from as high as 18% compared with conventional "blind" thoracentesis [13, 14]. Furthermore, use of ultrasound adds an extra layer of security and confidence in difficult clinical situations such as morbid obesity, supine patient, mechanically ventilated patient *etc*. Ultrasound reduces the dry taps or unsuccessful thoracentesis attempts. In addition, as previously mentioned ultrasound is more sensitive than a Chest X-ray and relying simply on chest X-ray in regards to decision making on when to perform thoracentesis is likely to miss a significant number of pleural effusions that do need to be sampled.

In our practice, we evaluate the pleural space with ultrasound prior to draping the patient. Once an adequate fluid pocket is identified, the site is marked, cleaned and draped. If the patient position changes, it is not hard to imagine how the fluid pocket may shift; especially for smaller effusions and thus we recommend that ultrasound examination, site marking, and the procedure happen simultaneously or immediately sequentially. In mechanically ventilated patients or those with small windows, at times we do real-time ultrasound guidance, similar to that used for vascular access. The ultrasound probe is covered with a sterile sheath and entry into pleural space happens directly under sonographic "vision".

American College of Chest Physicians recommended in 2009 in a consensus statement that first objective should be the identification of pleural effusion with typical anatomic boundaries and dynamic findings [15]. In this context, it is notable that patients with ascites may sometimes present a challenge to a beginner, as it may be hard to differentiate pleural fluid from ascites. The fluid in the hepatorenal recess may appear as pleural effusion, and a beginner may mistake inferior margin of the liver as atelectatic lung; and the space between liver and kidney as pleural space. A similar mistake can be made on the left side in the splenorenal recess. Thus it is absolutely essential that a careful sonographic exam is done and the normal anatomy identified prior to starting an invasive procedure. Finally, it must be remembered that ultrasound guidance does not obviate the need to avoid the neurovascular bundle which runs along the inferior margin of the rib. Thus, the needle entry should happen along the superior margin of the lower rib in a particular intercostal space.

Note should be made of the nature of effusion (Anechoic, hypoechoic, septated, debris *etc.*). Pre and post-procedure assessment of lung sliding should be done as the presence of lung sliding post procedure obviates the need for routine X-ray for pneumothorax.

Ultrasound guidance is also useful for chest tube placement including pigtail catheters and indwelling tunneled chest tubes for malignant pleural effusions. Once an adequate site is selected, a needle is inserted into pleural space similar to performing thoracentesis through which a wire is placed. Using serial dilators, a chest tube or an introducer for medical thoracoscope can be placed in the pleural space over the wire. We have used ultrasound to visualize the wire in pleural space prior to further dilatation or dissection to further enhance safety. Ultrasound is also useful as an easily available, cheap and repeatable bedside tool to follow the progress of more complicated effusions and/or to troubleshoot a chest tube which is not draining anymore. Given poor sensitivity of chest X-ray and obvious drawback of CT scans (cost, time, radiation, +/- IV contrast); use of ultrasound in this regard is clearly appealing to the interventional pulmonologist. Ease of visualizing the presence of complex septations makes ultrasound an effective tool in the decision making of administering or re-dosing intra-pleural thrombolytics.

POINT OF CARE ULTRASOUND USE FOR PERCUTANEOUS DILATATIONAL TRACHEOSTOMY

Percutaneous dilatation tracheostomy is being increasingly done at the bedside by intensivists and interventional pulmonologists. As the name suggests, this is done by percutaneously inserting a wire into the trachea in the appropriate location followed by some blunt dissection and then serial dilatation. Finally, the tracheostomy tube is deployed over a dilator into the trachea. Most often, this is done with real-time bronchoscopic visualization. Although safe, known complications of tracheostomy include bleeding. Ultrasound can be used prior to the procedure in studying anatomy and to also look for any aberrant vasculature. Since tracheal landmarks and the vasculature in question are superficial, a high-frequency vascular probe is used. This can easily visualize tracheal rings, cricoid cartilage, thyroid cartilage, cricothyroid membrane, thyroid gland and the adjacent vasculature. Ultrasound can also be used to see if any thyroidal blood vessels or brachiocephalic vessels are aberrantly located in the path of planned percutaneous entry into the trachea. If so, the anticipated site of entry can be changed or the patient referred for surgical tracheostomy. In fact, in our practice, we always use ultrasound prior to the procedure to identify the patients with aberrant vasculature or high-risk anatomy and this has also been favored by others based on their experience [16]. Over last several years, in addition, there has been data to show that percutaneous tracheostomy can be completely done with real-time ultrasound alone and without bronchoscope. In a recent trial real-time ultrasound-guided percutaneous tracheostomy was shown to be non-inferior to bronchoscopy guided percutaneous tracheostomy in mechanically ventilated patients in the ICU [17]. However, we should note that bronchoscopy and ultrasound are not mutually exclusive and both can be used in combination to improve the ease and safety of percutaneous tracheostomy.

SUMMARY

Ultrasound is rapidly becoming the standard of care both in the intensive care unit and in procedure suites. Though it has a steep learning curve; once adequate skills are acquired; ultrasound provides an easy, cost-effective, reproducible and a safe way of evaluating and also accessing pleural space for diagnostic and therapeutic procedures. Commonly available bedside ultrasound machines with a body probe are adequate for thoracic ultrasonography. Ultrasound is also being increasingly used - both alone and in concert with bronchoscopy for percutaneous dilatational tracheostomy. Point of care ultrasound is an invaluable tool for Interventional Pulmonologist.

CONFLICT OF INTEREST

The authors declare no conflict of interest, financial or otherwise.

ACKNOWLEDGEMENTS

Declared none.

REFERENCES

[1] Lichtenstein D. Lung Ultrasound in the Critically Ill Yearbook of Intensive Care and Emergency Medicine. Berlin, Germany: Springer- Verlag 2004; pp. 625-44.

[2] Lichtenstein DA, Mezière GA. Relevance of lung ultrasound in the diagnosis of acute respiratory failure: the BLUE protocol. Chest 2008; 134(1): 117-25. [http://dx.doi.org/10.1378/chest.07-2800] [PMID: 18403664]

[3] Lichtenstein DA, Mezière GA, Lagoueyte JF, Biderman P, Goldstein I, Gepner A. A-lines and B-lines: lung ultrasound as a bedside tool for predicting pulmonary artery occlusion pressure in the critically ill. Chest 2009; 136(4): 1014-20. [http://dx.doi.org/10.1378/chest.09-0001] [PMID: 19809049]

[4] McLoud TC, Flower CD. Imaging the pleura: sonography, CT, and MR imaging. AJR Am J Roentgenol 1991; 156(6): 1145-53. [http://dx.doi.org/10.2214/ajr.156.6.2028857] [PMID: 2028857]

[5] Chen HJ, Tu CY, Ling SJ, *et al.* Sonographic appearances in transudative pleural effusions: not always an anechoic pattern. Ultrasound Med Biol 2008; 34(3): 362-9. [http://dx.doi.org/10.1016/j.ultrasmedbio.2007.09.009] [PMID: 17996356]

[6] Yang PC, Luh KT, Chang DB, Wu HD, Yu CJ, Kuo SH. Value of sonography in determining the nature of pleural effusion: analysis of 320 cases. AJR Am J Roentgenol 1992; 159(1): 29-33. [http://dx.doi.org/10.2214/ajr.159.1.1609716] [PMID: 1609716]

[7] Qureshi NR, Rahman NM, Gleeson FV. Thoracic ultrasound in the diagnosis of malignant pleural effusion. Thorax 2009; 64(2): 139-43. [http://dx.doi.org/10.1136/thx.2008.100545] [PMID: 18852159]

[8] Lichtenstein DA, Menu Y. A bedside ultrasound sign ruling out pneumothorax in the critically ill. Lung sliding. Chest 1995; 108(5): 1345-8. [http://dx.doi.org/10.1378/chest.108.5.1345] [PMID: 7587439]

[9] Lichtenstein DA, Mezière G, Lascols N, *et al.* Ultrasound diagnosis of occult pneumothorax. Crit Care Med 2005; 33(6): 1231-8. [http://dx.doi.org/10.1097/01.CCM.0000164542.86954.B4] [PMID: 15942336]

[10] Lichtenstein D, Mezière G, Biderman P. "lungpoint":an ultrasound sign specific to pneumothorax. Intensive Care Med 2000; 26(10): 1434-40. [http://dx.doi.org/10.1007/s001340000627] [PMID: 11126253]

[11] Yang PC, Luh KT, Lee YC, *et al.* Lung abscesses: US examination and US-guided transthoracic aspiration. Radiology 1991; 180(1): 171-5. [http://dx.doi.org/10.1148/radiology.180.1.2052687] [PMID: 2052687]

[12] Bandi V, Lunn W, Ernst A, Eberhardt R, Hoffmann H, Herth FJ. Ultrasound vs. CT in detecting chest wall invasion by tumor: a prospective study. Chest 2008; 133(4): 881-6. [http://dx.doi.org/10.1378/chest.07-1656] [PMID: 17951616]

[13] Raptopoulos V, Davis LM, Lee G, Umali C, Lew R, Irwin RS. Factors affecting the development of pneumothorax associated with thoracentesis. AJR Am J Roentgenol 1991; 156(5): 917-20. [http://dx.doi.org/10.2214/ajr.156.5.2017951] [PMID: 2017951]

[14] Jones PW, Moyers JP, Rogers JT, Rodriguez RM, Lee YC, Light RW. Ultrasound-guided thoracentesis: is it a safer method? Chest 2003; 123(2): 418-23. [http://dx.doi.org/10.1378/chest.123.2.418] [PMID: 12576360]

[15] Mayo PH, Beaulieu Y, Doelken P, *et al.* American College of Chest Physicians/La Société de Réanimation de Langue Française statement on competence in critical care ultrasonography. Chest 2009; 135(4): 1050-60.
[http://dx.doi.org/10.1378/chest.08-2305] [PMID: 19188546]

[16] Sooby P, Pocock L, King T, Manjaly G. An anterior jugular vein variant in a patient requiring tracheostomy, demonstrating the importance of preoperative/procedural ultrasound. BMJ Case Rep 2016; 2016: bcr2016214599.
[http://dx.doi.org/10.1136/bcr-2016-214599] [PMID: 27033293]

[17] Gobatto AL, Besen BA, Tierno PF, *et al.* Ultrasound-guided percutaneous dilational tracheostomy *versus* bronchoscopy-guided percutaneous dilational tracheostomy in critically ill patients (TRACHUS): a randomized noninferiority controlled trial. Intensive Care Med 2016; 42(3): 342-51.
[http://dx.doi.org/10.1007/s00134-016-4218-6] [PMID: 26831676]

[18] Chichra A, Makaryus M, Chaudhri P, Narasimhan M. Ultrasound for the Pulmonary consultant. Clin Med Insights Circ Respir Pulm Med 2016; 10: 1-9.
[http://dx.doi.org/10.4137/CCRPM.S33382] [PMID: 27398039]

[19] Koenig SJ, Narasimhan M, Mayo PH. Thoracic ultrasonography for the pulmonary specialist. Chest 2011; 140(5): 1332-41.
[http://dx.doi.org/10.1378/chest.11-0348] [PMID: 22045878]

CHAPTER 14

Management of Malignant Pleural Effusion

Rosmadi Ismail[1,*], Abdul Aziz Marwan[2] and Jamalul Azizi Abdul Rahaman[1]

[1] *Pulmonology Unit, Department of Medicine, Serdang Hospital, Selangor, Malaysia*

[2] *Faculty of Medicine and Health Sciences, Universiti Sains Islam Malaysia, Negeri Sembilan, Malaysia*

Abstract: Malignant pleural effusion (MPE) is common and the management options available for MPE are often limited. The key goal in the management of MPE is to relieve patient's symptoms with the least invasive means and in the most cost-effective manner. The approach to the management of MPE should be tailored according to patient's overall prognosis, symptoms, functional status, social support, treatment availability, and financial situation.

Pleurodesis has been the standard of care for the management of MPE for years and talc continues to be the most effective sclerosant available for pleurodesis in MPE. However, it is also associated with more invasive procedure and longer hospitalization.

Most clinical studies on MPE treatments in the past were focused on the creation of successful pleurodesis in an attempt to stop reaccumulation of pleural fluid rather than patient-related outcome measures (PROM). The current trend of incorporating indwelling pleural catheter (IPC) in the management of MPE has been shown to be as equally effective as talc pleurodesis with significantly fewer hospitalization days and may be less costly compared to pleurodesis .

Keywords: Indwelling pleural catheter (IPC), Malignant Pleural Effusion (MPE), Pleurodesis, Pleuroscopy, Thoracentesis, Thoracoscopy.

INTRODUCTION

Malignant pleural effusion (MPE) is one of the most distressing complications of advanced malignancies. In most cases, the diagnosis of MPE indicates incurable disease with short median survival that measures in months and majority of these patients are symptomatic at presentation with breathlessness and cough as the most common symptoms. Given the short life expectancy and grave prognosis of the illness, clinicians now recognize that the key management options for MPEs should focus on therapy that alleviates patient symptoms with the least invasive

* **Corresponding author Rosmadi Ismail:** Pulmonology Unit, Department of Medicine, Serdang Hospital, Malaysia; Tel: +603-89475555; +60351036193; Fax: +60389475050; +603-89475210; E-mail: rismacc@yahoo.com

Ali I. Musani (Ed.)

means, preferably out-patient care and in the most cost-effective manner. The choice of therapies must address the patient's current functional status, life expectancy, or prognosis and their social support. Therapies that remove excess fluid from the pleural cavity (*i.e.* chest tube insertion) as well as sclerotherapy (*i.e.* pleurodesis) have been the cornerstone in the management of MPE for years. Newer and less invasive therapeutic options such as indwelling pleural catheter (IPC) and medical pleuroscopy have been successfully integrated as the standard of care in MPE. These procedures can be performed as out of hospital care and may cause less discomfort to the patient.

INCIDENCE

In the United States, the estimated incidence of MPEs is reported between 150,000 to 175,000 cases a year [1, 2], whereas in Europe, it is estimated that more than 125,000 patients suffer from MPE secondary to lung malignancies alone [3]. The most common causes of MPE are lung cancer in men and breast cancer in women which account for 50% to 65% of all MPE, followed by hematological malignancies, unknown primary, genitourinary and gastrointestinal malignancies [2, 4 - 9]. Carcinoma of the lung, breast or ovary, or lymphoma causes more than 75% of MPEs cases [10, 11]. Malignant pleural mesothelioma is the most common primary malignancy of the pleura, the second most common overall malignancy of the pleura after metastatic disease and is associated with asbestos exposure in approximately 80% of patients [12]. Metastatic adenocarcinoma is the most common histological phenotype associated with MPE [13]. In one case series, 19% of lung cancer patients had MPE at presentation and the incidence increased to 40% as their illness progressed [14]. Morgensztern and colleagues analyzed data of 57,000 patients with Non-Small Cell Lung Carcinoma extracted from Surveillance, Epidemiology, and End Results (SEER) registry which showed that 9,170 subjects (15.9%) had MPE and were associated with larger primary tumors, mediastinal nodal metastasis, as well as adenocarcinoma [15]. Meanwhile, chylothorax is most commonly associated with lymphomas [16]. Approximately 20% to 30% of patients with non- Hodgkin's lymphoma and Hodgkin's disease develop pleural effusions during their course of illness [17].

PATHOGENESIS

Physiologically, the pleural space contains a small amount of fluid (~10-20 ml) that acts as a lubricant to aid the normal breathing process. Pleural fluid is normally generated in the pleural space through the systemic capillaries of both the pleural surfaces and subsequently removed by lymphatic drainage through the stomata of the parietal pleura, by the absorptive pressure gradients through the parietal pleura, and by cellular mechanisms [18]. Pleural effusion is usually caused by a disturbance of the normal Starling forces regulating reabsorption of fluid in the pleural space as well as due to an increased production of fluid in the pleural cavity. MPE is diagnosed by identification of malignant cells in the pleural fluid or by pleural biopsy. However, not all malignancies involving the pleura will result in MPE. Based on autopsy studies, only 60% of patients with pleural malignancies have MPE [19, 20].

Paramalignant pleural effusion is defined by cytology-negative effusions occurring in patients with confirmed malignancy and the effusion is not the direct result of neoplastic involvement of the pleura [1]. The mechanism of fluid accumulation in these patients is likely from one or more of these factors- obstruction of the thoracic duct, obstruction of superior vena cava, post-obstructive atelectasis, low oncotic pressure from poor nutrition status, trapped lung, related to chemotherapy or radiation treatment, pneumonia, or pulmonary embolism [1, 8, 21]. Paramalignant effusion can be present in up to 50% of patients with known malignancy during their course of illness [10].

It is a known fact that seeding of the cancer cells to the pleura occurs via lymphatic or hematogenous routes, or by direct invasion, but the exact mechanism of the cancer cells generating excess fluid in the pleura remains poorly understood. The well-established mechanism of MPE accumulation is attributed to impaired reabsorption process of the fluid due to tumor-associated blockage of the local lymphatic outflow [22]. Blockade of the lymphatic network by dissemination of tumor cells to pleural stomata and mediastinal lymph nodes causes impairment of fluid drainage from the pleural cavity [19]. Further support for this mechanism is provided by the observation that no direct relationship was found between the extent of pleural involvement with the occurrence of pleural effusion, and pleural effusions do not generally develop when the pleura is involved by sarcoma due to its characteristically absence of lymphatic metastases [19].

Another recognized mechanism in MPE accumulation is an increase in vascular permeability leading to enhanced fluid production through excessive plasma leakage [23]. Studies have shown that tumor cells secreted an excessive amount of several vasoactive mediators which contributed to the development of MPE by increasing blood vessel permeability. Several probable mediators have been identified which include vascular endothelial growth factor (VEGF) and angiopoietins [23, 24], as well as host-elaborated transforming growth factor-β (TGF-β) secretion that induces the production of VEGF by mesothelial cells [25], contributing to MPE formation.

Several preclinical studies have identified several pro-inflammatory mediators associated with MPE, such as, interleukin (IL)-6 [26], tumor necrosis factor-alpha (TNF-α) [27], chemokine ligand 2 (CCL2) [28], and secreted phosphoprotein-1 (SPP1) [29]. These molecules are likely to play important roles in MPE formation in more than one way, as they are potent inducers of vascular hyperpermeability, angiogenesis and inflammation. It is likely that the formation of MPE is mediated by multiple molecules, back up redundancy, cross-talk between mediators, and tumor-host interaction [30].

CLINICAL FEATURES, DIAGNOSIS AND OUTCOME

MPE patients most commonly present with breathlessness, cough as well as constitutional symptoms such as weight loss which further worsen the underlying condition and severely affect the quality of life [11]. Dyspnea in MPE is caused by reduced compliance of the chest wall, depression of the ipsilateral diaphragm, mediastinal shift and reduction in lung volume, ultimately restricting ventilation [31]. The pleural effusion also causes ventilatory asynchrony between the lungs and in some patients, paradoxical ventilation [32]. Patients with malignant pleural effusion are more likely to experience dull chest pain, as compared to benign diseases which is associated with pleuritic chest pain [33]. Presence of chest pain usually signifies tumor invasion of the parietal pleura as the visceral pleura is devoid of pain fibers. Constitutional symptoms such as anorexia, weight loss, and fever as well as symptoms specific to primary malignancy are common and sometimes difficult to distinguish from the effect of MPE. The presence of a massive pleural effusion, which is defined as complete or almost complete opacification of a hemithorax on chest radiograph, is commonly associated with malignancies, and usually symptomatic [34]. Up to 25% of MPE patients are asymptomatic at diagnosis with an incidental finding of pleural effusion on chest radiograph or during physical examination [8].

Pleural fluid from MPE has a preponderance for being exudative via Light's criteria. However, up to 5% of MPE can be transudative [35]. Grossly bloody pleural fluid is usually associated with malignancy (up to 50%), however several other conditions such as pulmonary embolus with infarction, trauma, benign asbestos pleural effusions, or post-cardiac injury syndrome may cause hemorrhagic appearance as well [36, 37]. Interestingly, 56% to 89% of MPE do not appear bloody [37, 38]. Pleural fluid cell proportions are helpful in narrowing the differential diagnosis but none are specific for MPE, thus the presence or absence of specific cell type does not alter the likelihood of malignancy [39].

Pleural fluid cytology is a quick and minimally invasive way to diagnose MPE; approximately 60% of MPE can be diagnosed by pleural fluid cytology alone

[39]. Submission of a 60 ml pleural fluid sample has been found to produce a significantly better sensitivity for the diagnosis of malignancy than a 10 ml sample [30]. The positive yield from sending more than two specimens (taken on different occasions) is very low and should be avoided [39]. There is no significant difference in sensitivity of positive cytology with bloody or non-bloody effusion [38].

In a cytology positive sample, immunohistochemistry stains of malignant cells are used to confirm a diagnosis and to specify tumor type, with many new markers being used in panels for optimal diagnostic efficacy [40 - 42]. With adequate tumour cellularity in effusion sample, cytology alone from MPE is enough to provide molecular profiling in 59% of cases [43]. This includes *epidermal growth factor receptor* (EGFR) mutation, *anaplastic lymphoma kinase* (ALK) activating mutations, and *Kristen ras proto-oncogene* (KRAS) mutation [43 - 45]. It is important to bear in mind that many cancer patients have comorbidities, and that pleural effusion may have other etiology and thus a complete work up of the collected fluid is warranted (Table **1**).

Table 1. Types of pleural fluid investigations.

Test	Notes
Biochemistry: LDH and Protein	Blood should be sent simultaneously to biochemistry for total protein and LDH for application of Light's criteria
Microscopy and Culture	Culture for aerobic and anaerobic organism
Cytological and differential cell count	Minimum 60 ml of fluid is recommended and should be analyzed
pH	To be handled in a similar manner of blood gas analysis with Arterial Blood Gas machine. Low pH (< 7.3) may provide prognostic information.
Glucose	Concentration above or below simultaneous blood concentration may have diagnostic and prognostic implication.
AFB and MAC culture	Clinical suspicion of tuberculosis or dual pathology (TB and malignancy) especially in high burden TB countries
Optional test depending on condition described in the notes	
TG and Cholesterol	If milky effusions are encountered, to distinguish chylothorax from pseudochylothorax.
Amylase	If pancreatitis-related effusion or rupture of esophagus suspected
Hematocrit	If hemothorax suspected, Pleural fluid to serum haematocrit> 50%.
Immunohistochemistry and molecular essay	In cytology confirmed sample. Help to identify specific cell and activating mutation types

The poor survival of patients with MPE and lung cancer is reflected in the 7th edition of the TNM staging classification of lung cancer in 2007 [46]. The median length of survival of patients following the diagnosis of MPE varies greatly between 3 to 12 months depending on the type of primary malignancy. Earlier studies showed that the shortest median survival time was observed in MPE associated with lung malignancies, longest with ovarian cancer, and MPE secondary to an unknown primary had intermediate survival time [6, 47 - 49]. However, data from the LENT study group reported that the lowest median survival time in MPE is observed in urological cancer, sarcoma and melanoma, the longest median survival time was observed in patients with mesothelioma, while patients with lung malignancy had a median survival of 74 days [4].

Several prognostic factors have been identified and may help predict survival of patients with MPE such as; tumor characteristics [50, 51], comorbidities [52], low Karnofsky performance status [51, 53], and the composition of the effusion (high LDH, low pH, low glucose level) [50, 51]. Low pH has been associated with shorter survival, more extensive disease and a lower chance of successful pleurodesis [54]. A meta-analysis of 417 patients with malignant pleural effusions by Heffner *et al* found that a pleural pH of <7.28 was associated with a shorter median survival time (2.5 months vs 4.5 months) and a lower 3-month survival rate (38.9% vs 61.6%) [55].

A study by Pilling *et al.* on 278 MPE patients undergoing palliative surgical procedures identified three factors significantly associated with a poor prognosis; leukocytosis, hypoxemia, and hypoalbuminemia [52]. Clive *et al.* have validated the LENT score (pleural fluid **l**actate dehydrogenase, **E**astern Cooperative Oncology Group (ECOG) performance score (PS), **n**eutrophil-to-lymphocyte ratio, and **t**umour type) as the first validated risk-stratification system to predict survival in patients with MPE (Table **2**). LENT score performed significantly better than ECOG performance status alone at predicting mortality [4]. The study shows only 65% of patients with a high risk LENT score survived at 1 month from diagnosis and just 3% survived at 6 months [4]. The more accurate prognostication at presentation may help individualize treatment strategies as treatment may cause morbidity and necessitate an inpatient stay. Identifying patients with the poorest prognosis may help to minimize discomfort and inconvenience at the end of their lives.

MANAGEMENT OF MPE

In the setting of known MPE, the ideal management options would be the one that effectively controls fluid reaccumulation thus providing immediate and long term relief of symptoms, easing distress and ultimately improving quality of life (QoL).

Table 2. The LENT score calculation and expected prognosis.

	Variable	Score	Total Score	Risk Category	Median Survival in Days (IQR)
	LDH level in pleural fluid (IU/L)	0			
L	<1500	1			
	>1500				
			0-1	Low risk	319 (228–549)
	ECOG PS				
	0	0			
E	1	1			
	2	2			
	3–4	3			
	Neutrophil –to-lymphocyte ratio				
N	<9	0			
	>9	1	2-4	Moderate risk	130 (47–467)
	Tumour type				
	Lowest risk tumour types				
T	▸ Mesothelioma	0			
	▸ Haematological malignancy				
	Moderate risk tumour types				
	▸ Breast cancer				
	▸ Gynaecological cancer	1	5-7	High Risk	44 (22–77)
	▸ Renal cell carcinoma				
	Highest risk tumour types				
	▸ Lung cancer	2			
	▸ Other tumour types				

These treatments ideally should be well tolerated, had limited potential side effects, minimally invasive, cost effective, and preferentially can be delivered as out of hospital care. Several factors need to be taken into consideration to help guide the treatment decisions such as tumor type, patient's functional status, patient's preference, symptomatic improvement following initial fluid removal, rate of reaccumulation of pleural effusion and choices of management option available in a particular center. Asymptomatic patients do not require treatment following their diagnosis of MPE and can be observed for progression of disease. However, most of patients with MPE are symptomatic and have some degree of impairment in their quality of life In the past, most clinical studies on MPE treatments were focused on generation of successful pleurodesis in an attempt to stop reaccumulation of pleural fluid rather than 'patient-related outcome measures' (PROM) such as improvement in QoL, avoidance of invasive procedures, and hospitalization [56]. We will review the current available options for patients with MPE which include; recurrent thoracentesis, pleurodesis, indwelling pleural catheter, pleuroperitoneal shunt and pleurectomy.

RECURRENT THORACENTESIS

Therapeutic thoracentesis is a common starting point employed in the management of MPE. It is simple, gives immediate relief of the breathlessness and can be done as out of hospital setting, although the benefit may be temporary. Removal of the fluid restores the mechanical advantage of the diaphragmatic muscles and improves dyspnea. Alleviation of the symptoms post-procedure may be the most direct way to determine relative contribution of the effusion to the overall symptoms and help to decide which patients may benefit from subsequent removal of the fluid. Dyspnea in MPE patients is often multifactorial as up to 50% of them may not have significant symptomatic improvement following thoracentesis [2]. Concurrent lung pathologies such as pneumonia, underlying comorbidities, and cancer related complications such as pulmonary embolism, trapped or entrapped lung, and diaphragmatic paralysis secondary to phrenic nerve palsy can all contribute to dyspnea in MPE patients [57]. Adequate lung expansion confirmed radiographically post-evacuation of the fluid is vital in ensuring pleurodesis success [58, 59]. Thoracentesis is generally a safe procedure and there are no absolute contraindications, but caution should be advised for patients with bleeding tendencies, on positive pressure ventilation, or small amount of fluid detected radiographically. Several known morbidities have been associated with thoracentesis such as iatrogenic infection, pain (5%), cough (24%), shortness of breath (15%), vasovagal reaction (3%), and pneumothorax (20% to 39%) [60]. The incidence of pneumothorax can be reduced down to 9% by performing the procedure under ultrasound guidance [61, 62].

Reexpansion pulmonary edema is a well-known but rare complication (< 1% risk) associated with large volume thoracentesis and carries up to 20% mortality [63]. Monitoring of intrapleural pressure with pleural manometry during large-volume thoracentesis and maintaining the pressure less than -20 cmH_2O has been shown to be safe [64]. There is no well documented safe amount of fluid that can be drained in each session and manometry device is not always readily available. Practically, removal of 1 to1.5 liter of fluid is advised on each thoracentesis session and to discontinue aspiration if the patient develops dyspnea, chest pain or cough (signs of rapid pulmonary expansion) [65].

Thoracentesis can be the treatment of choice in selected group of patients with underlying malignancies that are susceptible to personalized targeted therapy (*e.g.* adenocarcinoma with EGFR mutation) or systemic chemotherapy (*e.g.* small cell carcinoma or lymphoma) while waiting for the treatment to work. Patients with primary lung adenocarcinoma associated with EGFR mutation presenting with MPE have favorable response to tyrosine kinase inhibitor compounds (*e.g.* Erlotinib, Gefitinib) [66, 67].

Therapeutic thoracentesis is suitable for symptomatic patients that require immediate short-term measures and is not a reliable option in patients whose life expectancy is measured in months rather than weeks as fluid reaccumulation can occur very fast [65]. Repeated therapeutic thoracentesis may be preferable especially those with short expected survival, or because of patient preference or after failed pleurodesis and intercostal drainage.

PLEURODESIS

Pleurodesis has been the standard of care for the management of MPE for many years. It is an iatrogenic intervention to provoke a rapid and widespread inflammatory reaction intended to obliterate the pleural space. The establishment of pleurodesis hinges on symphysis of both the visceral and parietal pleurae through the formation of extensive adhesion. The aim of the procedure is to prevent re-accumulation of either air or fluid in the pleural space.

Pleurodesis has other roles outside MPE management, such as pneumothorax and in selected cases of non-malignant pleural effusions. In pneumothoraces, pleurodesis is indicated in patients with a second ipsilateral pneumothorax, first contralateral pneumothorax, synchronous pneumothoraces, continuous air leak, or a spontaneous hemopneumothorax as well as in those with job restrictions (*e.g.* airline staff, diver) [68]. For benign conditions, successful chemical pleurodesis has been reported in cases such as heart failure [69, 70], yellow nail syndrome [71], hepatic hydrothorax [72, 73], chronic ambulatory peritoneal dialysis [74], lupus pleuritis [75], and chylothorax [72, 76].

MECHANISM OF PLEURODESIS

Pleurodesis can be achieved through intrapleural instillation of chemical sclerosant, by mechanical abrasion during thoracoscopy or open thoracotomy, or by pleurectomy/decortication surgery.

All these procedures will lead to the formation of fibrin and fibrotic tissues within the pleural cavity. However, the exact mechanism involved in the development of pleurodesis is poorly understood.

The traditional belief of pleurodesis process describes the induction of an acute inflammation of the pleura that results in denudation of mesothelial cells. This causes activation of inflammatory pathway which eventually leads to the formation of pleural fibrosis and obliteration of the pleural space. Inflammation triggers recruitment of neutrophils into the pleural space and they secrete a variety of chemokines such as interleukin-8 (IL-8) for the continuation of inflammatory pathway [77, 78], a pathway that is potentially inhibited by concurrent corticosteroid use [77, 79 - 81]. The inflammation may resolve prematurely, resulting in failed pleurodesis. As such, the likelihood of successful pleurodesis is increased through producing more injury to the pleura that will result in more inflammation. This however is at the expense of more adverse effect from severe pleuritis such as pain and fever.

Instillation of a sclerosing agent is responsible for an increase in the pleural coagulation and a decrease in fibrinolytic activity which is responsible for the formation of fibrin mesh and the subsequent proliferation of fibroblast leading to collagen production in the pleural space [77]. Several fibroblast growth factors such as platelet-derived growth factor, *basic fibroblast growth factor* (bFGF) and *transforming growth factor- β* (TGF- β) have been found in the pleural fluid of patients receiving sclerosing agents [77]. Some researchers believe that an intact mesothelium is critical for a successful pleurodesis [82, 83]. As such, tumors such as malignant mesothelioma or extensive tumor burden of the pleura, in which the normal mesothelial cells are scarce will have a poorer response to pleurodesis [77].

TYPES OF PLEURODESIS

Chemical Pleurodesis

Chemical pleurodesis is the application of chemical sclerosant intrapleurally. The chemical irritant can be introduced into the pleura either through a chest tube or via medical thoracoscopy or during video-assisted thoracoscopic surgery (VATS). There are over 30 different chemical irritants that have been proposed as pleurodesis agents since 1935. All of these chemical irritants have varying degree of efficacy and side effect profiles. Ideal pleurodesis agents should be inexpensive, available worldwide and free of adverse effects. Till today, no chemical agent is able to fulfill these criteria completely. Chemical pleurodesis via tube thoracotomy has comparable success rates to surgical pleurodesis and is not associated with risk of general anesthetic.

CHOICE OF SCLEROSANT AGENTS

Talc

Talc, a trilayered, magnesium sheet silicate [$Mg_3(Si_2O_5)$] is the most well-established and widely used sclerosant agent for chemical pleurodesis. It was first introduced as far back as 1935 [84]. Talc pleurodesis technique is used to manage persistent pneumothorax and pleural effusion in benign or malignant disease. Talc is considered the best agent because of its effectiveness, ease of use, availability, lack of side effects, low cost, and can be administered via chest tube or during thoracoscopy [85]. Only correctly sterilised talc should be used for pleurodesis to avoid the incidence of empyema [68]. Adverse reactions such as acute respiratory distress syndrome (ARDS) [86], acute pneumonitis, respiratory failure, and treatment-related mortality due to systemic absorption of talc particles have also been reported after talc pleurodesis [87]. This is most likely related to the smaller particle size of the talc preparation and unlikely to occur with the use of graded talc (where most particles size < 10 μm removed or reduced to less than 10%) [88, 89]. Systematic review and meta-analyses showed that talc was the chemical agent that most frequently resulted in successful pleurodesis and preventing recurrence MPE or other causes of pleural effusion, with success rate over 90% [90 - 93].

Chemical pleurodesis with talc can be accomplished through powder insufflation (poudrage) via thoracoscopy or during thoracotomy, or as slurry (talc mixed with saline solution to form a suspension) form via a chest drain. Both methods have comparable efficacy.

Other Sclerosant Agents

Although sterile talc is the most commonly used agent worldwide, there are other substances that have been used for induction of pleurodesis such as antibiotics (tetracycline hydrochloride, minocycline, doxycycline, erythromycin), cytotoxic agents (bleomycin, cisplatin, cytarabine, etoposide), biological agents (streptococcus pyogenes A3 [OK-432], *Corynebacterium parvum*), antiseptics (iodine povidone, silver nitrate), 50% glucose, autologous blood and many others.

Cytotoxic agents such as nitrogen mustard, bleomycin, cytarabine and dacarbazine have been tested with variable success rates ranges from 25% to 85% [94]. However, the use of cytotoxic agent such as bleomycin is now uncommon due to its low efficacy, systemic toxicity and high cost [85]. Cyclins (tetracycline, minocycline and doxycycline) have been used for chemical pleurodesis with a success rate ranging from 65% to 87% [95, 96] and has been the agent of choice for a significant proportion of pulmonologists [97]. Parenteral tetracycline is no longer available in many countries due to cessation of its production. However, oral forms of tetracycline derivatives doxycycline dissolved in normal saline can be used for pleurodesis. Pleurodesis with minocycline, another tetracycline derivative has shown comparable success rate compared to pleural abrasion for primary spontaneous pneumothorax [98] and talc pleurodesis for secondary pneumothorax [99].

The use of Povidone–iodine as pleurodesis agent has been reported in case series and small randomised trial with success rate between 72% and 96% [100 - 102]. Povidone-iodine advantages include low cost, availability, safety and effectiveness for chemical pleurodesis in patients with pleural effusions and recurrent pneumothoraces [103].

Silver nitrate (SN) as a chemical pleurodesis agent has been the subject of few studies, mainly involving cohort of MPE patients. A systematic review showed that SN is an effective agent in inducing pleurodesis in patients with either MPE or primary spontaneous pneumothorax with comparable success rate to talc pleurodesis and potentially fewer side effects [104].

MECHANICAL PLEURODESIS

Mechanical pleurodesis is carried out in the operating room by a surgeon and done under general anesthesia. There are several different mechanical techniques to obtain pleurodesis which include abrasion (with swabs, scraper or dry gauze), by pleural cauterization (with electrocautery or laser), and by pleurectomy (partial or total) to activate an inflammatory process and create adherences between pleural layers. Surgical pleurodesis can also be combined with application of chemical sclerosant. The approach of mechanical pleurodesis can either be via VATS, open thoracotomy, or transaxillary mini-thoracotomy. VATS is now the procedure of choice amongst surgeons and is associated with a shorter hospital stay and lower postoperative morbidity [68].

In the treatment of pneumothoraces, surgical pleurodesis technique is performed in isolation or combined with resection of bullae and blebs of the lung parenchyma depending on the surgical findings. For pneumothoraces, VATS approach is better tolerated by patients but carries a higher rate of recurrence (5% vs 1%) [68]. However, a randomized trial by Joshi *et al.* showed that once the learning curve of VATS is surpassed, the recurrence rate of pneumothorax is comparable between the two options [105]. The use of surgical pleurodesis in MPE is typically limited to VATS combined with talc poudrage, largely due to morbidity associated with pleurectomy, and open thoracotomy may greatly reduce the palliative benefits in patients with MPE.

The use of non-steroidal anti-inflammatory drugs (NSAIDs) as a pain control postoperatively may have an effect on the pleurodesis process and rate of pneumothorax recurrence. Available data from several studies were conflicting with some studies showing that systemic use of NSAIDs postoperatively (for pain control) may reduce adhesion formation [106, 107] while others showed no detrimental effect to pleurodesis success [108, 109].

PRACTICAL ASPECT OF CHEMICAL PLEURODESIS

Chemical Pleurodesis via Chest Tube

Chemical pleurodesis is usually performed as an inpatient case in a minor procedure room, bronchoscopy suite, or at bedside with proper aseptic technic. An informed written consent must be obtained prior to the procedure. Oxygen saturation, blood pressure and pulse are continuously monitored during the procedure for safety purposes especially in patients that receive opiate premedication and conscious sedation. Adequate pain control is delivered via intrapleural administration of lidocaine 3mg/kg with maximum dosage of 250mg follow by instillation of sclerosant agent (*e.g.*; talc, doxycycline) via the chest tube. Cessation of pleural fluid drainage by clamping of the chest tube for one to two hours following administration of the chemical irritant is recommended. No study has been done to address the optimal chest tube clamping time to assess whether prolonged contact of a pleurodesing agent with the pleural surfaces is required to induce successful pleurodesis. Some clinicians may rotate their patient who undergo talc slurry pleurodesis due to the belief of sclerosant agent's poor distribution in the pleural cavity. However, there is no evidence that patient rotation improves the likelihood of pleurodesis and may be associated with discomfort [90, 110, 111]. After the chest tube clamping has been released, the amount of passive fluid drainage is recorded on daily basis. Some clinicians may opt for high volume low pressure suction (-20 cm H_2O) of the chest tube over 24 hours duration. Majority of the chest tube can be taken out at 48 hours following pleurodesis procedure. Traditionally, the chest tube will be kept in place until the drainage is less than approximately 150 ml per 24 hours, whereas some pulmonologists may opt to remove the drain at specific time after pleurodesis procedure regardless of the fluid volume [97]. The largest randomized trial comparing chest tube removal at 24 hours *versus* 72 hours following pleurodesis in MPE patients showed no significant difference in success of pleurodesis rates [112]. A summary of recommendation of chemical pleurodesis procedure is listed in Table **3**.

Chest Tube Size for Pleurodesis

The British Thoracic Society (BTS) guideline advocates the use of smaller tubes for pleurodesis especially in the cases of pneumothoraces mainly due to equivalent success compared to the use of larger drains [68, 113]. The use of smaller chest tube is also associated with less pain [114]. For MPE, result from the TIME1 randomised clinical trial showed that small bore chest tubes failed to meet non-inferiority criteria for pleurodesis efficacy and is associated with higher rate of pleurodesis failure [114]. It is probable that smaller chest tubes may be associated with incomplete drainage of the effusion and increase in the frequency of blockage, thereby preventing adequate drainage after pleurodesis.

Table 3. Summary of recommendations for patient undergoing chemical pleurodesis via chest drain.

1) Use small-bore (10–14 F) chest tubes as the initial choice for pneumothorax drainage and pleurodesis (MPE patients may benefit from larger bore chest tubes).
2) Lidocaine (3 mg/kg; maximum 250 mg) should be administered intrapleurally immediately prior to administration of chemical irritant.
3) Premedication should be considered to alleviate anxiety and pain associated with pleurodesis.
4) Patient rotation is not necessary after intrapleural instillation of the sclerosant.
5) The intercostal tube should be clamped for 1 hour after sclerosant administration.
6) In the absence of excessive fluid drainage (> 150 mL/ day), the intercostal tube should be removed within 24–48 hours of sclerosant administration.
7) NSAIDs are equally effective as opiates post-procedure analgesic and would not hinder pleurodesis success.

Pain Control Following Pleurodesis

Chest tube insertion and pleurodesis are painful procedures, presumably from the iatrogenic skin and soft tissue injuries as well as intense pleural inflammation provoked. Premedication with narcotic analgesia and/or conscious sedation and instillation of intrapleural analgesia has been recommended for better pain management during pleurodesis procedure. Following pleurodesis procedure, most physician use opiates instead of non-steroidal anti-inflammatory drugs (NSAIDs) [97]. The avoidance of NSAIDs in pleurodesis may likely due to concerns that these drugs may impair the success of pleurodesis by suppressing acute inflammation caused by sclerosant agents. TIME1 randomised clinical trial showed that there was no clinically significant difference in pleurodesis efficacy when comparing NSAIDS with opioids as well as no significant difference in pain scores; but the use of NSAIDs was associated with more usage of rescue medication [114].

Effect of Prednisolone on Pleurodesis

There is no randomized clinical trial assessing the effect of prednisolone on the success or failure of pleurodesis. Animal studies have shown that concomitant administration of high dose corticosteroids reduced effectiveness of pleurodesis process [79 - 81]. In the absence of high quality evidence, the use of high dose systemic corticosteroids should be avoided in patients undergoing pleurodesis procedure.

Dosage of Sclerosing Agent

The dosage of the same sclerosing agent may vary according to indications of the pleurodesis- either for pneumothorax or pleural effusion. Dosages of different sclerosing agents are listed in the Table **4**.

Table 4. Dosage of sclerosant agents.

Sclerosant Agent	Dosage and Preparation
Talc	- 4g for talc insufflation - 5g for talc slurry
Cyclins - Tetracycline - Doxycycline - minocycline	 - 1500mg or 20mg/kg - 500mg - 300mg
Bleomycin	- 1 unit/kg, 15-240 units
Iodopovidone	- 100ml of 2% solution
Autologous blood	- 100- 120ml

Successful Pleurodesis

There are no universally accepted criteria for pleurodesis success. Clinical studies on pleurodesis have often defined success of pleurodesis as no fluid reaccumulation or recurrence at one month post-procedure. However, many studies have shown that the longer the patient survives the more likelihood that the fluid will re-accumulate [114, 115]. From the patient's point of view, a successful pleurodesis is the one that provides lifelong control of the fluid, amelioration of symptoms, and improvement in quality of life.

Failed Pleurodesis

Failure of pleurodesis may occur and the likely cause is the presence of trapped lung. At this moment, there is no reliable marker or way to predict pleurodesis failure in patient with pleural effusion. Patients with pleurodesis failure should have further evacuation of the pleural fluid followed by either a repeat pleurodesis or insertion of indwelling pleural catheter, depending on the presence of trapped lung [65].

COMPLICATION OF PLEURODESIS

Common complications of chemical pleurodesis are fever and chest pain, likely due to intense inflammation provoked by sclerosant agent. Other rare complications include empyema [93, 116], arrhythmias, cardiac arrest, myocardial infarction, and hypotension [89, 117]. Talc pleurodesis using small size talc particle is associated with respiratory failure and ARDS as a result of systemic absorption [88]. Observational study using only talc preparations of large particle size on patients undergoing thoracoscopic talc poudrage found no cases of ARDS, however, it was observed that oxygenation deteriorated in the first few days after pleurodesis [118].

PLEUROSESIS IN MPE

The main indication for pleurodesis in MPE is to relieve dyspnea and improve quality of life. It should only be attempted following improvement of dyspnea after therapeutic thoracentesis, and pleurodesis can be done simultaneously or sequentially. Patients with MPE who are symptomatic from pleural effusion that is rapidly re-accumulating following the initial thoracentesis (*e.g.* less than one month), whose life expectancy is more than one month, and without evidence of trapped lung may benefit from a pleurodesis procedure [65]. Dyspnea that is not relieved by thoracentesis may suggest other underlying causes such as lymphangitic carcinomatosis, atelectasis, thromboembolism, and tumor embolism. When pleurodesis is indicated, it should be performed as early as possible.

The most important requirement for a successful pleurodesis is satisfactory apposition of the parietal and visceral pleurae that is radiologically confirmed. While it is not difficult to achieve this in patients with pneumothorax and patients with no persistent air leak, achieving satisfactory apposition in cases of MPE could be more problematic, as the visceral pleura can become very thick and/or the lung parenchyma is very stiff (due to diffuse tumor involvement), thus leading to incomplete lung reexpansion (trapped lung). Mediastinum position on chest radiograph may provide valuable information on the existence of trapped lung and is a useful information for the management of these patients. The presence of a large effusion with contralateral mediastinal shift requires an immediate therapeutic thoracentesis and is a good candidate for pleurodesis. If a patient has a large effusion where the mediastinum is shifted ipsilaterally or in a midline position, a more careful approach and further evaluations are needed for possible occurrence of a trapped lung (Fig. **1**).

Talc is the most commonly used and most potent sclerosant agent for chemical pleurodesis in MPE patients [91]. Both talc poudrage and talc slurry have comparable efficacy in achieving pleurodesis in MPE [115, 119]. Talc pleurodesis in MPE has a success rate of approximately 75% at 1 month, but it was progressively reduced to approximately 50% by 6 months [115]. Several other agents have been used for chemical pleurodesis over the years including bleomycin [120, 121], silver nitrates [122], tetracycline, mistletoe extract [123], povidone-iodine [102, 124, 125], and doxycycline [126 - 128] (Table 5).

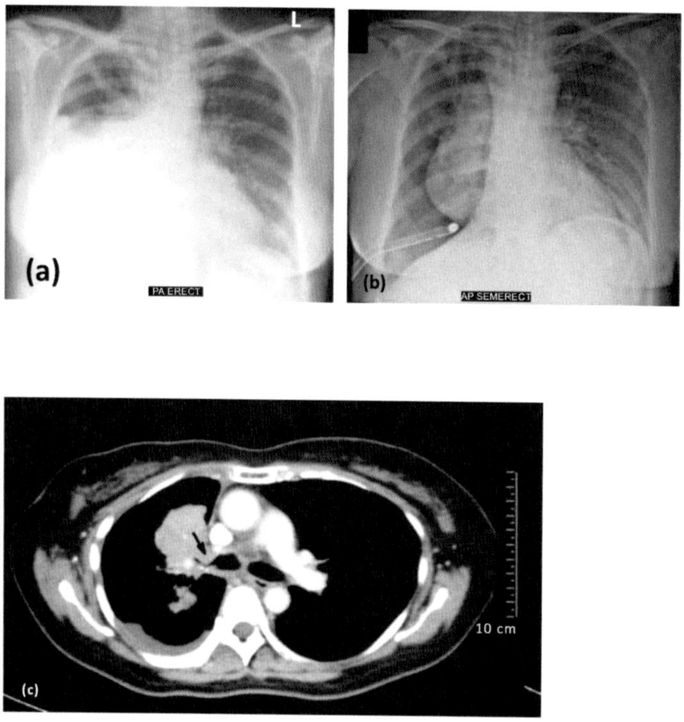

Fig. (1). (a) Chest x-ray of a patient with advanced non-small cell carcinoma showing a large right malignant pleural effusion. (b) Underlying trapped lung was revealed after drainage of pleural fluid with chest tube. (c) Chest CT showing endoluminal mass as the cause of the trapped lung (arrow).

Table 5. Prospective randomized trials comparing talc with other agents in MPE patients.

Author	Number of Patient	Outcome Measure	Result
Talc Slurry vs Bleomycin Hadad *et al*. 2004 [120] Ong *et al*. 2000 [121]	71 50	recurrence of pleural effusion Radiological control > 1month	There was no significant difference between groups Favored talc (89% v 79%)
Talc slurry vs talc poudrage Dresler *et al*. 2005 [115]	501	radiological recurrence at 1 month	There was no significant difference between groups
Silver nitrate vs talc slurry Paschoalini *et al*. 2005 [122]	60	Symptoms control and recurrence of effusion	There was no significant difference between groups for effectiveness of pleurodesis, underpowered to detect symptomatic differences.

(Table 5) contd.....

Author	Number of Patient	Outcome Measure	Result
Talc slurry vs Doxycycline Kuzdzal *et al.* 2003 [128]	33	recurrence of pleural effusion	Favored talc
Talc vs Iodopovidone Mohsen *et al.* 2011 [125]	42	Radiological recurrence and symptom control	There was no significant difference between groups

INDWELLING PLEURAL CATHETER

Indwelling pleural catheter (IPC) is a soft silicone tube placed within the pleural cavity and tunneled subcutaneously prior to exiting the skin with a one-way valve and protective cap at the distal end. PleurX 15.5 Fr-diameter catheter is the most widely used IPC worldwide, manufactured by CareFusion (McGaw, Ill., USA) and was approved by the Food and Drug Administration in 1997 for use in MPE to relieve breathlessness and to achieve pleurodesis. It has a multi-fenestrated chest drain made from a soft and flexible silicone elastomer, with a small polyester cuff enveloping the medial portion of the tube. The middle portion of the tube is tunneled through a short section of subcutaneous tissue before the proximal portion enters the pleural space, the cuff then acts as a focal point for fibrous growth to allow the drain to stay in place and reduce the risk of pathogen entering the pleural space, analogous to long-term vascular access. At the external end is a one-way access valve with a protective cap designed to be attached to proprietary vacuum drainage bottles.

INDWELLING PLEURAL CATHETER IN MALIGNANT PLEURAL EFFUSIONS

IPC has revolutionized the way MPE is treated by providing immediate symptom relief and effective long term control of recurrent effusion. The use of IPC has grown exponentially, partly due to increase in indications, from initially being reserved for patients with trapped lung or as a second-line management of MPE refractory to chemical pleurodesis, to currently as one of the first line therapies in MPE. The fact that IPC-related therapies can be done in outpatients setting is appealing to physicians who provide the care and to patients who already suffer tremendously from their advanced malignancies. This strategy enables the patients with MPE to be more independent, spending more time with their family members and less time in hospital to maximize their remaining QoL.

IPC allows ambulatory drainage by patients or their home support and typically the drainage is done every other day or as per needed, based on their symptoms, showing that pleurodesis is unnecessary to achieve the goal of symptomatic relief.

Patients treated with IPC are usually capable to carry on with their social activities and maintaining good QoL due to infrequent (x3/week) and typically short intervals of drainage session as well as IPC dressing that is invisible under clothing which is not cosmetically intrusive.

As in all types of therapy, it is imperative to choose the right patient that will benefit the most from IPC therapy. IPC therapy should only be a choice in patients whose life expectancy is more than 1 month, who show evidence that the fluid re-accumulates after thoracentesis and have subjective improvement in symptoms with drainage of the fluid. IPC placement should be avoided in patients with no anticipated benefit especially those with large parenchymal tumor burden or endobronchial lesion.

INDICATIONS

The main indication for inserting an IPC is recurrent pleural effusions due to malignancy that are unlikely to respond to medical management (*e.g.* trapped lung) or failed pleurodesis [39].

Although current management guidelines for MPE advocate talc slurry pleurodesis as a first-line treatment for symptomatic patients [65], data from several published studies showed that insertion of IPC is an equally acceptable therapeutic option [127, 129 - 132]. Data from TIME-2 trial showed equivalent efficacy in the control of dyspnea and maintenance of patient's quality of life between first-line pleurodesis and IPC use for MPE [129].

The use of IPC in patients with symptomatic recurrent pleural effusion in non-malignant cases is steadily increasing and evidence now exists to suggest that IPC insertion may also be appropriate in these groups of patients. A review by Bhatnagar *et al.* on 57 IPC insertions in five large UK centers showed that the commonest indications for IPC insertion in non-MPE were hepatic hydrothorax (33%) and inflammatory pleuritis (26%) [133]. Several case series showed that IPC insertion may be beneficial in patients with recurrent symptomatic chylothorax [134, 135], and cardiogenic pleural effusion [136] that are refractory to usual medical therapy. From our experience, the use of IPC in these groups of patients must be done on a case-by-case basis and should remain a consideration for carefully selected patients only.

CONTRAINDICATIONS

There are few absolute contraindications for IPC insertion in adult, which include uncorrected coagulopathic state, extensive cutaneous disease resulting from local tumor infiltration, cutaneous infection over the planned insertion site, inability for patient, family or health care services to manage the device, extensive loculated pleural collection, and short predicted survival time (< 1 month).

TECHNICAL ASPECT OF IPC

Insertion of an IPC

The insertion of IPC is usually performed as an out of hospital setting in a minor procedure room or bronchoscopy suite thereby avoiding hospital admission. However, IPC can also be done at the bedside. Anticoagulant and anti-platelet medication should be omitted temporarily beforehand according to manufacturer's recommendation and an informed written consent must be obtained prior to the procedure. In our practice, oxygen saturation and pulse are continuously monitored during the procedure for safety purposes.

Stepwise Approach in IPC Insertion

We recommend the following method of IPC insertion:

1. Place patient on a lateral decubitus position with the affected hemithorax in the upmost position (Fig. **2a**). Administer intravenous midazolam or fentanyl for conscious sedation as needed.
2. Perform thoracic ultrasound to identify the ideal insertion site and mark 'X'. Identify the location of the catheter exit site, approximately 5 cm inferior and lateral / medial to the guidewire insertion site. Consideration should be given to the patient's ease of access and comfort in determining the location of the catheter exit site (*e.g.* in women, the position of their bra in relation to the exit site).
3. Create a sterile field with liberal application of sterilizing agent (*e.g.* chlorhexidine) over the hemithorax, axilla and upper arm, and place proper sterile drape.
4. Infiltrate local anesthetic agent, lidocaine 1% or 2% subcutaneously and downward into the pleural cavity until fluid is obtained (Fig. **2b**).
5. Enter the pleura cavity with standard needle thoracentesis and pass the guide wire using Seldinger technique (Fig. **2c**).
6. Make a 1 to 1.5 cm horizontal incision at the site of thoracentesis (Fig. **2c**).
7. A second horizontal incision is made approximately 5 cm inferomedially or laterally after application of local anesthesia to the vertical tract that intersects these 2 incisions (Fig. **2d**).
8. Create subcutaneous tunnel between these points with the aid of a trocar attached to the fenestrated end of IPC tube and pull the tube through the tunnel until the polyester cuff sits 1 cm from the distal incision within the tract (Fig. **2e**). The fenestrated end of the catheter can be shortened to accommodate the

patient's anatomy.

9. Insert the dilator with Teflon 'peel-away' sheath into the thorax over the guidewire. Leaving the Teflon sheath in situ, remove the guidewire and dilator (Fig. **2f**).
10. Feed the fenestrated end of the catheter through the sheath into the pleural cavity while the operator splitting and withdrawing the sheath simultaneously with one finger keeping the IPC secure in the thorax (Fig. **2g**).
11. Apply one simple interrupted suture in the distal incision and another adjacent to the tube exit port after straightening the tubing at the pleural insertion site with a gentle pull of the IPC. An optional stay suture can be applied at the exit site to secure the tube.
12. Apply the sterile gauze and waterproof dressing provided in the packaging.
13. Following a successful insertion, drainage of pleural fluid can be performed immediately with a standard vacuum container connected to the proprietary connector supplied with the IPC kit, typically 1000-1500 ml can be drained or until the patient experiences chest pain or discomfort.
14. Document the drainage, perform chest radiograph to evaluate for trapped lung and pneumothorax.

Drainage Technique

Typical initial drainage frequency might be 3 times per week, with subsequent adjustment based upon volumes and symptoms. A recent trial suggested that daily drainage resulted in higher rate and shorter time of achieving auto-pleurodesis [137]. The drainage of IPC is usually achieved *via* a proprietary drainage container set that is primed with a vacuum in order to draw out the pleural contents, usually to a maximum of 500–1,000 ml at a time. The drainage of IPC can also be done through a standard underwater seal with the use of a correct adapter set if the patient requires more sustained periods of pleural access such as in patients with pleural infections, or following instillation of chemical pleurodesis agents through the catheter.

Removal of IPC

Removal of an IPC can be considered once the patient has achieved spontaneous pleurodesis or on the patient's request. Uncontrolled catheter-related pleural infection not responding to antibiotic therapy, severe persistent catheter-related pain, catheter misplacement or failure to achieve symptomatic improvement are other factors that may necessitate removal of the catheter. The process of IPC removal can be challenging mainly due to intense and extensive fibrotic reaction over the polyester cuffing especially with the catheter that has been in situ for long periods of time. Furthermore, aggressive malignant pleural processes can lead to the development of fibrotic bands growing through IPC fenestrations or along its surface, leading to painful and problematic extraction.

Fig. (2). Stepwise approach of IPC insertion.

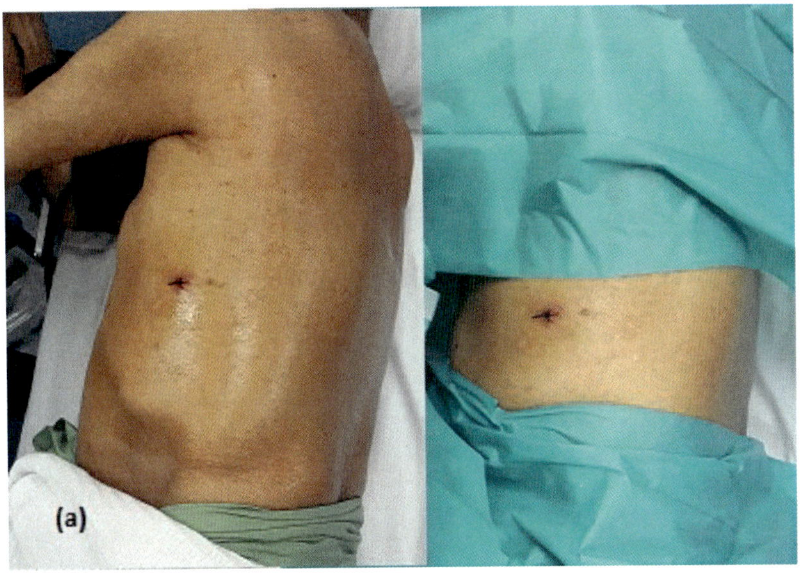

Fig. (2a). Patient positioning and initial draping.

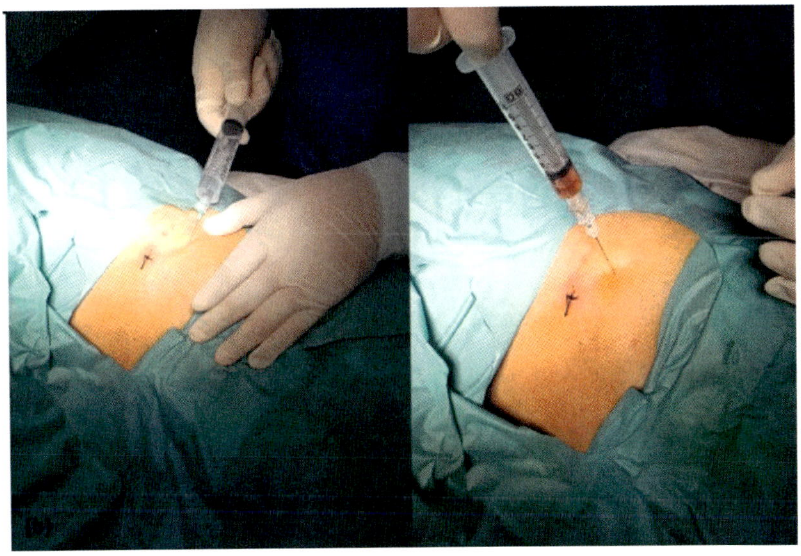

Fig. (2b). Infiltration of LA and aspiration of fluids.

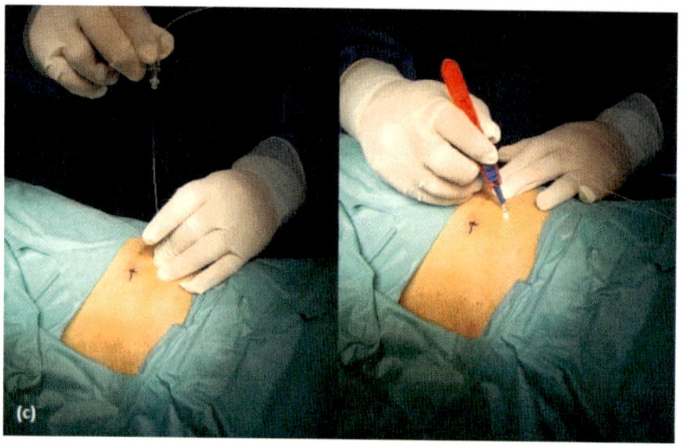

Fig. (2c). Insertion of guidewire and small incision at the point of insertion.

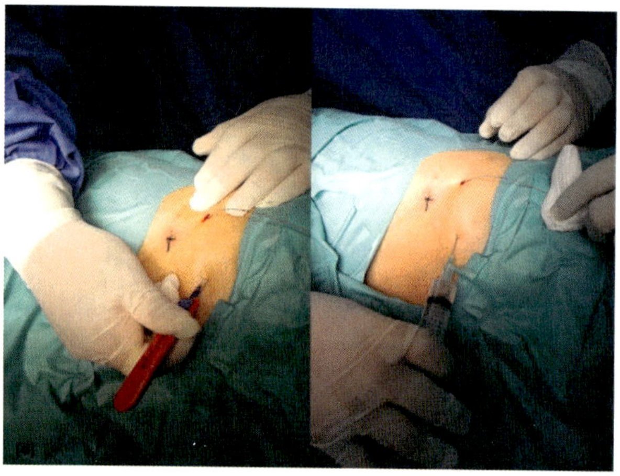

Fig. (2d). Identify exit site and apply LA vertically intersecting the two incisions.

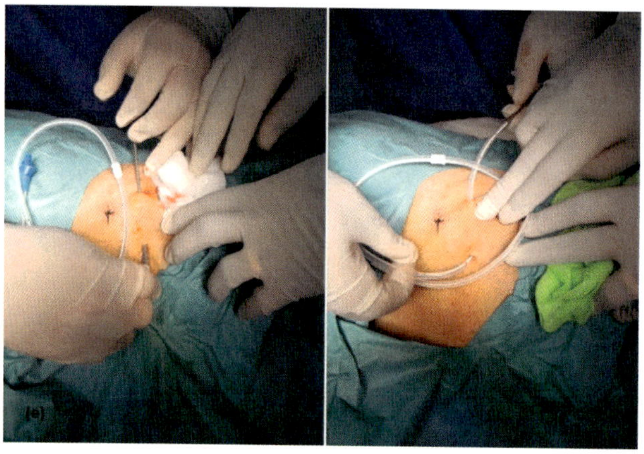

Fig. (2e). Passing the trocar and tube through the subcutaneous tract.

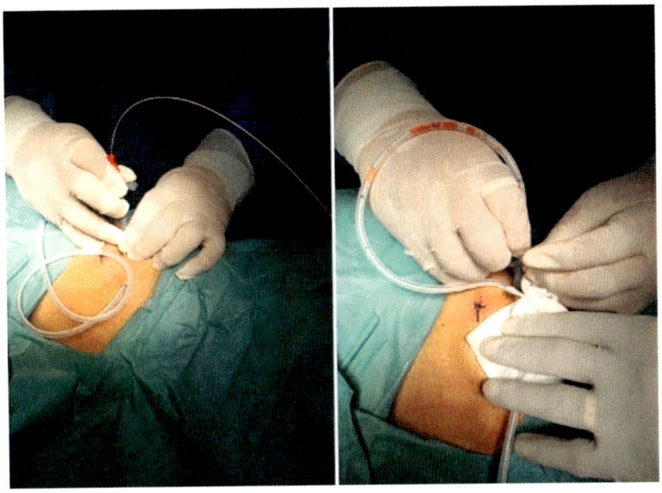

Fig. (2f). Insert peel-away sheath in to pleural cavity and push the catheter through it.

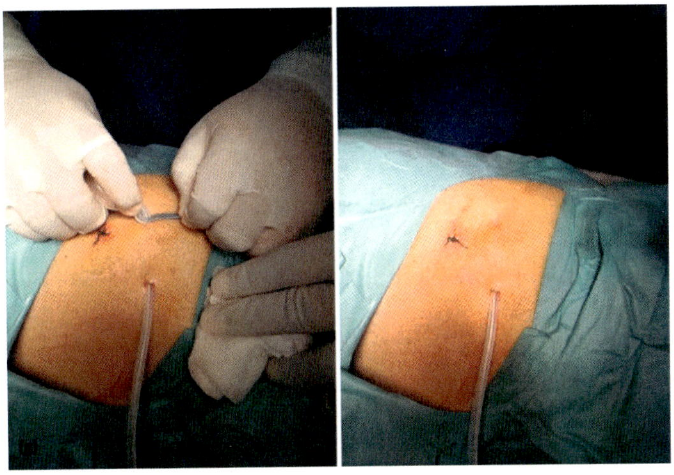

Fig. (2g). Splitting-withdrawing peel-away sheath while simultaneously inserting the catheter.

IPC removal can be performed on an outpatient basis after obtaining a written consent from the patient. Prior to the procedure, the patient should be informed of all the possible complications related to the removal, which include incomplete removal (catheter fracture), pain, infection and bleeding. The removal of the catheter can be done with the patient placed in any position preferred by the operator or the one that gives more comfort to the patient. The use of conscious sedation is optional. Here is the usual stepwise approach to IPC removal employed in our center.

1. Create a sterile field with liberal application of a sterilizing agent (*e.g.* chlorhexidine) over the hemithorax surrounding the catheter site and apply a

proper sterile drape after positioning the patient.
2. Infiltrate local anesthetic agent (Lidocaine 1% or 2%) subcutaneously along the tunneled catheter as this will help with pain control as well as ease the removal process by separating the tissue from the tunneled catheter.
3. Make a small horizontal incision to extend the length of the exit port, and perform a blunt dissection alongside the tunneled catheter, within the tract, with simultaneous application of gentle traction on the IPC.
4. Liberate the adhesions surrounding the cuff with curved forceps, occasionally with a scalpel, to allow catheter withdrawal. Avoid vigorous pulling on the tube as it may result in IPC fracture.
5. Once the catheter is removed, apply 1 to 2 simple interrupted sutures over the wound and it should be removed in 7 days.

CLINICAL ASPECTS OF IPC

Post Insertion Management

Patients and their family members or careers are usually able to manage the long term care of IPC after minimal amount of supervised training. They should also be educated on what IPC is, how and when to use it, possible complications related to IPC and when to notify the doctor to maximize the benefits, and promptly address any concerns. Further assistance on the care of the catheter can be provided by the community nursing programme as well as supplemental written and pictorial guidance. We recommend a routine follow up of 10 to 14 days post catheter placement with repeat chest radiograph followed by every 4 to 8 weeks thereafter or as needed.

Patient Related Outcome Measure (PROM) with IPC

Managing MPE patients with IPC has been shown to reduce the length of hospital stay which is an important patient related outcome measure (PROM) [129 - 131, 138]. In TIME-2 trial, the initial hospitalization was significantly shorter in IPC, with median of 0 days compared to 4 days in the talc slurry group [129]. The benefit seen with IPC-treated group was maintained in the long term where the median number of days spent in hospital for drainage over the following 12 months was significantly lower compared to the talc pleurodesis group (1 vs 4.5 days) [129].

Similar outcome was reported from a study on MPE patients done by Fysh *et al* which showed shorter number of hospital stay in the IPC group (6.5 days) compared to the pleurodesis group (18 days) and more importantly, the patients in the IPC group also spent a smaller percentage of their remaining lives in hospital compared to those in the pleurodesis group (8.0% vs 11.2%) [130].

Repeated procedures done on patients already suffering from end-stage illness greatly hamper the quality of life, but the placement of IPC has been shown to avoid further pleural interventions in a majority of the patients (>90%) [129, 131, 139].

A systematic review by Van Meter *et al.* shows that IPC provides improvement for over 95% of cases evaluated and 100% experienced QoL improvement from studies that include its measurement [140]. The first randomized clinical trial on IPC by Putnam *et al.* shows that IPC is equal compared to pleurodesis with doxycycline in symptom improvement as it did not demonstrate a significant difference in Borg Dyspnea Score and Guyatt Chronic Respiratory Questionnaire score between groups [127]. The TIME-2 trial also found that both therapies improved dyspnea with no significant difference in the first 42 days on visual analog scale, although improved symptoms became significant at the 6 months' time point in favor of the IPC group [129]. Up to 90% of patients with underlying trapped lung have shown symptomatic benefit from IPC placement [141]. In one prospective non-randomized trial, IPC provided more rapid improvements in dyspnea and QoL, and patients spent fewer days in hospital compared to talc pleurodesis [130]. The use of IPC in patients with non-malignant pleural effusions offers several additional benefits apart from symptomatic benefit when compared to traditional medical therapy as they also have reduction in their required drainage frequency over time, reduced frequency of hospitalizations and negate the need for repeated pleural procedures in the majority of patients [133, 142].

Spontaneous Pleurodesis with IPC

Although the principal aim of IPC treatment is to provide symptom relief from recurrent pleural effusion, spontaneous symphysis of pleura or pleurodesis does occur in a significant proportion of patients while on IPC therapy. Spontaneous pleurodesis is arbitrarily defined as minimal IPC drainage of less than 50 ml on three consecutive attempts despite catheter patency and confirmed using sequential imaging assessment. A systematic review of IPC efficacy and safety in MPE (n=1370) reported an overall spontaneous pleurodesis rate of 45% [140]. Data from later published studies showed spontaneous pleurodesis rate can be up to 57% [129, 130, 139, 143, 144]. For patients with non-malignant pleural effusion, spontaneous pleurodesis is seen in 29–64.3% of patients [133, 134, 145]. IPC-related spontaneous pleurodesis has been reported to occur between mean/median of 29 to 59 days following catheter insertion for MPE [139, 146, 147] and usually takes a longer duration in benign pleural effusion [133, 136, 145]. A small percentage of patients (3.8%- 8.7%) who have their IPC removed because of spontaneous pleurodesis will require additional ipsilateral intervention later on [129, 139, 146, 147]. The exact mechanism of IPC-related pleurodesis is unknown. It is possible that the presence of the tube invokes chronic inflammatory reaction through mechanical means with subsequent pleural fibrosis formation.

Cost Saving in IPC

The issue of whether IPC treatment ultimately contributes to cost saving has been subjected to ongoing debate and clinical trials. IPC allows patients with effusion to be managed almost entirely on outpatient basis, thus reflecting positively on patient's general physical and emotional well-being and, inferentially, on healthcare economics compared to conventional treatments that are usually associated with prolonged or repeated hospital admissions. There is little disagreement that IPC treatment is associated with a significant reduction in the number of inpatient days for management of pleural effusions in MPE cohort [129, 130, 148]. However, translating this into direct cost savings to a particular healthcare system can be tricky due to highly divergent life expectancies and expected time IPC needed to be in place, heterogeneity of illness that can be treated with IPC (individual types of malignancy vs non-malignant effusion), cost of IPC alone compared when combined with other therapy as well as different countries' healthcare system.

IPC plus Chemical Pleurodesis Hybrid Therapy

Approach to combine both IPC treatment and instillation of chemical sclerosant together sequentially may provide additional benefit compared with when they are done separately. The idea of combining both therapies was mooted following the success of pleurodesis through small bore catheter (≤ 14 French) [149 - 151]. A pilot study combining talc pleurodesis by medical thoracoscopy with simultaneous insertion of an IPC in 30 patients with MPE demonstrated high success rate of pleurodesis (92% at 6 months), short hospital stay (median of 1.79 days) as well as universal improvement of dyspnea and QoL [152]. The result was reproducible in a subsequent smaller study [153]. Another hybrid approach is the subject of a recently completed randomized controlled trial, the IPC-PLUS trial (EudraCT number: 2012-000599-40) [154] comparing the efficacy of IPC alone vs IPC plus talc through IPC as an outpatient in a MPE cohort, results are anticipated. The third hybrid approach of combining drug eluting (silver nitrate) IPC to deliver sclerosing agent to the pleural space over time has been tested in animal model but has not been replicated in human subject [155, 156]. To date, there is no published data on the use of combination therapy for non-malignant pleural effusion patients.

IPC and Chemotherapy

Historically, there has been a concern of an excess risk of IPC-related infection in patients who have a catheter in situ receiving immunosuppressive chemotherapy. Up to the present time, there is no randomized controlled data available to guide the practice. However, a retrospective review and case series analysis of MPE patients with IPC receiving immunosuppressive chemotherapy did not demonstrate a significant difference in pleural infection rates when compared to those who had IPC and did not receive chemotherapy [157 - 159]. Hence immunosuppressive systemic chemotherapy should not be withheld in patients with IPC in situ.

COMPLICATIONS AND MANAGEMENT

Complications related to IPC therapy can be divided into early and late or long term complications. Early complications in IPC are usually directly due to IPC insertion procedure such as; pain and discomfort, bleeding, pneumothorax, catheter dislodgement and cutaneous infection while pleural infection, catheter blockage, loculated effusion, loss of nutrients through regular drainage of effusion, catheter tract metastasis, fractures of catheter are uncommon complications associated with long term usage of IPC. Based on the largest review of IPC safety and efficacy, a majority (87.5%) of the patients who received IPC treatment did not experience any complications and in those patients that required catheter removal, only 8.5% were due to complications [140]. A later review documented the rate of complications following IPC management for MPE is up to 29% with the most common complication noted as empyema (up to 15%) [160].

Early Complications

Most of early complications if not all are not unique to IPC procedure but rather are risks associated with small bore catheter insertion using the Seldinger technique (although technically IPC may not be considered as small bore catheter ≤ 14 French). Major complications directly associated with IPC procedure are rare and there has been no reported case of death with IPC insertion in any patient groups [139, 140]. Some degree of discomfort with IPC insertion is expected, adequate local anesthesia and minimal amount of sedation may suffice in the majority of the patients. Pain associated with IPC insertion has been reported in 5.6% of patients in one large systematic review [140]. One case series reported transient occurrence of pain lasting < 3 days in 35% of patients undergoing IPC insertion with VATS [141], this is most likely related to the VATS procedure rather than IPC itself. Discomfort during the initial fluid drainage may indicate complete emptying of the pleural fluid or occurrence of trapped lung and should prompt cessation of drainage session. Severe persistent pain post catheter insertion may indicate intercostal nerve injury and may require catheter removal.

The presence of a small amount of free air in the pleura detected on post procedure X-ray immediately following catheter insertion is common. It should not cause any harm and will resolve spontaneously without any further intervention. The presence of a trapped lung may be uncovered by the removal of the fluid and its presence may simulate incidence of pneumothorax. Further radiologic examination with computed tomography may aid the diagnosis and will not warrant further pleural procedures. Large and symptomatic collection of air may indicate iatrogenic injury to the visceral structure, a connection of IPC to standard underwater seal through appropriate adapter and hospitalization is warranted till the pneumothorax completely resolves.

The other known immediate complications of IPC procedure are cellulitis (3.4%), catheter dislocation or dislodgement (2.2%) and bleeding (0.4%) [140]. Cellulitis can be prevented with proper maintaining of sterile field and application of universal precaution.

A quality improvement intervention study by Gilbert *et al.* found that cellulitis rates drop to 0% from 1.5% with preoperative antibiotics, full-body sterile draping, and limiting placement of IPC to a single defined location [161]. The infections that result in cellulitis can easily be treated with proper oral antibiotic on an outpatient basis. Some degree of bruises is a common occurrence post IPC insertion, especially along the tunneled tract and it should resolve spontaneously after a few days. Persistent hematoma, continuous oozing from incision site and frank hemorrhagic effusion may necessitate further evaluation as well as review of medications. Dislodgement of the catheter can be prevented by applying stay suture, proper dressing application, appropriate placement of polyester cuff (1 to 2 cm from the skin exit), and control of patient's cough. Improving physician training on IPC insertion with didactic lectures, practical training session and supervised insertion as well as improve site selection using pleural ultrasound may reduce immediate complication rates from IPC insertion [162].

Late Complications

IPC-related pleural infection remains a major concern for patients and treating clinicians, especially among oncologists who administer immunosuppressive chemotherapy. A review of IPC-related complications by Lui *et al.* has found that the incidence of IPC-related infection ranges from 0% to 12% [163]. The two earlier largest collections of IPC data, one a systematic review of 19 studies [140] and another from a multicenter trial in Europe, North America and Australasia [164], reported pleural infection rates of 2.8% and 4.7% respectively with typical time to infection around 4 to 8 weeks post IPC insertion. Therefore, it is unlikely that the IPC-related pleural infections were the results of insertion procedure. Hence, education as well as practice of proper handling and aftercare of the catheter are the best options to prevent IPC-related pleural infection.

The most common organisms involved in IPC-related infection are *Staphylococcus spp* (especially *S. aureus*), followed by *Pseudomonas Aeruginosa* and Enterobacteriaceae [164]. Most of reported cases of IPC-related infections have been mild and resolve with antibiotic treatment without requiring surgical intervention [164]. Based on the only large study that includes mortality data on its analysis showed that IPC-related infection has a mortality of 0.29% in all patients treated with IPC and 6% among those who had IPC-related infection [164]. Interestingly, the rate of mortality in IPC-related pleural infection is lower than mortality in an earlier reported large case series of community-acquired pleural infection [165]. The low mortality rate has been hypothesized to be due to regular care received by IPC-treated patients allowing earlier detection of infection and the presence of IPC that provides ready access to drainage of infected effusion as well as enables the use of intrapleural tissue plasminogen activator/DNase therapy [163]. Catheter removal is not necessary in IPC-related pleural infection due to reasons stated earlier, unless in cases of persistent infection that fails to respond to antibiotic therapy.

Other commonly reported IPC-related complication is catheter blockage which has been reported to range up to 18% and is defined as a sudden reduction to less than 10 ml in pleural fluid drainage with fluid visualized in the thorax on ultrasound or radiography [162, 166]. Formation of fibrous tissue around or within the fenestrated part of the catheter may contribute to catheter blockage. The instillation of a fibrinolytic agent through the catheter has been shown to be safe and effective in restoring function of an obstructed IPC without an increased risk of bleeding [166]. Other available management strategies for IPC-related blockage include flushing the catheter with saline, retrograde mechanical instrumentation of the catheter and catheter removal. Catheter removal may be the preferred option in patients with blocked catheter with radiologically confirmed little residual fluid left in the pleura [163].

A reduction in catheter drainage might be due to IPC-related symptomatic loculation which is defined by residual pleural effusion that fails to evacuate through a patent catheter confirmed by chest radiography, residual effusion causing breathlessness and it's not due to infection [167].

It has been reported to range up to 14% of IPC-treated patients, and typically occurs at about 2 months after IPC insertion [130, 147, 167]. Instillation of a fibrinolytic agent through the catheter has been shown to be safe and effective in restoring function of an IPC-related loculated effusion with risk of pleural bleeding in a small percentage of patients [167]. Other management options include pleural aspiration, removal of the ineffective IPC and insertion of a second catheter targeting the residual locules can be considered in selected cases [163].

Catheter tract metastases (CTM) may complicate patients with IPC, typically presenting with a new and frequently painful subcutaneous mass or nodules near the IPC insertion site. CTM is caused by seeding of pleural tumor along the IPC tract, commonly associated with malignant mesothelioma but can arise with any underlying pleural malignancy [168, 169]. The risk of developing CTM is increased with time and usually develops late (median 280 days) after IPC insertion [168]. CTM can be treated with external beam radiotherapy and analgesia to relieve the associated pain without the need for catheter removal [163, 168]. External beam radiation is not associated with any detrimental effect on the catheter [168].

Loss of proteins, electrolytes and other nutrients through drained pleural fluid is possible especially with exudative, voluminous and long term use of IPC [163]. However, there is no documented conclusive evidence that the loss of nutrients causes significant detrimental effect to patients [135].

Table 6. Summary of IPC-related late complications and management options.

Complication	Management
Pleural Infection	- Intravenous antibiotic - May require hospitalization in moderate to severe cases
Symptomatic loculation	- Instillation of fibrinolytic agent +/- DNase - Percutaneous aspiration of locules
Catheter tract metastases	- Analgesia - External beam radiation as prophylaxis and treatment
Blockage	- Instillation of saline solution - fibrinolytic agent - manual manipulation - removal of catheter
Nutrition loss	- observation and improvement in overall nutritional status
Fractured catheter	- conservative management

Fracture of catheter may occur during the removal process leaving a portion of the catheter inside the pleura. It may happen due to forceful traction applied during removal process or intentional iatrogenic severing to free-up completely embedded IPC [170]. Retained catheter fragment inside the pleural cavity is not associated with any adverse consequences [170]. Table **6** summarizes the late complications of IPC and its management.

PLEUROPERITONEAL SHUNT

Pleuroperitoneal shunt (PPS) is a device tunneled beneath the skin with its ends connecting the pleural space and peritoneal cavity. The mid portion of the tunneled PPS tube is a pump that could operate manually (Denver shunt) or operated by passive drainage (LaVeen shunt). The indications for use of PPS in MPE patients is almost the same as for IPC; that is to treat patients with trapped lung, in those who have failed chemical pleurodesis, or for patients who cannot undergo surgery. Aside from similarities in indications with IPC, high incidence of complications such as catheter blockage and infection [171, 172], and the fact that the device needs to be operated manually have led to the management with PPS falling out of favor compared to IPC.

There are limited studies done on the role of PPS in the management of MPE and the majority of these studies were retrospective reviews involving small number of cases. A retrospective review by Schulze *et al.* of PPS performed in a single center in Germany comparing PPS *vs* talc pleurodesis, showed a longer operative time (55 *vs* 35 minutes), shorter hospital stay (8.1 *vs* 10.7 days), higher complication rates (14.3% *vs* 2.8%), lower success rates (57.1% *vs* 92.3%), and shorter survival length (4.3 *vs* 6.7 months) than talc pleurodesis [173]. Another retrospective review by Genc *et al.* on 160 cases of PPS done at 2 centers in United Kingdom showed higher pleurodesis rate of 95%, mean hospital stay of 6.2 days, complication rate of 14.8% and mean survival length of 7.7 months [174]. All of the PPS procedures in this study were performed by surgeons following rigid bronchoscopy and VATS.

TREATMENT ALGORITHM FOR MPE

There are many management options available in patients with MPE and several different treatment algorithms have been proposed [65]. Fig. (**3**) illustrated our preferred algorithm for management of patient with MPE.

CONCLUSION

MPE signifies far advanced stage of malignancy and the most important goal of MPE treatment should be aimed at controlling patient's symptoms and improving QoL. More emphasis should be placed on patient reported outcome measures such as symptoms relief, hospitalization and objective QoL assessment.

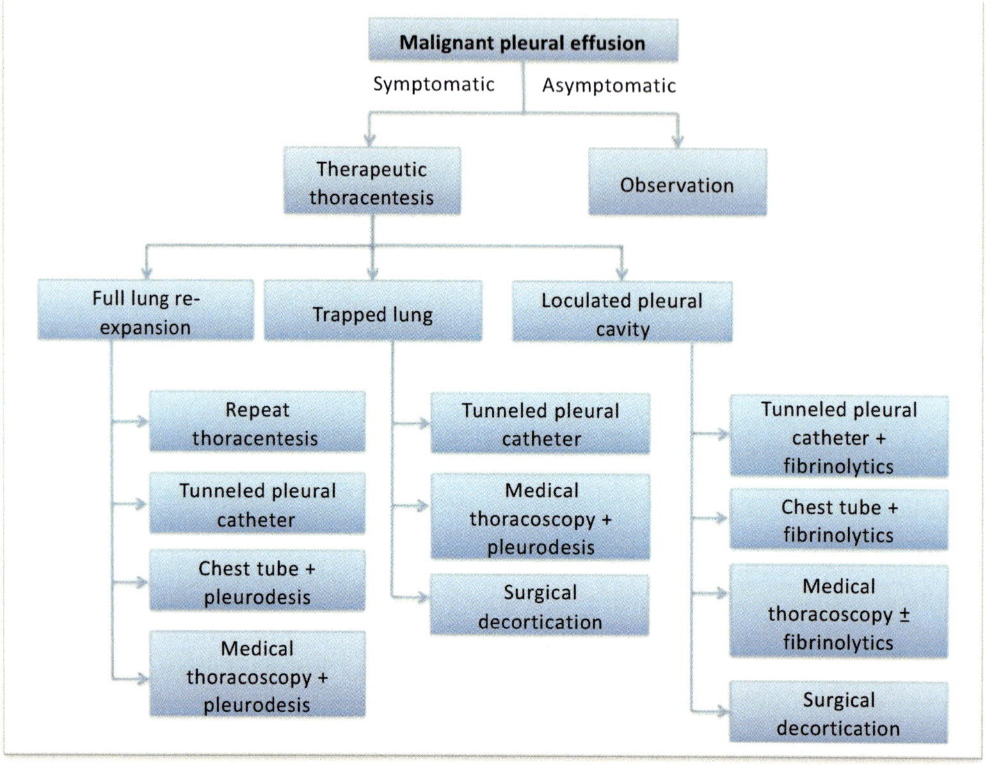

Fig. (3). Treatment algorithm for MPE (permission obtained from the author) [2].

While pleurodesis has been the standard of care for the management of MPE for many years, reports on IPC treatment for MPE have increased over the past 15 years, and international guidelines on MPE treatment now include both modalities as viable approaches. There is no clear superiority of either option that has been established and both remain valid therapeutic options for patients with MPE. It is of utmost importance to consider the patient's overall prognosis, symptoms, functional status, and social and financial situation when selecting the modality of treatment and combination of several treatment modalities may be beneficial in certain groups of patients. In managing MPE cases, it is advisable to select the most cost-effective, least invasive and most likely modality to lead to fewer hospitalisation days.

CONFLICT OF INTEREST

The authors declare no conflict of interest, financial or otherwise.

ACKNOWLEDGEMENTS

Declared none.

REFERENCES

[1] American Thoracic Society. Management of malignant pleural effusions. Am J Respir Crit Care Med 2000; 162(5): 1987-2001. [http://dx.doi.org/10.1164/ajrccm.162.5.ats8-00] [PMID: 11069845]

[2] Thomas JM, Musani AI. Malignant pleural effusions: a review. Clin Chest Med 2013; 34(3): 459-71. [http://dx.doi.org/10.1016/j.ccm.2013.05.004] [PMID: 23993817]

[3] Mishra EK, Davies HE, Lee YC. Malignant pleural disease in primary lung cancer.Thoracic malignancies European respiratory monograph Sheffield, UK: European Respiratory Society Journals Ltd. 2009; pp. 318-35. [http://dx.doi.org/10.1183/1025448x.00044019]

[4] Clive AO, Kahan BC, Hooper CE, *et al.* Predicting survival in malignant pleural effusion: development and validation of the LENT prognostic score. Thorax 2014; 69(12): 1098-104. [http://dx.doi.org/10.1136/thoraxjnl-2014-205285] [PMID: 25100651]

[5] Hsu C. Cytologic detection of malignancy in pleural effusion: a review of 5,255 samples from 3,811 patients. Diagn Cytopathol 1987; 3(1): 8-12. [http://dx.doi.org/10.1002/dc.2840030103] [PMID: 3568976]

[6] Sears D, Hajdu SI. The cytologic diagnosis of malignant neoplasms in pleural and peritoneal effusions. Acta Cytol 1987; 31(2): 85-97. [PMID: 3469856]

[7] Johnston WW. The malignant pleural effusion. A review of cytopathologic diagnoses of 584 specimens from 472 consecutive patients. Cancer 1985; 56(4): 905-9. [http://dx.doi.org/10.1002/1097-0142(19850815)56:4<905::AID-CNCR2820560435>3.0.CO;2-U] [PMID: 4016683]

[8] Chernow B, Sahn SA. Carcinomatous involvement of the pleura: an analysis of 96 patients. Am J Med 1977; 63(5): 695-702. [http://dx.doi.org/10.1016/0002-9343(77)90154-1] [PMID: 930945]

[9] Salyer WR, Eggleston JC, Erozan YS. Efficacy of pleural needle biopsy and pleural fluid cytopathology in the diagnosis of malignant neoplasm involving the pleura. Chest 1975; 67(5): 536-9. [http://dx.doi.org/10.1378/chest.67.5.536] [PMID: 1126189]

[10] Heffner JE. Diagnosis and management of malignant pleural effusions. Respirology 2008; 13(1): 5-20. [PMID: 18197908]

[11] Light RW. Pleural Diseases. Wolters Kluwer Health 2013.

[12] Nickell LT Jr, Lichtenberger JP III, Khorashadi L, Abbott GF, Carter BW. Multimodality imaging for characterization, classification, and staging of malignant pleural mesothelioma. Radiographics 2014; 34(6): 1692-706. [http://dx.doi.org/10.1148/rg.346130089] [PMID: 25310424]

[13] Awasthi A, Gupta N, Srinivasan R, Nijhawan R, Rajwanshi A. Cytopathological spectrum of unusual malignant pleural effusions at a tertiary care centre in north India. Cytopathology 2007; 18(1): 28-32. [http://dx.doi.org/10.1111/j.1365-2303.2007.00382.x] [PMID: 17250600]

[14] Porcel JM, Gasol A, Bielsa S, Civit C, Light RW, Salud A. Clinical features and survival of lung cancer patients with pleural effusions. Respirology 2015; 20(4): 654-9. [http://dx.doi.org/10.1111/resp.12496] [PMID: 25706291]

[15] Morgensztern D, Waqar S, Subramanian J, Trinkaus K, Govindan R. Prognostic impact of malignant

pleural effusion at presentation in patients with metastatic non-small-cell lung cancer. Journal of thoracic oncology : official publication of the International Association for the Study of Lung Cancer 2012; 7(10): 1485-9.
[http://dx.doi.org/10.1097/JTO.0b013e318267223a]

[16] Valentine VG, Raffin TA. The management of chylothorax. Chest 1992; 102(2): 586-91.
[http://dx.doi.org/10.1378/chest.102.2.586] [PMID: 1643953]

[17] Das DK. Serous effusions in malignant lymphomas: a review. Diagn Cytopathol 2006; 34(5): 335-47.
[http://dx.doi.org/10.1002/dc.20432] [PMID: 16604559]

[18] Zocchi L. Physiology and pathophysiology of pleural fluid turnover. Eur Respir J 2002; 20(6): 1545-58.
[http://dx.doi.org/10.1183/09031936.02.00062102] [PMID: 12503717]

[19] Meyer PC. Metastatic carcinoma of the pleura. Thorax 1966; 21(5): 437-43.
[http://dx.doi.org/10.1136/thx.21.5.437] [PMID: 5969243]

[20] Light RW, Hamm H. Malignant pleural effusion: would the real cause please stand up? Eur Respir J 1997; 10(8): 1701-2.
[http://dx.doi.org/10.1183/09031936.97.10081701] [PMID: 9272907]

[21] Jennings N, John H, Matthew LD, *et al.* A Systematic Review For Identifiable Causes Of Paramalignant Pleural Effusions.C46 PLEURAL DISEASES: DIAGNOSIS AND MANAGEMENT edn. American Thoracic Society 2013; pp. A4317-7.

[22] Sahn SA. Pleural diseases related to metastatic malignancies. Eur Respir J 1997; 10(8): 1907-13.
[http://dx.doi.org/10.1183/09031936.97.10081907] [PMID: 9272937]

[23] Yano S, Shinohara H, Herbst RS, *et al.* Production of experimental malignant pleural effusions is dependent on invasion of the pleura and expression of vascular endothelial growth factor/vascular permeability factor by human lung cancer cells. Am J Pathol 2000; 157(6): 1893-903.
[http://dx.doi.org/10.1016/S0002-9440(10)64828-6] [PMID: 11106562]

[24] Moschos C, Psallidas I, Kollintza A, *et al.* The angiopoietin/Tie2 axis mediates malignant pleural effusion formation. Neoplasia 2009; 11(3): 298-304.
[http://dx.doi.org/10.1593/neo.81480] [PMID: 19242611]

[25] Gary Lee YC, Melkerneker D, Thompson PJ, Light RW, Lane KB. Transforming growth factor beta induces vascular endothelial growth factor elaboration from pleural mesothelial cells in vivo and in vitro. Am J Respir Crit Care Med 2002; 165(1): 88-94.
[http://dx.doi.org/10.1164/ajrccm.165.1.2104006] [PMID: 11779736]

[26] Yeh HH, Lai WW, Chen HH, Liu HS, Su WC. Autocrine IL-6-induced Stat3 activation contributes to the pathogenesis of lung adenocarcinoma and malignant pleural effusion. Oncogene 2006; 25(31): 4300-9.
[http://dx.doi.org/10.1038/sj.onc.1209464] [PMID: 16518408]

[27] Stathopoulos GT, Kollintza A, Moschos C, *et al.* Tumor necrosis factor-alpha promotes malignant pleural effusion. Cancer Res 2007; 67(20): 9825-34.
[http://dx.doi.org/10.1158/0008-5472.CAN-07-1064] [PMID: 17942913]

[28] Stathopoulos GT, Psallidas I, Moustaki A, *et al.* A central role for tumor-derived monocyte chemoattractant protein-1 in malignant pleural effusion. J Natl Cancer Inst 2008; 100(20): 1464-76.
[http://dx.doi.org/10.1093/jnci/djn325] [PMID: 18840818]

[29] Psallidas I, Stathopoulos GT, Maniatis NA, *et al.* Secreted phosphoprotein-1 directly provokes vascular leakage to foster malignant pleural effusion. Oncogene 2013; 32(4): 528-35.
[http://dx.doi.org/10.1038/onc.2012.57] [PMID: 22370646]

[30] Spella M, Giannou AD, Stathopoulos GT. Switching off malignant pleural effusion formation-fantasy or future? J Thorac Dis 2015; 7(6): 1009-20.
[PMID: 26150914]

[31] Judson MA, Sahn SA. Pulmonary Physiologic Abnormalities Caused by Pleural Disease. Semin Respir Crit Care Med 1995; 16(04): 346-53.
[http://dx.doi.org/10.1055/s-2007-1009846]

[32] Alves SH, Amato MB, Terra RM, Vargas FS, Caruso P. Lung reaeration and reventilation after aspiration of pleural effusions. A study using electrical impedance tomography. Ann Am Thorac Soc 2014; 11(2): 186-91.
[http://dx.doi.org/10.1513/AnnalsATS.201306-142OC] [PMID: 24308560]

[33] Marel M, Stastny B, Melínová L, Svandová E, Light RW. Diagnosis of pleural effusions. Experience with clinical studies, 1986 to 1990. Chest 1995; 107(6): 1598-603.
[http://dx.doi.org/10.1378/chest.107.6.1598] [PMID: 7781353]

[34] Maher GG, Berger HW. Massive pleural effusion: malignant and nonmalignant causes in 46 patients. Am Rev Respir Dis 1972; 105(3): 458-60.
[PMID: 4501503]

[35] Ashchi M, Golish J, Eng P, O'Donovan P. Transudative malignant pleural effusions: prevalence and mechanisms. South Med J 1998; 91(1): 23-6.
[http://dx.doi.org/10.1097/00007611-199801000-00004] [PMID: 9438397]

[36] Light RW, Erozan YS, Ball WC Jr. Cells in pleural fluid. Their value in differential diagnosis. Arch Intern Med 1973; 132(6): 854-60.
[http://dx.doi.org/10.1001/archinte.1973.03650120060011] [PMID: 4757257]

[37] Villena V, López-Encuentra A, García-Luján R, Echave-Sustaeta J, Martínez CJ. Clinical implications of appearance of pleural fluid at thoracentesis. Chest 2004; 125(1): 156-9.
[http://dx.doi.org/10.1378/chest.125.1.156] [PMID: 14718435]

[38] Ozcakar B, Martinez CH, Morice RC, *et al.* Does pleural fluid appearance really matter? The relationship between fluid appearance and cytology, cell counts, and chemical laboratory measurements in pleural effusions of patients with cancer. J Cardiothorac Surg 2010; 5: 63.
[http://dx.doi.org/10.1186/1749-8090-5-63] [PMID: 20718978]

[39] Hooper C, Lee YC, Maskell N, Group BT. Investigation of a unilateral pleural effusion in adults: British Thoracic Society Pleural Disease Guideline 2010. Thorax 2010; 65 (Suppl. 2): ii4-ii17.
[http://dx.doi.org/10.1136/thx.2010.136978] [PMID: 20696692]

[40] Ordóñez NG. What are the current best immunohistochemical markers for the diagnosis of epithelioid mesothelioma? A review and update. Hum Pathol 2007; 38(1): 1-16.
[http://dx.doi.org/10.1016/j.humpath.2006.08.010] [PMID: 17056092]

[41] Westfall DE, Fan X, Marchevsky AM. Evidence-based guidelines to optimize the selection of antibody panels in cytopathology: pleural effusions with malignant epithelioid cells. Diagn Cytopathol 2010; 38(1): 9-14.
[PMID: 19626629]

[42] Fetsch PA, Abati A. Immunocytochemistry in effusion cytology: a contemporary review. Cancer 2001; 93(5): 293-308.
[http://dx.doi.org/10.1002/cncr.9044] [PMID: 11668464]

[43] Carter J, Miller JA, Feller-Kopman D, Ettinger D, Sidransky D, Maleki Z. Molecular Profiling of Malignant Pleural Effusion in Metastatic Non-Small-Cell Lung Carcinoma. The Effect of Preanalytical Factors. Ann Am Thorac Soc 2017; 14(7): 1169-76.
[PMID: 28557526]

[44] Bellevicine C, Malapelle U, de Luca C, Iaccarino A, Troncone G. EGFR analysis: current evidence and future directions. Diagn Cytopathol 2014; 42(11): 984-92.
[http://dx.doi.org/10.1002/dc.23142] [PMID: 24619906]

[45] Wang W, Tang Y, Li J, Jiang L, Jiang Y, Su X. Detection of ALK rearrangements in malignant pleural effusion cell blocks from patients with advanced non-small cell lung cancer: a comparison of Ventana

immunohistochemistry and fluorescence in situ hybridization. Cancer Cytopathol 2015; 123(2): 117-22.
[http://dx.doi.org/10.1002/cncy.21510] [PMID: 25529354]

[46] Goldstraw P, Crowley J, Chansky K, *et al.* International Association for the Study of Lung Cancer International Staging C. The IASLC Lung Cancer Staging Project: proposals for the revision of the TNM stage groupings in the forthcoming (seventh) edition of the TNM Classification of malignant tumours. Journal of thoracic oncology : official publication of the International Association for the Study of Lung Cancer 2007; 2(8): 706-14.

[47] Abbruzzese JL, Abbruzzese MC, Hess KR, Raber MN, Lenzi R, Frost P. Unknown primary carcinoma: natural history and prognostic factors in 657 consecutive patients. J Clin Oncol 1994; 12(6): 1272-80.
[http://dx.doi.org/10.1200/JCO.1994.12.6.1272] [PMID: 8201389]

[48] van de Molengraft FJ, Vooijs GP. Survival of patients with malignancy-associated effusions. Acta Cytol 1989; 33(6): 911-6.
[PMID: 2588923]

[49] Bonnefoi H, Smith IE. How should cancer presenting as a malignant pleural effusion be managed? Br J Cancer 1996; 74(5): 832-5.
[http://dx.doi.org/10.1038/bjc.1996.444] [PMID: 8795590]

[50] Bielsa S, Salud A, Martínez M, *et al.* Prognostic significance of pleural fluid data in patients with malignant effusion. Eur J Intern Med 2008; 19(5): 334-9.
[http://dx.doi.org/10.1016/j.ejim.2007.09.014] [PMID: 18549935]

[51] Ozyurtkan MO, Balci AE, Cakmak M. Predictors of mortality within three months in the patients with malignant pleural effusion. Eur J Intern Med 2010; 21(1): 30-4.
[http://dx.doi.org/10.1016/j.ejim.2009.09.012] [PMID: 20122610]

[52] Pilling JE, Dusmet ME, Ladas G, Goldstraw P. Prognostic factors for survival after surgical palliation of malignant pleural effusion. Journal of thoracic oncology : official publication of the International Association for the Study of Lung Cancer 2010; 5(10): 1544-50.
[http://dx.doi.org/10.1097/JTO.0b013e3181e95cb8]

[53] Burrows CM, Mathews WC, Colt HG. Predicting survival in patients with recurrent symptomatic malignant pleural effusions: an assessment of the prognostic values of physiologic, morphologic, and quality of life measures of extent of disease. Chest 2000; 117(1): 73-8.
[http://dx.doi.org/10.1378/chest.117.1.73] [PMID: 10631202]

[54] Sahn SA, Good JT Jr. Pleural fluid pH in malignant effusions. Diagnostic, prognostic, and therapeutic implications. Ann Intern Med 1988; 108(3): 345-9.
[http://dx.doi.org/10.7326/0003-4819-108-3-345] [PMID: 3341671]

[55] Heffner JE, Nietert PJ, Barbieri C. Pleural fluid pH as a predictor of pleurodesis failure: analysis of primary data. Chest 2000; 117(1): 87-95.
[http://dx.doi.org/10.1378/chest.117.1.87] [PMID: 10631204]

[56] Davies HE, Lee YC. Management of malignant pleural effusions: questions that need answers. Curr Opin Pulm Med 2013; 19(4): 374-9.
[http://dx.doi.org/10.1097/MCP.0b013e3283615b67] [PMID: 23673450]

[57] Thomas R, Francis R, Davies HE, Lee YC. Interventional therapies for malignant pleural effusions: the present and the future. Respirology 2014; 19(6): 809-22.
[http://dx.doi.org/10.1111/resp.12328] [PMID: 24947955]

[58] Villanueva AG, Gray AW Jr, Shahian DM, Williamson WA, Beamis JF Jr. Efficacy of short term *versus* long term tube thoracostomy drainage before tetracycline pleurodesis in the treatment of malignant pleural effusions. Thorax 1994; 49(1): 23-5.
[http://dx.doi.org/10.1136/thx.49.1.23] [PMID: 7512285]

[59] Hausheer FH, Yarbro JW. Diagnosis and treatment of malignant pleural effusion. Semin Oncol 1985; 12(1): 54-75.
[PMID: 2579439]

[60] Duncan DR, Morgenthaler TI, Ryu JH, Daniels CE. Reducing iatrogenic risk in thoracentesis: establishing best practice via experiential training in a zero-risk environment. Chest 2009; 135(5): 1315-20.
[http://dx.doi.org/10.1378/chest.08-1227] [PMID: 19017865]

[61] Cavanna L, Mordenti P, Bertè R, *et al.* Ultrasound guidance reduces pneumothorax rate and improves safety of thoracentesis in malignant pleural effusion: report on 445 consecutive patients with advanced cancer. World J Surg Oncol 2014; 12: 139.
[http://dx.doi.org/10.1186/1477-7819-12-139] [PMID: 24886486]

[62] Jones PW, Moyers JP, Rogers JT, Rodriguez RM, Lee YC, Light RW. Ultrasound-guided thoracentesis: is it a safer method? Chest 2003; 123(2): 418-23.
[http://dx.doi.org/10.1378/chest.123.2.418] [PMID: 12576360]

[63] Echevarria C, Twomey D, Dunning J, Chanda B. Does re-expansion pulmonary oedema exist? Interact Cardiovasc Thorac Surg 2008; 7(3): 485-9.
[http://dx.doi.org/10.1510/icvts.2008.178087] [PMID: 18334522]

[64] Light RW, Jenkinson SG, Minh VD, George RB. Observations on pleural fluid pressures as fluid is withdrawn during thoracentesis. Am Rev Respir Dis 1980; 121(5): 799-804.
[PMID: 7406313]

[65] Roberts ME, Neville E, Berrisford RG, Antunes G, Ali NJ, Group BT. BTS Pleural Disease Guideline Group. Management of a malignant pleural effusion: British Thoracic Society Pleural Disease Guideline 2010. Thorax 2010; 65 (Suppl. 2): ii32-40.
[http://dx.doi.org/10.1136/thx.2010.136994] [PMID: 20696691]

[66] Wu SG, Yu CJ, Tsai MF, *et al.* Survival of lung adenocarcinoma patients with malignant pleural effusion. Eur Respir J 2013; 41(6): 1409-18.
[http://dx.doi.org/10.1183/09031936.00069812] [PMID: 23018906]

[67] Guo H, Wan Y, Tian G, *et al.* EGFR mutations predict a favorable outcome for malignant pleural effusion of lung adenocarcinoma with Tarceva therapy. Oncol Rep 2012; 27(3): 880-90.
[PMID: 22134479]

[68] MacDuff A, Arnold A, Harvey J, Group BT. BTS Pleural Disease Guideline Group. Management of spontaneous pneumothorax: British Thoracic Society Pleural Disease Guideline 2010. Thorax 2010; 65 (Suppl. 2): ii18-31.
[http://dx.doi.org/10.1136/thx.2010.136986] [PMID: 20696690]

[69] Davidoff D, Naparstek Y, Eliakim M. The use of pleurodesis for intractable pleural effusion due to congestive heart failure. Postgrad Med J 1983; 59(691): 330-1.
[http://dx.doi.org/10.1136/pgmj.59.691.330] [PMID: 6878108]

[70] Glazer M, Berkman N, Lafair JS, Kramer MR. Successful talc slurry pleurodesis in patients with nonmalignant pleural effusion. Chest 2000; 117(5): 1404-9.
[http://dx.doi.org/10.1378/chest.117.5.1404] [PMID: 10807829]

[71] Maldonado F, Tazelaar HD, Wang CW, Ryu JH. Yellow nail syndrome: analysis of 41 consecutive patients. Chest 2008; 134(2): 375-81.
[http://dx.doi.org/10.1378/chest.08-0137] [PMID: 18403655]

[72] Vargas FS, Milanez JR, Filomeno LT, Fernandez A, Jatene A, Light RW. Intrapleural talc for the prevention of recurrence in benign or undiagnosed pleural effusions. Chest 1994; 106(6): 1771-5.
[http://dx.doi.org/10.1378/chest.106.6.1771] [PMID: 7988198]

[73] Temes RT, Davis MS, Follis FM, Pett SB Jr, Wernly JA. Videothoracoscopic treatment of hepatic hydrothorax. Ann Thorac Surg 1997; 64(5): 1468-9.

[http://dx.doi.org/10.1016/S0003-4975(97)01061-8] [PMID: 9386726]

[74] Szeto CC, Chow KM. Pathogenesis and management of hydrothorax complicating peritoneal dialysis. Curr Opin Pulm Med 2004; 10(4): 315-9. [http://dx.doi.org/10.1097/01.mcp.0000127901.60693.d0] [PMID: 15220759]

[75] Breuer GS, Deeb M, Fisher D, Nesher G. Therapeutic options for refractory massive pleural effusion in systemic lupus erythematosus: a case study and review of the literature. Semin Arthritis Rheum 2005; 34(5): 744-9. [http://dx.doi.org/10.1016/j.semarthrit.2004.11.003] [PMID: 15846590]

[76] Akin H, Olcmen A, Isgorucu O, Denizkiran I, Dincer I. Approach to patients with chylothorax complicating pulmonary resection. Thorac Cardiovasc Surg 2012; 60(2): 135-9. [http://dx.doi.org/10.1055/s-0030-1270990] [PMID: 21557161]

[77] Rodriguez-Panadero F, Montes-Worboys A. Mechanisms of Pleurodesis. Respiration; international review of thoracic diseases 2012; 83(2): 91-8. [http://dx.doi.org/10.1159/000335419]

[78] Antony VB, Hott JW, Kunkel SL, Godbey SW, Burdick MD, Strieter RM. Pleural mesothelial cell expression of C-C (monocyte chemotactic peptide) and C-X-C (interleukin 8) chemokines. Am J Respir Cell Mol Biol 1995; 12(6): 581-8. [http://dx.doi.org/10.1165/ajrcmb.12.6.7766422] [PMID: 7766422]

[79] Xie C, Teixeira LR, McGovern JP, Light RW. Systemic corticosteroids decrease the effectiveness of talc pleurodesis. Am J Respir Crit Care Med 1998; 157(5 Pt 1): 1441-4. [http://dx.doi.org/10.1164/ajrccm.157.5.9708032] [PMID: 9603121]

[80] Teixeira LR, Vargas FS, Acencio MM, *et al.* Influence of antiinflammatory drugs (methylprednisolone and diclofenac sodium) on experimental pleurodesis induced by silver nitrate or talc. Chest 2005; 128(6): 4041-5. [http://dx.doi.org/10.1378/chest.128.6.4041] [PMID: 16354879]

[81] Teixeira LR, Wu W, Chang D-S, Light RW. The effect of corticosteroids on pleurodesis induced by doxycycline in rabbits. Chest 2002; 121(1): 216-9. [http://dx.doi.org/10.1378/chest.121.1.216] [PMID: 11796454]

[82] Genofre EH, Vargas FS, Antonangelo L, *et al.* Ultrastructural acute features of active remodeling after chemical pleurodesis induced by silver nitrate or talc. Lung 2005; 183(3): 197-207. [http://dx.doi.org/10.1007/s00408-004-2536-x] [PMID: 16078041]

[83] Marchi E, Vargas FS, Acencio MM, Antonangelo L, Genofre EH, Teixeira LR. Evidence that mesothelial cells regulate the acute inflammatory response in talc pleurodesis. Eur Respir J 2006; 28(5): 929-32. [http://dx.doi.org/10.1183/09031936.06.00037906] [PMID: 16870666]

[84] Bethune N. Pleural poudrage: new technique for deliberate production of pleural adhesions as preliminary to lobectomy. J Thorac Surg 1935; 4: 251.

[85] Dikensoy O, Light RW. Alternative widely available, inexpensive agents for pleurodesis. Curr Opin Pulm Med 2005; 11(4): 340-4. [http://dx.doi.org/10.1097/01.mcp.0000166587.24127.91] [PMID: 15928503]

[86] Rinaldo JE, Owens GR, Rogers RM. Adult respiratory distress syndrome following intrapleural instillation of talc. J Thorac Cardiovasc Surg 1983; 85(4): 523-6. [PMID: 6834872]

[87] Azzopardi M, Porcel JM, Koegelenberg CF, Lee YC, Fysh ET. Current controversies in the management of malignant pleural effusions. Semin Respir Crit Care Med 2014; 35(6): 723-31. [http://dx.doi.org/10.1055/s-0034-1395795] [PMID: 25463163]

[88] Janssen JP, Collier G, Astoul P, *et al.* Safety of pleurodesis with talc poudrage in malignant pleural effusion: a prospective cohort study. Lancet 2007; 369(9572): 1535-9.

[http://dx.doi.org/10.1016/S0140-6736(07)60708-9] [PMID: 17482984]

[89] Maskell NA, Lee YC, Gleeson FV, Hedley EL, Pengelly G, Davies RJ. Randomized trials describing lung inflammation after pleurodesis with talc of varying particle size. Am J Respir Crit Care Med 2004; 170(4): 377-82.
[http://dx.doi.org/10.1164/rccm.200311-1579OC] [PMID: 15142871]

[90] Tan C, Sedrakyan A, Browne J, Swift S, Treasure T. The evidence on the effectiveness of management for malignant pleural effusion: a systematic review. European journal of cardio-thoracic surgery : official journal of the European Association for Cardio-thoracic Surgery 2006; 29(5): 829-38.
[http://dx.doi.org/10.1016/j.ejcts.2005.12.025]

[91] Shaw P, Agarwal R. Pleurodesis for malignant pleural effusions. Cochrane Database Syst Rev 2004; (1): CD002916.
[PMID: 14973997]

[92] Xia H, Wang XJ, Zhou Q, Shi HZ, Tong ZH. Efficacy and safety of talc pleurodesis for malignant pleural effusion: a meta-analysis. PLoS One 2014; 9(1): e87060.
[http://dx.doi.org/10.1371/journal.pone.0087060] [PMID: 24475222]

[93] Kennedy L, Sahn SA. Talc pleurodesis for the treatment of pneumothorax and pleural effusion. Chest 1994; 106(4): 1215-22.
[http://dx.doi.org/10.1378/chest.106.4.1215] [PMID: 7924497]

[94] Marchi E, Vargas FS, Teixeira LR, *et al.* Comparison of nitrogen mustard, cytarabine and dacarbazine as pleural sclerosing agents in rabbits. Eur Respir J 1997; 10(3): 598-602.
[PMID: 9072991]

[95] Heffner JE, Standerfer RJ, Torstveit J, Unruh L. Clinical efficacy of doxycycline for pleurodesis. Chest 1994; 105(6): 1743-7.
[http://dx.doi.org/10.1378/chest.105.6.1743] [PMID: 8205870]

[96] Almind M, Lange P, Viskum K. Spontaneous pneumothorax: comparison of simple drainage, talc pleurodesis, and tetracycline pleurodesis. Thorax 1989; 44(8): 627-30.
[http://dx.doi.org/10.1136/thx.44.8.627] [PMID: 2799742]

[97] Lee YC, Baumann MH, Maskell NA, *et al.* Pleurodesis practice for malignant pleural effusions in five English-speaking countries: survey of pulmonologists. Chest 2003; 124(6): 2229-38.
[http://dx.doi.org/10.1378/chest.124.6.2229] [PMID: 14665505]

[98] Alayouty HD, Hasan TM, Alhadad ZA, Omar Barabba R. Mechanical *versus* chemical pleurodesis for management of primary spontaneous pneumothorax evaluated with thoracic echography. Interact Cardiovasc Thorac Surg 2011; 13(5): 475-9.
[http://dx.doi.org/10.1510/icvts.2011.270280] [PMID: 21828109]

[99] Ng CK, Ko FW, Chan JW, *et al.* Minocycline and talc slurry pleurodesis for patients with secondary spontaneous pneumothorax. The international journal of tuberculosis and lung disease : the official journal of the International Union against Tuberculosis and Lung Disease 2010; 14(10): 1342-6.

[100] Ibrahim IM, Dokhan AL, El-Sessy AA, Eltaweel MF. Povidone-iodine pleurodesis *versus* talc pleurodesis in preventing recurrence of malignant pleural effusion. J Cardiothorac Surg 2015; 10: 64.
[http://dx.doi.org/10.1186/s13019-015-0270-5] [PMID: 25947235]

[101] Agarwal R, Aggarwal AN, Gupta D. Efficacy and safety of iodopovidone pleurodesis through tube thoracostomy. Respirology 2006; 11(1): 105-8.
[http://dx.doi.org/10.1111/j.1440-1843.2006.00792.x] [PMID: 16423210]

[102] Olivares-Torres CA, Laniado-Laborín R, Chávez-García C, León-Gastelum C, Reyes-Escamilla A, Light RW. Iodopovidone pleurodesis for recurrent pleural effusions. Chest 2002; 122(2): 581-3.
[http://dx.doi.org/10.1378/chest.122.2.581] [PMID: 12171835]

[103] Agarwal R, Khan A, Aggarwal AN, Gupta D. Efficacy & safety of iodopovidone pleurodesis: a systematic review & meta-analysis. Indian J Med Res 2012; 135: 297-304.

[PMID: 22561614]

[104] Bucknor A, Harrison-Phipps K, Davies T, Toufektzian L. Is silver nitrate an effective means of pleurodesis? Interact Cardiovasc Thorac Surg 2015; 21(4): 521-5. [http://dx.doi.org/10.1093/icvts/ivv182] [PMID: 26188199]

[105] Joshi V, Kirmani B, Zacharias J. Thoracotomy *versus* VATS: is there an optimal approach to treating pneumothorax? Ann R Coll Surg Engl 2013; 95(1): 61-4. [http://dx.doi.org/10.1308/003588413X13511609956138] [PMID: 23317731]

[106] Lardinois D, Vogt P, Yang L, Hegyi I, Baslam M, Weder W. Non-steroidal anti-inflammatory drugs decrease the quality of pleurodesis after mechanical pleural abrasion. European journal of cardio-thoracic surgery : official journal of the European Association for Cardio-thoracic Surgery 2004; 25(5): 865-71. [http://dx.doi.org/10.1016/j.ejcts.2004.01.028]

[107] Hunt I, Teh E, Southon R, Treasure T. Using non-steroidal anti-inflammatory drugs (NSAIDs) following pleurodesis. Interact Cardiovasc Thorac Surg 2007; 6(1): 102-4. [http://dx.doi.org/10.1510/icvts.2006.140400] [PMID: 17669782]

[108] Lizardo RE, Langness S, Davenport KP, *et al.* Ketorolac does not reduce effectiveness of pleurodesis in pediatric patients with spontaneous pneumothorax. J Pediatr Surg 2015; 50(12): 2035-7. [http://dx.doi.org/10.1016/j.jpedsurg.2015.08.017] [PMID: 26385568]

[109] Ben-Nun A, Golan N, Faibishenko I, Simansky D, Soudack M. Nonsteroidal antiinflammatory medications: efficient and safe treatment following video-assisted pleurodesis for spontaneous pneumothorax. World J Surg 2011; 35(11): 2563-7. [http://dx.doi.org/10.1007/s00268-011-1207-3] [PMID: 21882030]

[110] Dryzer SR, Allen ML, Strange C, Sahn SA. A comparison of rotation and nonrotation in tetracycline pleurodesis. Chest 1993; 104(6): 1763-6. [http://dx.doi.org/10.1378/chest.104.6.1763] [PMID: 8252959]

[111] Mager HJ, Maesen B, Verzijlbergen F, Schramel F. Distribution of talc suspension during treatment of malignant pleural effusion with talc pleurodesis. Lung Cancer 2002; 36(1): 77-81. [http://dx.doi.org/10.1016/S0169-5002(01)00475-5] [PMID: 11891037]

[112] Goodman A, Davies CW. Efficacy of short-term *versus* long-term chest tube drainage following talc slurry pleurodesis in patients with malignant pleural effusions: a randomised trial. Lung Cancer 2006; 54(1): 51-5. [http://dx.doi.org/10.1016/j.lungcan.2006.06.004] [PMID: 16920219]

[113] Chen JS, Chan WK, Tsai KT, *et al.* Simple aspiration and drainage and intrapleural minocycline pleurodesis *versus* simple aspiration and drainage for the initial treatment of primary spontaneous pneumothorax: an open-label, parallel-group, prospective, randomised, controlled trial. Lancet 2013; 381(9874): 1277-82. [http://dx.doi.org/10.1016/S0140-6736(12)62170-9] [PMID: 23489754]

[114] Rahman NM, Pepperell J, Rehal S, *et al.* Effect of opioids vs nsaids and larger vs smaller chest tube size on pain control and pleurodesis efficacy among patients with malignant pleural effusion: The time1 randomized clinical trial. JAMA 2015; 314(24): 2641-53. [http://dx.doi.org/10.1001/jama.2015.16840] [PMID: 26720026]

[115] Dresler CM, Olak J, Herndon JE II, *et al.* Cooperative Groups Cancer and Leukemia Group B; Eastern Cooperative Oncology Group; North Central Cooperative Oncology Group; Radiation Therapy Oncology Group. Phase III intergroup study of talc poudrage vs talc slurry sclerosis for malignant pleural effusion. Chest 2005; 127(3): 909-15. [http://dx.doi.org/10.1378/chest.127.3.909] [PMID: 15764775]

[116] Abraham G, Cherian JH, Gopalakrishnan TJ. Pyopneumothorax with bronchofleural fistula following tetracycline pleurodesis in a patient on CAPD. Peritoneal dialysis international : journal of the International Society for Peritoneal Dialysis 1992; 12(3): 327-8.

[117] Kennedy L, Rusch VW, Strange C, Ginsberg RJ, Sahn SA. Pleurodesis using talc slurry. Chest 1994; 106(2): 342-6.
[http://dx.doi.org/10.1378/chest.106.2.342] [PMID: 7774299]

[118] Janssen JP, Collier G, Astoul P, *et al.* Safety of pleurodesis with talc poudrage in malignant pleural effusion: a prospective cohort study. Lancet 2007; 369(9572): 1535-9.
[http://dx.doi.org/10.1016/S0140-6736(07)60708-9] [PMID: 17482984]

[119] Yim AP, Chan AT, Lee TW, Wan IY, Ho JK. Thoracoscopic talc insufflation *versus* talc slurry for symptomatic malignant pleural effusion. Ann Thorac Surg 1996; 62(6): 1655-8.
[http://dx.doi.org/10.1016/S0003-4975(96)00808-9] [PMID: 8957368]

[120] Haddad FJ, Younes RN, Gross JL, Deheinzelin D. Pleurodesis in patients with malignant pleural effusions: talc slurry or bleomycin? Results of a prospective randomized trial. World J Surg 2004; 28(8): 749-53.
[http://dx.doi.org/10.1007/s00268-004-7269-8] [PMID: 15457352]

[121] Ong KC, Indumathi V, Raghuram J, Ong YY. A comparative study of pleurodesis using talc slurry and bleomycin in the management of malignant pleural effusions. Respirology 2000; 5(2): 99-103.
[http://dx.doi.org/10.1046/j.1440-1843.2000.00235.x] [PMID: 10894097]

[122] Paschoalini MdaS, Vargas FS, Marchi E, *et al.* Prospective randomized trial of silver nitrate vs talc slurry in pleurodesis for symptomatic malignant pleural effusions. Chest 2005; 128(2): 684-9.
[http://dx.doi.org/10.1378/chest.128.2.684] [PMID: 16100154]

[123] Cho JS, Na KJ, Lee Y, *et al.* Chemical Pleurodesis Using Mistletoe Extraction (ABNOVAviscum® *Injection*) for Malignant Pleural Effusion. Annals of Thoracic and Cardiovascular Surgery 2015. advpub

[124] Wang X, Wang G, Zhang H, Zhang W. Pleurodesis with povidone-iodine *versus* talc in malignant pleural effusion: A retrospective study. Chest 2016; 149(4_S): A442-2.
[http://dx.doi.org/10.1016/j.chest.2016.02.460]

[125] Mohsen TA, Zeid AA, Meshref M, *et al.* Local iodine pleurodesis *versus* thoracoscopic talc insufflation in recurrent malignant pleural effusion: a prospective randomized control trial. European journal of cardio-thoracic surgery : official journal of the European Association for Cardio-thoracic Surgery 2011; 40(2): 282-6.

[126] Porcel JM, Salud A, Nabal M, Vives M, Esquerda A, Rodríguez-Panadero F. Rapid pleurodesis with doxycycline through a small-bore catheter for the treatment of metastatic malignant effusions. Support Care Cancer 2006; 14(5): 475-8.
[http://dx.doi.org/10.1007/s00520-005-0001-x] [PMID: 16404570]

[127] Putnam JB Jr, Light RW, Rodriguez RM, *et al.* A randomized comparison of indwelling pleural catheter and doxycycline pleurodesis in the management of malignant pleural effusions. Cancer 1999; 86(10): 1992-9.
[http://dx.doi.org/10.1002/(SICI)1097-0142(19991115)86:10<1992::AID-CNCR16>3.0.CO;2-M] [PMID: 10570423]

[128] Kuzdzał J, Sładek K, Wasowski D, *et al.* Talc powder vs doxycycline in the control of malignant pleural effusion: a prospective, randomized trial. Med Sci Monit 2003; 9(6): PI54-9.
[PMID: 12824959]

[129] Davies HE, Mishra EK, Kahan BC, *et al.* Effect of an indwelling pleural catheter vs chest tube and talc pleurodesis for relieving dyspnea in patients with malignant pleural effusion: the TIME2 randomized controlled trial. JAMA 2012; 307(22): 2383-9.
[http://dx.doi.org/10.1001/jama.2012.5535] [PMID: 22610520]

[130] Fysh ET, Waterer GW, Kendall PA, *et al.* Indwelling pleural catheters reduce inpatient days over pleurodesis for malignant pleural effusion. Chest 2012; 142(2): 394-400.
[http://dx.doi.org/10.1378/chest.11-2657] [PMID: 22406960]

[131] Hunt BM, Farivar AS, Vallières E, *et al.* Thoracoscopic talc *versus* tunneled pleural catheters for palliation of malignant pleural effusions. Ann Thorac Surg 2012; 94(4): 1053-7. [http://dx.doi.org/10.1016/j.athoracsur.2012.01.103] [PMID: 22513274]

[132] Srour N, Amjadi K, Forster A, Aaron S. Management of malignant pleural effusions with indwelling pleural catheters or talc pleurodesis. Canadian respiratory journal : journal of the Canadian Thoracic Society 2013; 20(2): 106-10. [http://dx.doi.org/10.1155/2013/842768]

[133] Bhatnagar R, Reid ED, Corcoran JP, *et al.* Indwelling pleural catheters for non-malignant effusions: a multicentre review of practice. Thorax 2014; 69(10): 959-61. [http://dx.doi.org/10.1136/thoraxjnl-2013-204563] [PMID: 24343783]

[134] DePew ZS, Iqbal S, Mullon JJ, Nichols FC, Maldonado F. The role for tunneled indwelling pleural catheters in patients with persistent benign chylothorax. Am J Med Sci 2013; 346(5): 349-52. [http://dx.doi.org/10.1097/MAJ.0b013e31827b936c] [PMID: 23426083]

[135] Jimenez CA, Mhatre AD, Martinez CH, Eapen GA, Onn A, Morice RC. Use of an indwelling pleural catheter for the management of recurrent chylothorax in patients with cancer. Chest 2007; 132(5): 1584-90. [http://dx.doi.org/10.1378/chest.06-2141] [PMID: 17890482]

[136] Srour N, Potechin R, Amjadi K. Use of indwelling pleural catheters for cardiogenic pleural effusions. Chest 2013; 144(5): 1603-8. [http://dx.doi.org/10.1378/chest.13-0331] [PMID: 23807028]

[137] Wahidi MM, Reddy C, Yarmus L, *et al.* Randomized Trial of Pleural Fluid Drainage Frequency in Patients with Malignant Pleural Effusions. The ASAP Trial. Am J Respir Crit Care Med 2017; 195(8): 1050-7. [http://dx.doi.org/10.1164/rccm.201607-1404OC] [PMID: 27898215]

[138] Freeman RK, Ascioti AJ, Mahidhara RS. A propensity-matched comparison of pleurodesis or tunneled pleural catheter in patients undergoing diagnostic thoracoscopy for malignancy. Ann Thorac Surg 2013; 96(1): 259-63. discussion 263-254 [http://dx.doi.org/10.1016/j.athoracsur.2013.03.063]

[139] Suzuki K, Servais EL, Rizk NP, *et al.* Palliation and pleurodesis in malignant pleural effusion: the role for tunneled pleural catheters. Journal of thoracic oncology : official publication of the International Association for the Study of Lung Cancer 2011; 6(4): 762-7. [http://dx.doi.org/10.1097/JTO.0b013e31820d614f]

[140] Van Meter ME, McKee KY, Kohlwes RJ. Efficacy and safety of tunneled pleural catheters in adults with malignant pleural effusions: a systematic review. J Gen Intern Med 2011; 26(1): 70-6. [http://dx.doi.org/10.1007/s11606-010-1472-0] [PMID: 20697963]

[141] Efthymiou CA, Masudi T, Thorpe JA, Papagiannopoulos K. Malignant pleural effusion in the presence of trapped lung. Five-year experience of PleurX tunnelled catheters. Interact Cardiovasc Thorac Surg 2009; 9(6): 961-4. [http://dx.doi.org/10.1510/icvts.2009.211516] [PMID: 19638358]

[142] Krishnan M, Cheriyath P, Wert Y, Moritz TA. The Untapped Potential of Tunneled Pleural Catheters. Ann Thorac Surg 2015; 100(6): 2055-7. [http://dx.doi.org/10.1016/j.athoracsur.2015.05.086] [PMID: 26294344]

[143] Bertolaccini L, Viti A, Gorla A, Terzi A. Home-management of malignant pleural effusion with an indwelling pleural catheter: ten years experience. Eur J Surg Oncol (EJSO) 2012; 38(12): 1161-4. [http://dx.doi.org/10.1016/j.ejso.2012.08.021] [PMID: 22959168]

[144] Sabur NF, Chee A, Stather DR, *et al.* The impact of tunneled pleural catheters on the quality of life of patients with malignant pleural effusions. Respiration; international review of thoracic diseases 2013; 85(1): 36-42.

[http://dx.doi.org/10.1159/000342343]

[145] Chalhoub M, Harris K, Castellano M, Maroun R, Bourjeily G. The use of the PleurX catheter in the management of non-malignant pleural effusions. Chron Respir Dis 2011; 8(3): 185-91. [http://dx.doi.org/10.1177/1479972311407216] [PMID: 21636653]

[146] Warren WH, Kalimi R, Khodadadian LM, Kim AW. Management of malignant pleural effusions using the Pleur(x) catheter. Ann Thorac Surg 2008; 85(3): 1049-55. [http://dx.doi.org/10.1016/j.athoracsur.2007.11.039] [PMID: 18291195]

[147] Tremblay A, Michaud G. Single-center experience with 250 tunnelled pleural catheter insertions for malignant pleural effusion. Chest 2006; 129(2): 362-8. [http://dx.doi.org/10.1378/chest.129.2.362] [PMID: 16478853]

[148] Munson CF, West DG, Vasey L, Kirk AJ. 48 Indwelling pleural catheters reduce inpatient stay for patients with malignant pleural effusion. Lung Cancer 2011; 71: S16-7. [http://dx.doi.org/10.1016/S0169-5002(11)70048-4]

[149] Patz EF Jr, McAdams HP, Erasmus JJ, *et al.* Sclerotherapy for malignant pleural effusions: a prospective randomized trial of bleomycin vs doxycycline with small-bore catheter drainage. Chest 1998; 113(5): 1305-11. [http://dx.doi.org/10.1378/chest.113.5.1305] [PMID: 9596311]

[150] Patz EF Jr. Malignant pleural effusions: recent advances and ambulatory sclerotherapy. Chest 1998; 113(1) (Suppl.): 74S-7S. [http://dx.doi.org/10.1378/chest.113.1_Supplement.74S] [PMID: 9438694]

[151] Saffran L, Ost DE, Fein AM, Schiff MJ. Outpatient pleurodesis of malignant pleural effusions using a small-bore pigtail catheter. Chest 2000; 118(2): 417-21. [http://dx.doi.org/10.1378/chest.118.2.417] [PMID: 10936134]

[152] Reddy C, Ernst A, Lamb C, Feller-Kopman D. Rapid pleurodesis for malignant pleural effusions: a pilot study. Chest 2011; 139(6): 1419-23. [http://dx.doi.org/10.1378/chest.10-1868] [PMID: 20930006]

[153] Ahmed L, Ip H, Rao D, Patel N, Noorzad F. Talc pleurodesis through indwelling pleural catheters for malignant pleural effusions: retrospective case series of a novel clinical pathway. Chest 2014; 146(6): e190-4. [http://dx.doi.org/10.1378/chest.14-0394] [PMID: 25451360]

[154] Bhatnagar R, Kahan BC, Morley AJ, *et al.* The efficacy of indwelling pleural catheter placement *versus* placement plus talc sclerosant in patients with malignant pleural effusions managed exclusively as outpatients (IPC-PLUS): study protocol for a randomised controlled trial. Trials 2015; 16: 48. [http://dx.doi.org/10.1186/s13063-015-0563-y] [PMID: 25880969]

[155] Tremblay A, Stather DR, Kelly MM. Effect of repeated administration of low-dose silver nitrate for pleurodesis in a rabbit model. Respirology 2011; 16(7): 1070-5. [http://dx.doi.org/10.1111/j.1440-1843.2011.02007.x] [PMID: 21651643]

[156] Tremblay A, Dumitriu S, Stather DR, Maceachern P, Illanes O, Kelly MM. Use of a drug eluting pleural catheter for pleurodesis. Exp Lung Res 2012; 38(9-10): 475-82. [http://dx.doi.org/10.3109/01902148.2012.731715] [PMID: 23050934]

[157] Mekhaiel E, Kashyap R, Mullon JJ, Maldonado F. Infections associated with tunnelled indwelling pleural catheters in patients undergoing chemotherapy. J Bronchology Interv Pulmonol 2013; 20(4): 299 303. [http://dx.doi.org/10.1097/LBR.0000000000000001] [PMID. 24162111]

[158] Morel A, Mishra E, Medley L, *et al.* Chemotherapy should not be withheld from patients with an indwelling pleural catheter for malignant pleural effusion. Thorax 2011; 66(5): 448-9. [http://dx.doi.org/10.1136/thx.2009.133504] [PMID: 20880866]

[159] Sachdeva A, Dawson J, Lee H, Malhotra R, Shepherd R. RIsk of infectious complications with

tunneled pleural catheter in patients undergoing chemotherapy. Chest 2012; 142(4_MeetingAbstracts): 522A.

[160] Marks M, Dotson T, Bellinger C. An Update on Tunneled Pleural Catheters. Clin Pulm Med 2015; 22(4): 157-64.
[http://dx.doi.org/10.1097/CPM.0000000000000110]

[161] Gilbert CR, Lee HJ, Akulian JA, *et al.* A Quality Improvement Intervention to Reduce Indwelling Tunneled Pleural Catheter Infection Rates. Ann Am Thorac Soc 2015; 12(6): 847-53.
[http://dx.doi.org/10.1513/AnnalsATS.201411-511OC] [PMID: 25871702]

[162] Wrightson JM, Fysh E, Maskell NA, Lee YC. Risk reduction in pleural procedures: sonography, simulation and supervision. Curr Opin Pulm Med 2010; 16(4): 340-50.
[http://dx.doi.org/10.1097/MCP.0b013e32833a233b] [PMID: 20531083]

[163] Lui MM, Thomas R, Lee YC. Complications of indwelling pleural catheter use and their management. BMJ Open Respir Res 2016; 3(1): e000123.
[http://dx.doi.org/10.1136/bmjresp-2015-000123] [PMID: 26870384]

[164] Fysh ET, Tremblay A, Feller-Kopman D, *et al.* Clinical outcomes of indwelling pleural catheter-related pleural infections: an international multicenter study. Chest 2013; 144(5): 1597-602.
[http://dx.doi.org/10.1378/chest.12-3103] [PMID: 23828305]

[165] Rahman NM, Maskell NA, West A, *et al.* Intrapleural use of tissue plasminogen activator and DNase in pleural infection. N Engl J Med 2011; 365(6): 518-26.
[http://dx.doi.org/10.1056/NEJMoa1012740] [PMID: 21830966]

[166] Wilshire CL, Louie BE, Aye RW, Farivar AS, Vallières E, Gorden JA. Safety and Efficacy of Fibrinolytic Therapy in Restoring Function of an Obstructed Tunneled Pleural Catheter. Ann Am Thorac Soc 2015; 12(9): 1317-22.
[http://dx.doi.org/10.1513/AnnalsATS.201503-182OC] [PMID: 26214713]

[167] Thomas R, Piccolo F, Miller D, *et al.* Intrapleural Fibrinolysis for the Treatment of Indwelling Pleural Catheter-Related Symptomatic Loculations: A Multicenter Observational Study. Chest 2015; 148(3): 746-51.
[http://dx.doi.org/10.1378/chest.14-2401] [PMID: 25742001]

[168] Thomas R, Budgeon CA, Kuok YJ, *et al.* Catheter tract metastasis associated with indwelling pleural catheters. Chest 2014; 146(3): 557-62.
[http://dx.doi.org/10.1378/chest.13-3057] [PMID: 24676503]

[169] Janes SM, Rahman NM, Davies RJ, Lee YC. Catheter-tract metastases associated with chronic indwelling pleural catheters. Chest 2007; 131(4): 1232-4.
[http://dx.doi.org/10.1378/chest.06-2353] [PMID: 17426232]

[170] Fysh ET, Wrightson JM, Lee YC, Rahman NM. Fractured indwelling pleural catheters. Chest 2012; 141(4): 1090-4.
[http://dx.doi.org/10.1378/chest.11-0724] [PMID: 22474151]

[171] Reich H, Beattie EJ, Harvey JC. Pleuroperitoneal shunt for malignant pleural effusions: a one-year experience. Semin Surg Oncol 1993; 9(2): 160-2.
[http://dx.doi.org/10.1002/ssu.2980090216] [PMID: 7683822]

[172] Lee KA, Harvey JC, Reich H, Beattie EJ. Management of malignant pleural effusions with pleuroperitoneal shunting. J Am Coll Surg 1994; 178(6): 586-8.
[PMID: 7514936]

[173] Schulze M, Boehle AS, Kurdow R, Dohrmann P, Henne-Bruns D. Effective treatment of malignant pleural effusion by minimal invasive thoracic surgery: thoracoscopic talc pleurodesis and pleuroperitoneal shunts in 101 patients. Ann Thorac Surg 2001; 71(6): 1809-12.
[http://dx.doi.org/10.1016/S0003-4975(01)02586-3] [PMID: 11426752]

[174] Genc O, Petrou M, Ladas G, Goldstraw P. The long-term morbidity of pleuroperitoneal shunts in the

management of recurrent malignant effusions. European journal of cardio-thoracic surgery : official journal of the European Association for Cardio-thoracic Surgery 2000; 8(2): 143-6. [http://dx.doi.org/10.1016/S1010-7940(00)00422-X]

CHAPTER 15

Medical Pleuroscopy

Ioannis Psallidas[1], Maged Hassan[2] and Najib M. Rahman[1,*]

[1] *Oxford Centre for Respiratory Medicine and Oxford Respiratory Trials Unit, Oxford University Hospitals NHS Foundation Trust, Oxford, UK*

[2] *Chest Diseases Department, Alexandria Faculty of Medicine, Alexandria, Egypt*

Abstract: In recent years, an increasing trend has been recognized in the number of centers performing medical thoracoscopy across the world, mainly as a gold standard investigation for undiagnosed exudative effusion. It is a particularly useful diagnostic and therapeutic tool with a very low rate of complications that should be incorporated in the respiratory physicians' armamentarium. Pleural biopsies under direct vision, therapeutic evacuation of effusions, and pleurodesis can be performed in one sitting. This chapter summarizes the important literature relating to the equipment, clinical indications, safety, complications and technical aspects of the procedure. We also aim to inform the reader regarding the latest research advances and potential areas of that MT will have a role in the future.

Keywords: Pleurodesis, Pleuroscopy, Respiratory physicians, Therapeutic evacuation of effusions, Thoracoscopy.

INTRODUCTION

The first report in modern history of Medicine of medical pleuroscopy (MP) was presented in 1866 when an Irish physician used a cystoscope to perform the first "thoracoscopy" on an 11-year-old girl with empyema [1]. The more renowned report came more than half a century later when H. C. Jacobeus, a Swedish internist who is widely regarded as the father of thoracoscopy, published the details of his endeavour, where he used, again, a cystoscope to examine the pleura of a patient with tuberculosis [2]. During the procedure, he severed adhesions between visceral and parietal pleura aiming to facilitate lung collapse therapy, one of the few options of managing tuberculosis in the pre-antibiotic era [1]. This technique, later named "Jacobeus operation", gained popularity across Europe. The zeal for thoracoscopy waned significantly after the discovery of streptomycin in the 1950s [3].

* **Corresponding author Najib M. Rahman:** Oxford Centre for Respiratory Medicine and Oxford Respiratory Trials Unit, Oxford University Hospitals NHS Foundation Trust, Oxford, UK; Tel: +44 1865 225256; Fax: +44 1865 857109; E-mail: najib.rahman@ouh.nhs.uk

Ali I. Musani (Ed.)

The revival in the interest for thoracoscopy was brought by various technological breakthroughs in miniature cameras and lighting/video technologies in the late 1980s, especially in continental Europe [3]. The gained momentum extended interest in thoracoscopy from respiratory physicians to cardiothoracic surgeons who modified the procedure and called it video-assisted thoracoscopic surgery (VATS) [4, 5]. Respiratory physicians distinguished their technique by using the terms medical thoracoscopy, local anaesthetic thoracoscopy, or pleuroscopy (MP). MP is a procedure performed by respiratory physicians, on spontaneously breathing patients under local anaesthesia or analgo-sedation [6]. It is usually performed through a single port in order to investigate the pleural space, biopsy any abnormalities and conduct talc pleurodesis. In comparison to VATS, MP is less invasive and costly and better tolerated by patients who are not fit for general anaesthesia [7]. It allows comprehensive visualization of the pleural space besides acting as a port for passing forceps or catheters according to need. On the other hand, VATS is performed by thoracic surgeons, under general anaesthesia in operating theatres, with double-lumen intubation and single lung ventilation.

Respiratory physicians both in the UK and USA were more skeptical to take up MT, and it was only in the late 1990s that the technique started to be practiced in some specialist centres. Over the following years, MP gained wider popularity and was being offered by more centres. For example, in the UK the number of centres performing MP rose between 1999 and 2009 from 11 to 37 centers [6]. MP is now routinely used across the US, Europe and Asia as well as other parts of the world and has a central role in the diagnosis and treatment of pleural diseases [8].

TECHNICAL CONSIDERATIONS

Rigid Scope

The rigid thoracoscope is composed of a 9 mm stainless steel telescope with a working channel and a trocar (a cannula and blunt-tipped obturator) of varying outer diameters [9]. A trocar wider than 10 mm will usually limit the capacity of thorough inspection of the pleural space due to pain caused by compression on the intercostal nerves. There is a variety of thoracoscopes with different fields of vision (0, 50, and 90°). The technique requires a cold (xenon) light source for adequate visual exploration, an endoscopic camera attached to the eyepiece of the telescope, a video monitor and recorder. The working channel of the telescope can accommodate various instruments according to the indication, and these include forceps, catheters for fluid suction or talc insufflation and electrocautery probes for haemorrhage control. Based on the recent BTS guidelines, rigid thoracoscopy is the recommended equipment for pleural biopsy and talc insufflation [6].

Semi-rigid Scope

The semi-rigid thoracoscopy is a 7 mm scope developed by the Japanese Company Olympus with a design largely simulating their flexible video-bronchoscopies [10]. The handle is almost identical to that of the videoscope, the shaft is 27 cm in length and the working channel is 2.8 mm in diameter. The shaft is made up of two constituents; the first is a 22-cm rigid section followed by flexible 5-cm end. The flexible end is moved by means of the lever on the handle and has a range of motion of 160^0 upward and 130^0 downward. A single-use 8-mm plastic trocar is inserted into the intercostal space and guides the scope into the pleura. The semi-rigid thoracoscope is compatible with the processors used for video-bronchoscopy which decreases the acquisition cost of the machine. The flexible biopsy forceps, the needles and all other accessories used in bronchoscopy can be accommodated through its working channel [8]. These include electrocautery, cryosurgery and laser probes as well as the possibility of using narrow-band imaging and autoflouresence [7].

Current evidence suggest that although flexible forceps are smaller, pleural biopsies obtained by semi-rigid thoracoscopy are of adequate size to confirm the diagnosis [11]. In a randomized controlled trial, 90 patients with exudative pleural effusion underwent either rigid or semi-rigid thoracoscopy [12]. The diagnostic yield for rigid thoracoscopy was overall superior to semi-rigid technique (100% vs. 94%), but the diagnostic yield was similar in both techniques if pleural biopsy could be successfully performed. In order to improve the size and quality of biopsy obtained by the flexible forceps, cryoprobe technique has been suggested. In a recent study comparing the biopsies obtained by flexible forceps, rigid forceps and cryoprobe in the same patient undergoing MP, the size of the cryoprobe biopsy was larger than that obtained by the flexible forceps [13]. The two biopsy methods were, however, inferior to the rigid forceps both in terms of biopsy size and its diagnostic potential. Due to the small sample size within the previous clinical trials, a larger study is needed in the future to prove whether significant clinical and statistical differences are noticed between the 2 procedures and to establish the place of cryoprobe in MP.

INDICATIONS

Appropriate patient selection is a necessary part of any investigative process. In 75% of cases with pleural effusion the clinical history, physical examination, radiographic techniques and pleural fluid analysis will identify a cause for the pleural effusion, with the remaining 25% requiring further invasive diagnostic procedures most of the time with MP [14]. It is vital to ensure that any procedure offered to a patient is in their best interests, and not, as may be the temptation, simply because it is technically possible.

Undiagnosed Exudate Pleural Effusion

The two primary causes of undiagnosed exudative lymphocytic effusions that are not diagnosed by thoracentesis are malignancy and tuberculosis [15]. A pleural biopsy is almost always indicated to make the differentiation in the setting of a negative culture and cytology of pleural fluid. In 1958, Abrams and Cope simultaneously presented their simple and cheap technique to perform closed pleural biopsy [16, 17]. Through a small skin incision, and with the customized needle, a piece of pleural tissue could be obtained. While closed pleural biopsy has good results in tuberculous effusions, mainly due to the diffuse nature of the pleural affection in the disease, it was notoriously insensitive in malignant effusion [6]. In addition, it was merely a diagnostic procedure, since pleural fluid drainage was not done, unlike MP where both pleural biopsy under vision, evacuation of effusion and pleurodesis if necessary could be achieved.

Malignant Pleural Effusions

Involvement of the pleura in cancer patients is fairly common and results from autopsy revealed evidence of malignant pleural effusion in 15% of oncological patients [18]. The first step in the diagnostic algorithm of a suspected MPE is the cytological analysis of pleural fluid. Approximately 60% of cases will be diagnosed after single aspiration, and data suggest that second aspiration improves the yield a further 15% [15]. In mesothelioma, the diagnostic yield of cytology is even lower, approximately 32% for the first sample and could increase to around 50% with a repeat thoracentesis. Traditionally, the next step on the diagnostic algorithm was a closed biopsy, which only improved the yield by approximately 10% and lesions located on the visceral, diaphragmatic and mediastinal pleura are beyond the reach of such needles. The use of closed biopsy in suspected MPE has been abandoned after the widespread use of MP, which is more sensitive and also has the potential for combining diagnostic and therapeutic management [6, 8]. Some authorities even advocate resorting to MP after a single negative cytology if there is sufficient expertise in it [5]. It is noteworthy that even in the setting of positive pleural fluid cytology, MP has a place if further tissue is required for histological type differentiation or molecular testing [6].

Proper recognition of the normal anatomical markings is key to identifying the macroscopic picture of malignancy, which will result in providing representative samples to the pathologist. Also if malignancy is suspected from the gross picture, pleurodesis with talc poudrage will be instituted (Fig. **1**). Pooling results from tens of case series reporting on results of MP, the procedure had a collective sensitivity of >90% for diagnosing MPE [6]. It remains to be said that a significant proportion of pleural biopsies from MT (up to one third of cases in some series) reveals non-specific pleuritis. This group of patients required follow up (with cross sectional imaging) due to a 5-10% possibility to developing malignancy (especially mesothelioma) in a later stage [19, 20].

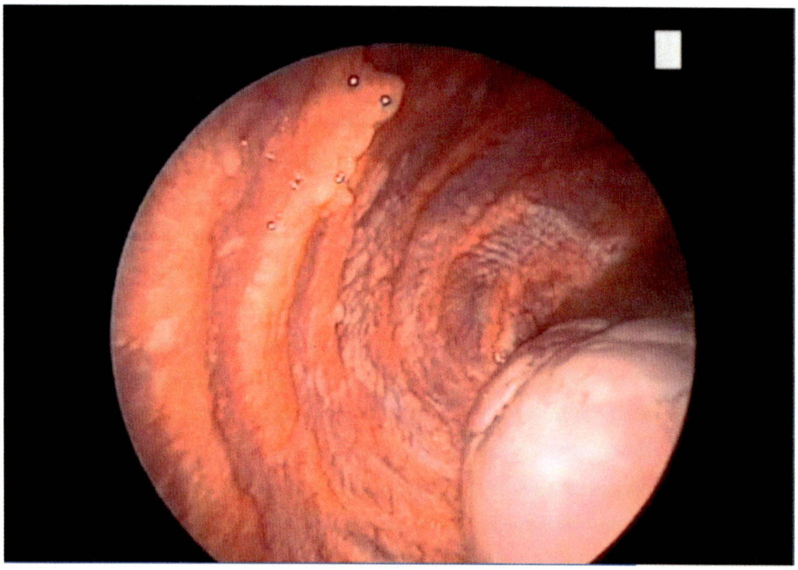

Fig. (1). Patient with gross pleural nodularity suggestive of an underlying malignant process.

A chest CT scan is not an absolute requirement prior to MP but is strongly recommended as valuable information can be provided [6]. Chest CT, especially when contrast-enhanced, is excellent in delineating pleural pathology. The presence of pleural nodules, irregular pleural thickening or smooth thickening more than 10 mm was fairly sensitive and highly specific for MPE [21]. It also provides with diagnostic information whether alternative procedures should be preferred *e.g.* an airway obstruction that can be approached bronchoscopically.

Thoracic ultrasound (TUS) could also be an asset prior MP for providing diagnostic information for the underlying cause of the effusion. Specifically, evidence of parietal pleural thickening, diaphragmatic thickening and presence of pleural or diaphragmatic nodules have good sensitivity and high specificity for MPE [22]. Bedside TUS is also of great value immediately before the MP to refine the choice for entry site and assess lung sliding and to successfully induce pneumothorax in cases with little or no fluid but other features concerning for pleural disease [23, 24]. Prior to introducing the scope, TUS is used to assess pleural sliding (to exclude lung tethering) and then pneumothorax is induced at the chosen spot usually using a Boutin needle. Additionally, on patients who are frail or when MP is not indicated (*e.g.* tethering lung) physician led TUS guided pleural biopsies could be an alternative technique with a diagnostic yield comparable to that obtained by radiologists [25, 26]. The procedure has also a good safety profile and can be performed on a day-case basis.

Pleural Tuberculosis

The nature of the pleural involvement in tuberculosis is diffuse in comparison to the patchy distribution in malignancy. This is why the diagnostic yield of closed pleural biopsy in cases of tuberculosis is approximately 80% [6]. In the setting of high tuberculosis prevalence, comparing closed pleural biopsy to MP; the former had 79% sensitivity while the latter had 100% sensitivity for pleural tuberculosis respectively [27]. For this reason in parts of the world where access (financial and geographical) to healthcare resources is limited with a high incidence of tuberculous pleuritis closed pleural biopsy is recommended as a diagnostic strategy and only resorting to MP when closed biopsy is non-diagnostic.

Pleurodesis

Pleurodesis aims at creating adhesion between the two layers of the pleura by instilling a sclerosant material inside the pleural space [28]. It is performed for the symptomatic control of patients with MPE and also for preventing the recurrence of spontaneous pneumothorax. The agent that had been most widely studied and used is sterile talc. Talc can be sprayed as powder *via* catheter through MP or as a slurry with saline and delivered through a chest drain [29].

In a recent meta-analysis of twenty trials involving 1525 patients with MPE, the relative risk for success of talc pleurodesis against other sclerosing agents in MPE was 1.21 (95% CI, 1.01–1.45; p=0.035) [30]. Additionally, talc poudrage was found to be more effective than talc slurry (relative risk 1.12; 95% CI, 1.01–1.23; p=0.026). A large randomized multicenter trial is currently in progress to elucidate the difference in efficacy between talc slurry and talc poudrage *via* MP in MPE [31]. What is established is that talc poudrage is at least as effective as talc slurry, and hence it is a very attractive option when MP is conducted to diagnose MPE, to perform pleurodesis at the same procedure.

The use of talc poudrage as a definitive management for pneumothorax by using MP is more popular in Europe than UK and USA. A recent European Respiratory Society task force on the management of primary spontaneous pneumothorax concluded that talc poudrage is cost effective and at least as effective as mechanical pleurodesis done through VATS [32].

Complicated Pleural Infections

The management of complicated parapneumonic effusion/empyema is based on two pillars; proper and timely use of antibiotics and thorough drainage of the pleural collection by a chest drain [33, 34]. When medical management fails, patients are referred for surgery. A few centres in Europe have advocated the use of MP in "early" empyema to interrupt pleural adhesions and facilitate complete drainage of the fluid by transforming a multi-loculated pleural cavity to a unified space (Fig. **2**). The available studies are all case series and despite showing very good results, these findings have not been confirmed with randomized trials [35, 36]. Such studies are required to probe the role of MP in managing pleural infection and setting a more defined limit for "early" intervention which is challenging, as the progression of infection is highly variable. Hence, the current management of failed simple drainage of empyema is still surgical and exploring the use of MP is, thus, investigational at best [3].

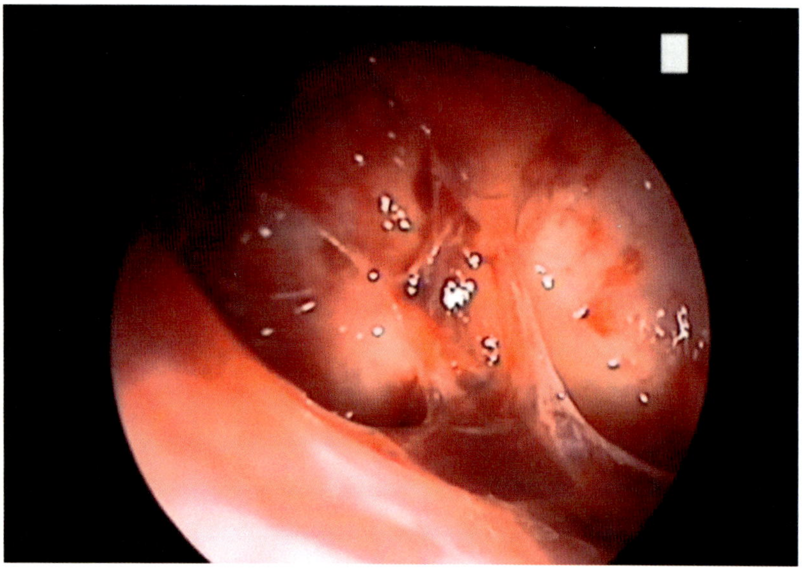

Fig. (2). Thoracoscopic findings of highly septated effusion on patients with pleural infection.

Other Conditions

Highly skilled practitioners of MP have reported to perform procedures that are usually only done by cardiothoracic surgeons like sympathectomy for hyperhidrosis, pericardial window, and forceps lung biopsy [3]. While in good hands these procedures were successful, routinely referring such patients for MP rather than surgery for these indications is beyond available evidence.

PROCEDURE

Contraindications

The absolute contraindications for MP are very few and inability to obtain informed consent and adherence of the lung to the chest wall are the most common. Uncontrollable cough, respiratory acidosis and severe respiratory distress are also cited as absolute contraindications [6]. Relative contraindications include: a bleeding diathesis, severe cardiovascular disease, intolerance to lie on one side and extreme obesity.

Preparation

Preoperative evaluation includes thorough medical history, physical examination and a chest X-ray. Chest CT with intravenous contrast on pleural phase and bedside TUS are also recommended [6]. Recent blood tests with full blood count, coagulation and basic biochemical profile are required prior to MP. Values below a platelet count of 50,000 or an INR higher than 1.5 render the procedure unsafe. Oxygen saturations more than 92% need to be retained during the procedure.

Setting

MP can be performed in the endoscopy suite or an operating theatre. Strict sterile precautions need to be taken by all personnels directly in charge of handling the patient or the equipment. At minimum, the thoracoscopist needs an assisting physician and a nurse for assistance during the procedure. Electrocardiogram, heart rate, blood pressure and oxygen saturations must be monitored during the whole procedure. Diathermy should be available and ready as well as equipment for resuscitation, intubation and assisted ventilation in case of need.

Anaesthesia

MP is usually performed under local anaesthesia with conscious sedation [6]. Local anaesthetic (*e.g.* 1% lidocaine) needs to be carefully infiltrated to the skin and parietal pleura. Conscious sedation is achieved by the use of one or more intravenous agents; conventionally a combination of a benzodiazepine (midazolam) and opioid (fentanyl or morphine). A recent trend towards replacing benzodiazepines with propofol especially when talc poudrage is planned has been reported [8]. Care should be taken when propofol is used due to its tendency to depress respiration and to cause more profound hypoxaemia compared to midazolam [37]. In cases where more advanced procedures are planned (*e.g.* talc pleurodesis for patients with pneumothorax, extensive adhesiolysis in empyema, lung biopsy), general anaesthesia is preferred.

Technique

The patient is placed on lateral decubitus position with the healthy lung down. The lead physician faces the patient, while the assistant stands either besides or at the opposite side of the table. Before injecting the local anaesthetic, it is strongly recommended to perform US examination to assess the anatomy of the area, the presence of septations and to evaluate the presence of sliding if pneumothorax induction is planned [6]. Air can be introduced into the pleura *via* a special atraumatic needle called the Boutin needle which has a blunt end that pierces the pleura and a side opening the creates communicates between the pleura and ambient air [38]. This needle is especially valuable when MP is performed in the absence of effusion but should only be used by practitioners with competency.

Depending on the TUS and the underlying anatomy the point of entry is usually in the mid-axillary line and a 1-2 cm skin incision is made in the middle of the intercostal space in the orientation of the ribs. Blunt dissection technique with curved mosquito forceps is used to dissect subcutaneous tissue, intercostal muscles and enter the pleural cavity. After ensuring entry of the trocar into the pleural cavity, the obturator is removed and suction catheter is passed through the cannula. During fluid evacuation, air is allowed to enter and leave the pleura freely. At most centres only one port is made for the scope to pass through. During some complex procedures, however, a second port using a 5-mm trocar can be inserted for passing accessory equipment to improve the manoeuver ability. Specifically, a two port MP is indicated when extensive adhesiolysis is needed or for the approach and biopsy and of areas not accessible with a single port.

The thoracic cavity should be meticulously inspected with the thoracoscope. The first visualized parts are usually the posterior chest wall directly ahead of the scope, the apex of the thoracic cavity at one side and the diaphragm on the other side. The ribs and the intervening intercostal vessels are easily identifiable except on the cases that the pleura is thickened. The lung can be viewed at the bottom of the image, and the major and minor fissures can be used as anatomical guidance. The costophrenic recess should be reached with a view to carefully assess whether there is evidence of nodularity or thickening. The scope should then be rotated to inspect the mediastinum, including the pericardium and great vessels.

Biopsies can be taken under vision from the parietal and visceral pleura, lung, diaphragm and mediastinum. It is always preferable to take biopsy from the pleura overlying ribs in order to avoid inadvertent trauma to the neurovascular bundle. A sweeping movement is done to strip or peel the tissue rather than snatch it. At least 8-12 biopsies are required from two different sites and obtaining deep biopsies until the level of extrapleural fat is recommended.

Rapid on-site pathological evaluation of pleural biopsies have been reported on a case series as a method to aid physician decisions for pleurodesis on cases with inconclusive macroscopic findings [39]. Talc poudrage can then be performed if malignancy is highly suspected based on the microscopic findings (Fig. **3**). After terminating the procedure, the scope and trocar are removed and a chest tube inserted through the same wound. The chest drain usually remains on site for a few hours until pneumothorax is drained which is confirmed with a chest X-ray. If pleurodesis was performed, the drain will be removed based on the current guidelines when the fluid output is minimal and the chest X- ray show lung expansion [29].

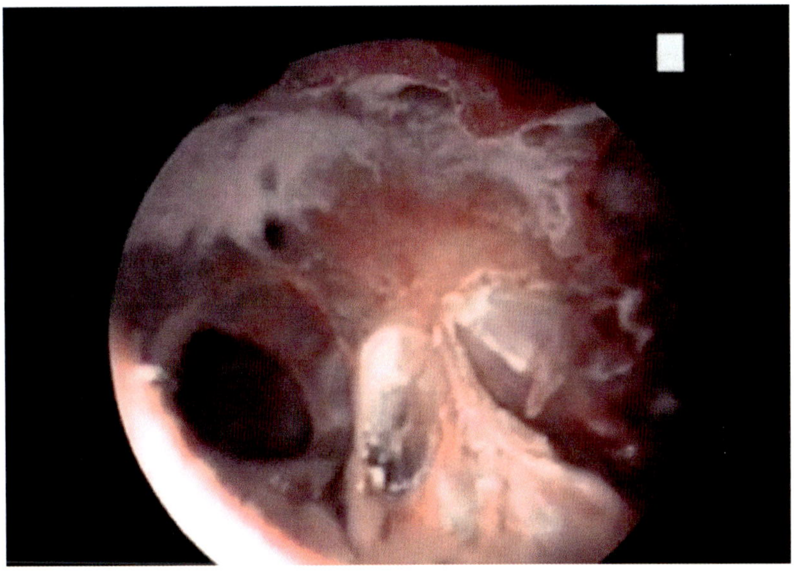

Fig. (3). Thoracoscopic image of talc pleurodesis on a patient with malignant pleural effusion from mesothelioma.

Complications

MP is generally a safe, minimally invasive procedure and mortality is a very rare event. Data from 47 studies reporting on complications of MP showed that death occurred in 0.34% of cases [6]. All reported deaths were subsequent to procedures where talc insufflation was done, and none in purely diagnostic procedures. Two thirds of these deaths were reported from centres that used for pleurodesis non-graded talc.

Major complications of MP include empyema, bronchopleural fistula, tumour growth in the thoracoscopy tract, major bleeding and pneumonia. The aforementioned 47 studies reporting on MP complications cited a combined rate of major complications of 1.8%, further confirming the acceptable safety profile of MP [6]. Minor complications (approximately 7%) can be in the form of wound infection, postoperative fever, surgical emphysema, hypotension and atrial fibrillation.

MEDICAL THORACOSCOPY IN RESEACRH

Much light was shed on the pathogenesis of primary spontaneous pneumothorax by the use of autofluorescence during MP. Patients with pneumothorax were examined with MP 10-30 minutes after inhaling nebulized fluorescein both with white light and autofluorescence [40]. In addition to apical emphysema-like changes seen with white light, scattered areas of fluorescein enhancement were seen all over the lung surface, denoting increased lung porosity at these spots. These findings challenged the long-standing theory that primary pneumothorax occurs in consequence to rupture of apical bullae/blebs, suggesting that the pathogenesis is likely more complex. Additionally, it is also justified why the rate of recurrence of primary spontaneous pneumothorax is less when pleurodesis is performed together with removing apical lung lesions rather than removing lesions only [32].

Fluorescence enhancement during MP was also used to better visualize lesions on the parietal pleura. In one study, patients being evaluated for MPE were asked to orally take 5-aminolaevulinic acid a few hours before MP. Subsequently, the pleura was examined both with white light and autofluorescence thoracoscopy [41]. Authors reported improved detection of the pleural lesions with autofluorescence which pointed out lesions that were not visible during white light examination leading to upstaging in 4 of 15 patients diagnosed with mesothelioma. In a subsequent study, researchers explored the use of autofluorescence during MP without extrinsic fluorescence enhancement with disappointing results hence questioning the added value of this new technique [42].

CONCLUSION

MP is an excellent tool to establish diagnosis in patients with exudative pleural effusion of unclear origin. It is highly valuable in clarifying the origin of pleural effusions in oncological patients, as the presence of a malignant pleural effusion is associated with poor survival and precludes the possibility of treatment with curative intention. Pleurodesis with talc poudrage is efficacious and well tolerated, especially with the use of large-particle talc. MP is a particularly useful diagnostic and therapeutic tool with a very low rate of complications that should be incorporated in the respiratory physicians' armamentarium.

CONFLICT OF INTEREST

The authors declare no conflict of interest, financial or otherwise.

ACKNOWLEDGEMENTS

Declared none.

REFERENCES

[1] Lee P, Mathur PN, Colt HG. Advances in thoracoscopy: 100 years since Jacobaeus. Respiration; international review of thoracic diseases 2010; 79(3): 177-86.

[2] Jacobaeus HC. The cauterization of adhesions in artificial pneumothorax treatment of pulmonary tuberculosis under thoracoscopic control. Proceedings of the Royal Society of Medicine. 45-62.

[3] Bhatnagar R, Corcoran JP, Maldonado F, *et al.* Advanced medical interventions in pleural disease. European respiratory review : an official journal of the European Respiratory Society 2016; 25(140): 199-213.
[http://dx.doi.org/10.1183/16000617.0020-2016]

[4] de Groot M, Walther G. Thoracoscopy in undiagnosed pleural effusions. South African medical journal = Suid-Afrikaanse tydskrif vir geneeskunde 1998; 88(6): 706-11.

[5] Harris RJ, Kavuru MS, Mehta AC, *et al.* The impact of thoracoscopy on the management of pleural disease. Chest 1995; 107(3): 845-52.
[http://dx.doi.org/10.1378/chest.107.3.845] [PMID: 7874962]

[6] Rahman NM, Ali NJ, Brown G, *et al.* British thoracic society pleural disease guideline group. Local anaesthetic thoracoscopy: British Thoracic Society Pleural Disease Guideline 2010. Thorax 2010; 65 (Suppl. 2): ii54-60.
[http://dx.doi.org/10.1136/thx.2010.137018] [PMID: 20696694]

[7] Shojaee S, Lee HJ. Thoracoscopy: medical *versus* surgical-in the management of pleural diseases. J Thorac Dis 2015; 7 (Suppl. 4): S339-51.
[PMID: 26807282]

[8] Lee P, Colt HG. Pleuroscopy in 2013. Clin Chest Med 2013; 34(1): 81-91.
[http://dx.doi.org/10.1016/j.ccm.2012.11.003] [PMID: 23411059]

[9] Menzies R, Charbonneau M. Thoracoscopy for the diagnosis of pleural disease. Ann Intern Med 1991; 114(4): 271-6.
[http://dx.doi.org/10.7326/0003-4819-114-4-271] [PMID: 1987873]

[10] McLean AN, Bicknell SR, McAlpine LG, Peacock AJ. Investigation of pleural effusion: an evaluation of the new Olympus LTF semiflexible thoracofiberscope and comparison with Abram's needle biopsy. Chest 1998; 114(1): 150-3.
[http://dx.doi.org/10.1378/chest.114.1.150] [PMID: 9674462]

[11] Yin Y, Eberhardt R, Wang XB, *et al.* Semi-rigid thoracoscopic punch biopsy using a hybrid knife with a high-pressure water jet for the diagnosis of pleural effusions. Respiration; international review of thoracic diseases 2016; 92(3): 192-6.
[http://dx.doi.org/10.1159/000448556]

[12] Dhooria S, Singh N, Aggarwal AN, Gupta D, Agarwal R. A randomized trial comparing the diagnostic yield of rigid and semirigid thoracoscopy in undiagnosed pleural effusions. Respir Care 2014; 59(5):

756-64.
[http://dx.doi.org/10.4187/respcare.02738] [PMID: 24106326]

[13] Wurps H, Schönfeld N, Bauer TT, *et al.* Intra-patient comparison of parietal pleural biopsies by rigid forceps, flexible forceps and cryoprobe obtained during medical thoracoscopy: a prospective series of 80 cases with pleural effusion. BMC Pulm Med 2016; 16(1): 98.
[http://dx.doi.org/10.1186/s12890-016-0258-5] [PMID: 27387441]

[14] Collins TR, Sahn SA. Thoracocentesis. Clinical value, complications, technical problems, and patient experience. Chest 1987; 91(6): 817-22.
[http://dx.doi.org/10.1378/chest.91.6.817] [PMID: 3581930]

[15] Hooper C, Lee YC, Maskell N, Group BT. BTS pleural guideline group. Investigation of a unilateral pleural effusion in adults: British Thoracic Society Pleural Disease Guideline 2010. Thorax 2010; 65 (Suppl. 2): ii4-ii17.
[http://dx.doi.org/10.1136/thx.2010.136978] [PMID: 20696692]

[16] Cope C. New pleural biopsy needle; preliminary study. J Am Med Assoc 1958; 167(9): 1107-8.
[http://dx.doi.org/10.1001/jama.1958.72990260005011a] [PMID: 13549237]

[17] Abrams LD. A pleural-biopsy punch. Lancet 1958; 1(7010): 30-1.
[http://dx.doi.org/10.1016/S0140-6736(58)92521-2] [PMID: 13492658]

[18] Rodrîguez-Panadero F, Borderas Naranjo F, López Mejîas J. Pleural metastatic tumours and effusions. Frequency and pathogenic mechanisms in a post-mortem series. Eur Respir J 1989; 2(4): 366-9.
[PMID: 2786818]

[19] Metintas M, Ak G, Cadirci O, Yildirim H, Dundar E, Metintas S. Outcome of patients diagnosed with fibrinous pleuritis after medical thoracoscopy. Respir Med 2012; 106(8): 1177-83.
[http://dx.doi.org/10.1016/j.rmed.2012.04.009] [PMID: 22608353]

[20] Davies HE, Nicholson JE, Rahman NM, Wilkinson EM, Davies RJ, Lee YC. Outcome of patients with nonspecific pleuritis/fibrosis on thoracoscopic pleural biopsies. European journal of cardio-thoracic surgery : official journal of the European Association for Cardio-thoracic Surgery 2010; 38(4): 472-7.

[21] Leung AN, Müller NL, Miller RR. CT in differential diagnosis of diffuse pleural disease. AJR Am J Roentgenol 1990; 154(3): 487-92.
[http://dx.doi.org/10.2214/ajr.154.3.2106209] [PMID: 2106209]

[22] Qureshi NR, Rahman NM, Gleeson FV. Thoracic ultrasound in the diagnosis of malignant pleural effusion. Thorax 2009; 64(2): 139-43.
[http://dx.doi.org/10.1136/thx.2008.100545] [PMID: 18852159]

[23] Corcoran JP, Psallidas I, Hallifax RJ, Talwar A, Sykes A, Rahman NM. Ultrasound-guided pneumothorax induction prior to local anaesthetic thoracoscopy. Thorax 2015; 70(9): 906-8.
[http://dx.doi.org/10.1136/thoraxjnl-2014-206676] [PMID: 25661112]

[24] Marchetti G, Valsecchi A, Indellicati D, Arondi S, Trigiani M, Pinelli V. Ultrasound-guided medical thoracoscopy in the absence of pleural effusion. Chest 2015; 147(4): 1008-12.
[http://dx.doi.org/10.1378/chest.14-0637] [PMID: 25188712]

[25] Hallifax RJ, Corcoran JP, Ahmed A, *et al.* Physician-based ultrasound-guided biopsy for diagnosing pleural disease. Chest 2014; 146(4): 1001-6.
[http://dx.doi.org/10.1378/chest.14-0299] [PMID: 24832701]

[26] Diacon AH, Schuurmans MM, Theron J, Schubert PT, Wright CA, Bolliger CT. Safety and yield of ultrasound-assisted transthoracic biopsy performed by pulmonologists. Respiration; international review of thoracic diseases 2004; 71(5): 519-22.
[http://dx.doi.org/10.1159/000080638]

[27] Diacon AH, Van de Wal BW, Wyser C, *et al.* Diagnostic tools in tuberculous pleurisy: a direct comparative study. Eur Respir J 2003; 22(4): 589-91.
[http://dx.doi.org/10.1183/09031936.03.00017103a] [PMID: 14582908]

[28] Rodriguez-Panadero F, Montes-Worboys A. Mechanisms of pleurodesis. Respiration; international review of thoracic diseases 2012; 83(2): 91-8. [http://dx.doi.org/10.1159/000335419]

[29] Roberts ME, Neville E, Berrisford RG, Antunes G, Ali NJ, Group BT. BTS Pleural Disease Guideline Group. Management of a malignant pleural effusion: British Thoracic Society Pleural Disease Guideline 2010. Thorax 2010; 65 (Suppl. 2): ii32-40. [http://dx.doi.org/10.1136/thx.2010.136994] [PMID: 20696691]

[30] Xia H, Wang XJ, Zhou Q, Shi HZ, Tong ZH. Efficacy and safety of talc pleurodesis for malignant pleural effusion: a meta-analysis. PLoS One 2014; 9(1): e87060. [http://dx.doi.org/10.1371/journal.pone.0087060] [PMID: 24475222]

[31] Bhatnagar R, Laskawiec-Szkonter M, Piotrowska HE, *et al.* Evaluating the efficacy of thoracoscopy and talc poudrage *versus* pleurodesis using talc slurry (TAPPS trial): protocol of an open-label randomised controlled trial. BMJ Open 2014; 4(11): e007045. [http://dx.doi.org/10.1136/bmjopen-2014-007045] [PMID: 25428632]

[32] Tschopp JM, Bintcliffe O, Astoul P, *et al.* ERS task force statement: diagnosis and treatment of primary spontaneous pneumothorax. Eur Respir J 2015; 46(2): 321-35. [http://dx.doi.org/10.1183/09031936.00219214] [PMID: 26113675]

[33] Psallidas I, Corcoran JP, Rahman NM. Management of parapneumonic effusions and empyema. Semin Respir Crit Care Med 2014; 35(6): 715-22. [http://dx.doi.org/10.1055/s-0034-1395503] [PMID: 25463162]

[34] Davies HE, Davies RJ, Davies CW, Group BT. BTS Pleural Disease Guideline Group. Management of pleural infection in adults: British Thoracic Society Pleural Disease Guideline 2010. Thorax 2010; 65 (Suppl. 2): ii41-53. [http://dx.doi.org/10.1136/thx.2010.137000] [PMID: 20696693]

[35] Ravaglia C, Gurioli C, Tomassetti S, *et al.* Is medical thoracoscopy efficient in the management of multiloculated and organized thoracic empyema? Respiration; international review of thoracic diseases 2012; 84(3): 219-24. [http://dx.doi.org/10.1159/000339414]

[36] Brutsche MH, Tassi GF, Györik S, *et al.* Treatment of sonographically stratified multiloculated thoracic empyema by medical thoracoscopy. Chest 2005; 128(5): 3303-9. [http://dx.doi.org/10.1378/chest.128.5.3303] [PMID: 16304276]

[37] Grendelmeier P, Tamm M, Jahn K, Pflimlin E, Stolz D. Propofol *versus* midazolam in medical thoracoscopy: a randomized, noninferiority trial. Respiration; international review of thoracic diseases 2014; 16(3): 479-86. [http://dx.doi.org/10.1159/000362797]

[38] Mathur PN, Astoul P, Boutin C. Medical thoracoscopy. Technical details. Clin Chest Med 1995; 16(3): 479-86. [PMID: 8521702]

[39] Porfyridis I, Georgiadis G, Michael M, *et al.* Rapid on-site evaluation with the Hemacolor rapid staining method of medical thoracoscopy biopsy specimens for the management of pleural disease. Respirology 2016; 21(6): 1106-12. [http://dx.doi.org/10.1111/resp.12799] [PMID: 27080382]

[40] Noppen M, Dekeukeleire T, Hanon S, *et al.* Fluorescein-enhanced autofluorescence thoracoscopy in patients with primary spontaneous pneumothorax and normal subjects. Am J Respir Crit Care Med 2006; 174(1): 26-30. [http://dx.doi.org/10.1164/rccm.200602-259OC] [PMID: 16627865]

[41] Baas P, Triesscheijn M, Burgers S, van Pel R, Stewart F, Aalders M. Fluorescence detection of pleural malignancies using 5-aminolaevulinic acid. Chest 2006; 129(3): 718-24.

[http://dx.doi.org/10.1378/chest.129.3.718] [PMID: 16537873]

[42] Chrysanthidis MG, Janssen JP. Autofluorescence videothoracoscopy in exudative pleural effusions: preliminary results. Eur Respir J 2005; 26(6): 989-92.
[http://dx.doi.org/10.1183/09031936.05.00027505] [PMID: 16319326]

CHAPTER 16

The Role of Palliative Care/ Hospice Medicine in Interventional Pulmonology

Muhammad Sajawal Ali* and **Lubna T. Sorathia**

Division of Pulmonary and Critical Care Medicine, Medical College of Wisconsin, WI 53226, USA

Abstract: Palliative care has been defined as "the active total care of patients whose disease is not responsive to curative treatment." The focus of palliative care/ hospice medicine according to the World Health Organization (WHO), is to prevent and relieve suffering by early identification, assessment, and treatment of pain and other debilitating symptoms. Unfortunately, lung cancer and chronic obstructive pulmonary disease are among the leading causes of death in the United States. Therefore, pulmonologists are often called upon to participate in the care of terminally ill patients. By incorporating components of palliative care, pulmonologists can help relieve their suffering. When conservative therapies fail, interventional pulmonologists can palliate the symptoms associated with disorders such as malignant pleural effusion, airway obstruction and hemoptysis. Commonly offered interventions in this regard include, indwelling pleural catheters (IPC), pleurodesis, endobronchial laser, electrocautery, argon plasma coagulation (APC), endobronchial brachytherapy, rigid bronchoscopy and airway stenting.

Keywords: Argon plasma coagulation, Endobronchial brachytherapy, Endobronchial stent, Hemoptysis, Hospice medicine, Indwelling pleural catheter (IPC), Interventional pulmonology, Lung cancer, Malignant airway obstruction, Malignant pleural effusion, Palliative care, Pleurodesis, Rigid bronchoscopy.

WHAT IS PALLIATIVE CARE/ HOSPICE MEDICINE?

World Health Organization (WHO) defines palliative care as "the active total care of patients whose disease is not responsive to curative treatment" [1]. The goal of palliative care is to provide symptomatic relief to terminally ill patients so that some of their suffering may be alleviated. Unfortunately, recent trends show that the proportion of patients getting aggressive treatments despite being close to the end of their lives, is increasing [2]. At times physicians continue to pursue aggressive therapies aimed at curing the underlying disease or prolonging life

* **Corresponding author Muhammad Sajawal Ali:** Division of Pulmonary and Critical Care Medicine, Medical College of Wisconsin, Wisconsin WI, 53226, USA; Tel: 267-241-9564; Fax: 414-805-0535; E-mail: muali@mcw.edu

Ali I. Musani (Ed.)

even though the end appears imminent. This not only exposes patients to a myriad of complications but also adds to their suffering through increased frequency of blood draws, investigations, frequent hospitalizations *etc*. Palliative care on the contrary focuses on improving the quality of life and making patients as comfortable as possible, even though this might not necessarily make them live longer. The philosophy of hospice medicine is centered on concepts of palliation as described above. There is some variation in the precise definition and timing of hospice care though. In the Unites States, Medicare deems patients in the last 6 months of their lives as being appropriate hospice candidates [3]. In the United Kingdom, the time frame is more liberal and patients with up to 1 year of life expectancy may be considered appropriate hospice care candidates.

Over the last few years, palliative care experts have also advocated moving away from a dichotomous system whereby life prolonging therapies and palliative care were considered mutually exclusive [4]. They have instead proposed an approach where by elements of palliative care such as pain control, minimizing dyspnea *etc*. may be incorporated in to the care of the patients who are otherwise being aggressively treated. The idea is to expose a greater proportion of patients to the benefits of palliative care. Another unique and often overlooked aspect of palliative care is the additional focus on the loved ones of the patient. Dame Cicely Mary Saunders who is considered the founder of modern palliative movement famously commented, “how people die lives on in the memories of those who live on”. By focusing on symptom management under the umbrella of palliative care, patients can be made more comfortable. For most people the knowledge that their loved one at least passed away peacefully, is an important factor that allows them to get through such trying times.

WHY DO PULMONOLOGISTS NEED TO UNDERSTAND PALLIATIVE CARE/ HOSPICE MEDICINE?

There are few medical specialties where a keen understanding of palliative care/ hospice medicine is more relevant than in pulmonary medicine. A quick look at the leading causes of death in the United States explains this. As per the Centers for Disease Control and Prevention (CDC), cancer is the second leading cause of death, followed by chronic lower respiratory diseases at number three [5]. Recent cancer statistics suggest that lung cancer is the most common cause of cancer deaths [6]. For pulmonologists, this means taking care of a large number of sick and complex patients with limited life expectancy due to a variety of benign and malignant lung disorders. Hence, it is crucial for these providers to incorporate various aspects of palliative/ hospice care into the treatment plan fairly early to help improve quality of life of patients and their care givers alike.

The American Thoracic Society in its official clinical policy statement released in April 2008 regarding palliative care for patients with respiratory diseases and critical illnesses, endorses that palliative care be available to patients at all stages of illness and should be tailored based on the individual patient needs and preferences. The statement endorses hospice care as an appropriate multidisciplinary system to provide palliative care to the patients and their families. It also discusses a number of "do's" and "don'ts" relevant to withholding and withdrawing life support for adults and children.

Lung Cancer

Data from the National Cancer Institute's Surveillance, Epidemiology and End Results (SEER) program suggests that 79% of lung cancer patients are diagnosed in third and fourth stages of their disease [7]. Unfortunately 5-year survival for such advanced disease is abysmal at 9.5 to 16.8% [4]. Majority of these patients suffer from disabling symptoms such as pain, dyspnea, cough and restlessness [8 - 10]. These patients often also suffer from a vicious cycle of deconditioning, isolation, respiratory symptoms and disability (Fig. **1**) [11]. Terminal secretions, also known as 'death rattle' are especially scary for those attending to these patients. They are caused by pooling of upper airway secretions at the back of the mouth and throat. As air passes through these secretions, the noise gives the impression that the patient is drowning [12].

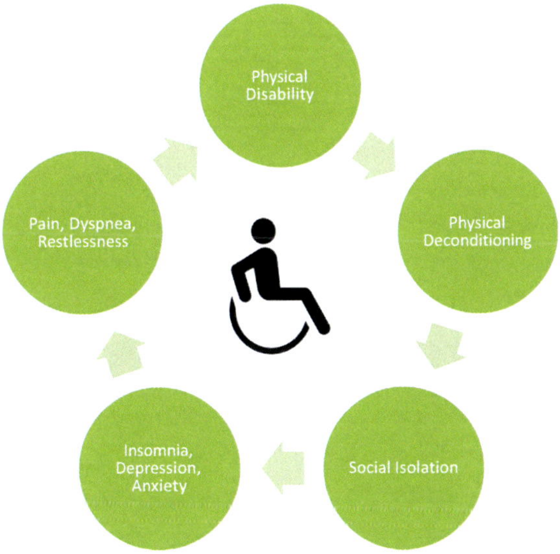

Fig. (1). The self-perpetuating vicious cycle of physical symptoms, physical disability and mood disorders.

Non-malignant Terminal Pulmonary Pathologies

Palliative care has traditionally focused on terminally ill cancer patients. However, the National Institute for Health and Care Excellence (NICE) has demanded that palliative care services be made available to all patients with chronic diseases, regardless of their malignant potential. Pulmonology is no exception; millions of people die each year of chronic non-malignant pulmonary disorders such as chronic obstructive pulmonary disease (COPD), cystic fibrosis (CF) and interstitial lung disease (ILD). The suffering from these diseases is comparable to lung cancer [1]. Yet, palliative care involvement and discussion of end of life care goals remains suboptimal [13]. A study evaluating patients dying in the intensive care units (ICU) found that patients with COPD and ILD, received fewer elements of palliative care as compared to patients suffering from lung cancer [14].

Non-interventional Palliative Strategies

A number of non-interventional strategies are available for addressing the distressing symptoms of advanced pulmonary diseases. Cough, dyspnea and pain are the most commonly reported symptoms. For productive cough with worsening dyspnea, antibiotics may be helpful, since infections are often responsible for causing exacerbation of symptoms in lung cancer, COPD, ILD, CF *etc*. In addition, nebulized saline, bronchodilators and mucolytic agents can be prescribed to promote clearance of the secretions. For dry cough, or if the patients are too frail or have a weak cough reflex, systemic opioids can be used to suppress cough [4]. For dyspnea without a reversible cause, opioids are the backbone of treatment [15, 16]. Opioids work by alleviating the perception of air hunger and decreasing the difference between the central ventilatory drive and the actual ventilation. Despite lack of strong evidence, benzodiazepines have also been used as second and third line agents for palliating dyspnea [17, 18]. For management of terminal secretions, atropine, hyoscine butylbromide and scopolamine can be used since they inhibit further production of secretions [19].

Non interventional palliative strategies for COPD closely overlap those for lung cancer. Opioids have a central role in the relief of dyspnea, just like in lung cancer. Evidence supporting the use of noninvasive ventilation (NIV) towards the end of life in COPD patients is equivocal, therefore NIV should be avoided [20]. Some authors have also recommended strategies such as upright positioning, cool air fans, deep breathing and relaxation exercises for alleviating distress in COPD patients.

Other non-pharmacological interventions include purse lip breathing, teaching relaxation techniques early in the disease course and referral to pulmonary rehabilitation programs. Having an action plan in place for recurrent exacerbations can also reduce frequent emergency room visits and hospitalizations.

INTERVENTIONAL PULMONOLOGY AND PALLIATIVE CARE/ HOSPICE MEDICINE

In addition to the above mentioned noninvasive interventions, interventional measures can be utilized to adequately relieve disabling symptoms towards the end of life. Recent advances in the field of interventional pulmonology have made it possible to offer these interventions with a very favorable risk benefit ratio. Most of these procedures with a palliative intent can be safely performed on an outpatient basis, thus minimizing the number of days patients spend in the hospital.

Some of the pulmonary pathologies that can be addressed by interventional pulmonology include malignant pleural effusions, hemoptysis, airway obstruction and, lobar and segmental lung collapse. These pathologies are responsible for the bulk of disabling symptoms experienced by advanced lung cancer patients, such as dyspnea, secretions, infections and fever. Thus, interventional pulmonology is revolutionizing the scope of palliative care in these patients.

Malignant Pleural Effusion

Introduction

Malignant pleural effusion (MPE) is defined as the accumulation of a significant amount of exudative fluid in the pleural space accompanied by malignant cells or tumor tissue [21]. Autopsy studies have revealed that tumor first spreads to the visceral pleura mostly through hematogenous route [22]. However, tumor can also spread through lymphangitic route or by direct extension. From the visceral pleura tumor subsequently spreads to the parietal pleura. The underlying mechanism behind MPE is believed to be a combination of increased fluid accumulation due to hyperpermeable pleura and decreased fluid clearance due to impaired lymphatic drainage [23].

About 150,000 cases of MPE are reported in the US each year [24]. Lung cancer is the single biggest cause of MPE and accounts for about 40% of all MPE cases [25]. Breast cancer is the second most common MPE etiology [26]. Unfortunately the presence of MPE is indicative of metastatic cancer and the median expected survival is only 4 to 6 months [27]. Patients with MPE due to mesothelioma have a slightly better survival at 9 to 12 months [28]. The incidence of MPE and associated health care costs are expected to further rise because of increased global cancer rates and advances in systemic therapies [29]. Therefore, MPE has been the focus of research over recent years, especially with regards to palliating some of the advanced lung cancer symptoms.

Diagnosing Malignant Pleural Effusions

Not all effusions seen in cancer patients are malignant. Patients with lung cancer can have effusions due to other etiologies such as pneumonia, pulmonary embolism or heart failure. Therefore, a reasonable amount of work-up must be performed before labelling a pleural effusion as malignant. Pleural thickening and nodularity on imaging suggest MPE [30, 31]. In particular circumferential pleural thickening, mediastinal pleural thickening and pleural thickening >1cm have been reported to be highly specific for MPE [32]. Positron emission tomography (PET) only has an 81% sensitivity and 74% specificity for MPE, therefore authors have recommended against its routine use for the diagnosis of MPE [33].

Ultrasound guided thoracentesis is typically the first procedure performed as part of suspected MPE work up. It serves both as a diagnostic procedure and also helps assess the impact of fluid drainage on symptom control. The latter is important since the amount of pleural fluid has been shown to poorly correlate with the level of dyspnea [24]. Complications are uncommon with ultrasound guided thoracentesis. One study reported a pneumothorax rate of 2.5% with chest tube insertion needed in only 0.8% of the cases [34, 35]. The mean sensitivity of cytological examination of pleural fluid is 60% [36]. However, the sensitivity goes up with subsequent taps. Despite the low sensitivity of the first pleural tap, it is invaluable since it also helps exclude competing diagnoses. Some investigators have also recommended using pleural manometry during thoracentesis for diagnosis of non-expandable lung and as a safeguard against re-expansion pulmonary edema [37]. However, others have argued against its usefulness [38].

If diagnostic uncertainty remains, medical thoracoscopy may be considered [39]. Medical thoracoscopy has a sensitivity of 91%, specificity of 100% and an overall accuracy of 93%. Only 1.9% of patients were reported to have major complications as per one study [40]. Mortality rate associated with medical thoracoscopy is very low at 0.3% [41]. At times, however, medical thoracoscopy may not be feasible if the patient has loculated pleural effusions or if the lung is tethered to the chest wall. In such cases physician based ultrasound guided pleural biopsy may be considered, which has an estimated sensitivity of 94% [42].

Management

Once the diagnosis of MPE has been established and it has been demonstrated that fluid drainage will improve symptoms, the next question is determining the optimal strategy for draining the pleural effusion on a long term basis. It is important to bear in mind that these patients have advanced malignancy and have a low life expectancy. So any intervention offered must be safe and shouldn't cause much discomfort for the patient, in line with the principles of palliative care. Over the years management of MPE has shifted from radical surgical procedures to minimally invasive procedures being offered by interventional pulmonologists [43]. Open thoracotomy was once the standard procedure for MPE, however it requires general anesthesia, large incisions and longer hospitalizations (5-7 days) [44]. Pain is a major issue post-thoracotomy, with a significant number of patients requiring further interventions for chronic pain [45, 46]. Open thoracotomy has therefore fallen out of favor and its place has been taken by other modalities being offered by interventional pulmonologists. These include indwelling pleural catheters (IPC), pleurodesis or repeat thoracentesis. It is worth noting here that there is no consensus about the timing of these interventions. Some investigators have proposed that early intervention reduces the risk of trapped lung [47]. However, other authors argue that all MPEs might not necessarily recur, therefore there should be no rush in terms of performing a definitive procedure for drainage.

Repeat Thoracentesis

Repeat thoracentesis is by no means an optimal strategy for long term management of MPE. Since each time the patient gets poked, it comes with additional pain and, risks of pneumothorax and infection. Therefore, repeat thoracentesis may only rarely be considered if the expected survival is so short that the patient is deemed unlikely to be able to draw significant benefit from more advanced procedures such as IPC insertion or pleurodesis [24].

Indwelling Pleural Catheters

Multiple studies have established the efficacy and safety profile of indwelling pleural catheters (IPCs). This has led to leading European and US guidelines advocating its use in the management of MPE [43, 48]. Van Meter *et al.* published a systematic review of IPC use in MPE. They reported symptomatic improvement in 95.6% of patients [49]. Second Therapeutic Intervention in Malignant Effusion Trial [TIME2] was a landmark trial comparing IPC with chest tube insertion and talc pleurodesis. Investigators reported significantly better symptom control in the IPC group at 6 weeks. Length of hospitalization was also significantly lower in the IPC group [50].

In a more recent prospective cohort trial in patients with MPE, Walker *et al.* compared four treatment options: IPC, video assisted thoracic surgery (VATS) and IPC; chest tube and talc slurry; and VATS talc poudrage [51]. Patient reported outcomes were assessed using functional assessment of chronic illness therapy–palliative (FACIT–PAL), London Chest Activity of Daily Living scale and FACIT–treatment satisfaction questionnaires. Authors concluded that while all treatment options addressed patients' symptoms and relieved dyspnea; IPC offered effective treatment with minimal discomfort and time in hospital, and with high patient satisfaction. Another advantage of IPC is that it can also lead to secondary pleurodesis in about half the patients [49]. If pleurodesis has been achieved, IPC can potentially be removed at that time.

IPC has also been deemed to be cost effective in multiple cost effectiveness analyses, especially if life expectancy is less than 6 weeks [52, 53] In another randomized study performed at multiple centers in Australia, New Zealand, Singapore and Hong Kong, authors compared IPC and pleurodesis (with talc slurry) in patients with MPE [54]. They found no significant difference in mortality or adverse event rates between the two groups, however, there was a mean reduction in the duration of hospitalization by 3.7 days/patient in the IPC group. The authors concluded that the use of IPC can reduce up to 555,000 hospital days over pleurodesis without adverse impact on mortality or complication rate.

Just like any other intervention, IPCs can be associated with a number of complications such as empyema, cellulitis, pneumothorax and catheter tract metastasis. The risk of IPC related pleural infection is low. In one study only 4.9% of patients developed infectious complications and 94% of these infections were controlled with antibiotics. Only one pleural infection related death was reported [55]. In another study, risks of cellulitis, empyema and pneumothorax were found to be 3.4%, 2.8% and 5.9%, respectively [49]. Catheter tract metastasis typically present as nodules along the IPC tract [56]. These respond well to radiation therapy. Davies *et al.* reported a 1.9% incidence of this complication in patients with IPC [50]. Severe pain requiring IPC removal is very rare [56]. Another complication associated with the use of IPCs is the development of pleural loculations, which can impede further fluid drainage. This has been reported in 14% of patients with IPCs [57]. Although instillation of a fibrinolytic agent in to the IPC can increase the pleural fluid drainage, there is no consensus as to which patients will benefit from its use [57].

Pleurodesis

Pleurodesis works by the introduction of a sclerosant in to the pleural space. This causes acute inflammation which in turn progresses to chronic inflammation and fibrosis. These changes eventually lead to apposition of the visceral and parietal pleural layers, therefore, obliterating the pleural space. Since the sclerosant works by inducing inflammation, patient will complain of pain, chills and malaise.

Stronger the sclerosant, greater will be the chances of success, but it will be at the expense of greater side effects [24]. Sclerosant is most often instilled via chest tube but can also potentially be introduced during thoracoscopy. Success rates are the same whether the sclerosant is introduced through a chest tube or during thoracoscopy [58 - 60]. Open pleurectomy has a high procedural morbidity and is rarely performed for this indication [43]. Various authors have looked at the factors that can predict failure of pleurodesis. Pleural fluid glucose levels < 60 mg/dL, pH < 7.20, lactate dehydrogenase (LDH) > 700 mg/dL, poor performance status and presence of radiographic abnormalities, have all been associated with increased risk of pleurodesis failure [25]. However, other investigators have advised caution when using these parameters as predictors of failure [27].

Talc is most commonly used sclerosant and was first described by Norman Bethune in 1935 [61]. Other investigators have also used iodopovidene, OK-432 (derived from Streptococcus Pyogenes) and Staphylococcal antigens for inducing pleurodesis and have reported good success rates [62 - 64]. Trials comparing talc with bleomycin, have found the former to be superior [65 - 68]. Similarly, talc has also been found to be superior to tetracycline derivatives [69, 70]. Interestingly, investigators have found no significant difference in the pleurodesis success rates whether a small bore catheter or a large one is used for the instillation of the sclerosant [71, 72].

If small sized talc particles are used there is a risk for systemic absorption which can in turn cause an intense pulmonary inflammatory response [73, 74]. This risk is minimal with the use of large sized talc particles. In one study 2.3% of patients died from respiratory failure attributable to systemic absorption of talc [58].

Hemoptysis

Introduction

Hemoptysis is another symptom commonly associated with advanced lung cancer. At least 30% of patients with lung cancer report hemoptysis at some stage; conversely lung cancer is responsible for 30% of all hemoptysis cases [75]. Lung cancer is also commonly associated with massive hemoptysis. Although there is no consensus about the precise volume of hemoptysis to qualify it as massive, it generally refers to hemoptysis that causes abnormal gas exchange and hemodynamic instability [76]. Just like MPE described previously, hemoptysis is often associated with advanced incurable disease. Majority of lung cancer patient with hemoptysis are candidates for palliative care and if conservative measures fail interventional pulmonologists can offer minimally invasive procedure to palliate their symptoms of bleeding.

Management

Initial management of massive hemoptysis begins with securing and maintaining adequate airway [48]. Single lumen cuffed endotracheal tube is preferred for this purpose, since a double lumen tube has narrow lumens which are more likely to get clogged up and can make bronchoscopic interventions difficult [77]. Flexible bronchoscopy is typically the first intervention performed. It can provide information about the bleeding's location and severity, and the feasibility of different treatment options. In one study bronchoscopy was able to localize bleeding in 90% of the cases [68]. When the source of bleeding is localized, management includes tamponading the effected segment by tightly wedging the scope in the airway leading to the affected segment and instilling cold saline to cause vasoconstriction [78]. If wedging, cold saline and topical epinephrine fail to control the bleeding, bronchial blockade balloons can be deployed [48].

If the above measures are not successful in stemming the blood loss, other modalities that can be offered by interventional pulmonologists include topical hemostatic tamponade (THT), argon plasma coagulation (APC) and neodymium-doped yttrium aluminum garnet (Nd:YAG) laser coagulation. THT is performed by placing oxidized regenerated cellulose (ORC) mesh over the bleeding site. Valipour *et al.* reported a 98% success rate for THT with ORC. All of the meshes were eventually resorbed without any foreign body reaction [79]. APC is a method of non-contact electrocoagulation using ionized argon gas [80]. Morice *et al.* reported employing APC in 31 patients with hemoptysis and 25 patients with hemoptysis and obstruction. Hemoptysis resolution was reported in all cases with no procedural complications [81]. Nd:YAG laser, on the other hand, has been shown to have a therapeutic response rate of 60% in hemoptysis [48]. In case bronchoscopic interventions fail or are unavailable, patient can also be referred to interventional radiology for bronchial artery embolization (BAE). In one study BAE was able to control hemoptysis in 77% cases [82]. Surgery is the last resort if all else fails.

Airway Obstruction

Introduction

Lung cancer can cause obstruction of trachea, main stem bronchi, lobar bronchi or smaller airways. Such lesions can in turn produce areas of lung collapse, atelectasis and post obstructive pneumonia. Patients will complain of dyspnea, cough, hemoptysis and increased secretions. In fact at least one third of lung cancer patients will develop obstruction of trachea or main stem bronchi at some point during their disease course [83]. Unfortunately, only one-fifth of lung cancer patients with malignant airway obstruction will be amenable to curative surgery [84]. For the rest the focus will be on palliating the symptoms. Advances in interventional pulmonology have made it possible to offer a number of interventions for airway obstructive lesions.

Management

Interventions for airway obstructing lesions include electrocautery, neodymium-doped yttrium aluminium garnet (Nd:YAG) laser, argon plasma coagulation (APC), high dose rate endobronchial brachytherapy (HDREB), rigid bronchoscopy and airway stenting. Electrocautery uses electricity to generate heat which causes tissue ablation [85, 86]. Boxem *et al.* retrospectively compared electrocautery and Nd:YAG laser for palliation of symptoms of airway obstruction [87]. Relief of dyspnea was the primary outcome studied. Overall relief of symptoms was achieved in 70% of the patients, with no significant differences in the outcomes between the two modalities. APC on the other hand causes tissue coagulation using ionized gas [80]. This is the same mechanism that makes APC a useful tool for bleeding pulmonary lesions as well. In one study APC was able to provide patency in about 90% of cases with malignant airway obstruction [80]. No significant complications were reported.

Brachytherapy involves bronchoscopic introduction of a radioactive isotope in close proximity of a tumor, which in turn allows for delivery of high dose radiotherapy [88]. Endobronchial brachytherapy has been studied and found to be effective in the management of non-small cell lung cancer (NSCLC) [89]. However, endobronchial brachytherapy appears to be losing ground to the previously discussed endobronchial modalities, as palliative procedure of choice for endobronchial obstruction. This is because the latter are not only more effective but also less costly. Ung *et al.* performed a systematic review of 29 trials of HDREB for palliation of lung cancer symptoms such as dyspnea, cough, chest pain and hemoptysis [90]. While external beam radiation (EBR) was superior to HDREB, HDREB plus EBR was superior to EBR alone. Therefore, the authors recommended considering HDREB for patients with recurrent endobronchial obstructing lesions, who have been previously treated with EBR. Also treatment adverse effects such as hemoptysis, tracheomalacia, fistulas *etc.* are a major limiting factor for endobronchial brachytherapy [91].

Rigid bronchoscopy with tumor debulking and airway stenting of larger airways has produced excellent results [92]. Furukawa *et al.* reported a review of 58 endobronchial stent placements in 40 patients with lung cancer [93]. These included Dumon silicone stents, self-expandable metallic stents (SEMS) and the Dynamic Stents. Significant improvement was noted on various functional and performance scales. Complication rate was 13% and included hemoptysis, fistulas, restenosis, secretions and stent migration. In another review of 12 patients with malignant tracheal obstruction who were treated with metallic expandable tracheal stents, Gaafar *et al*. reported that the procedure was tolerated well by all patients. All patients had significant improvement in their pulmonary function tests (PFTs) [94].

CONCLUSION

Discussion of advanced care planning, treatment options and end of life issues in patients with advanced chronic diseases like COPD is quite challenging. Major barriers are: i) chronic diseases are associated with quiet variable trajectories [95]. Even though prognosis of COPD is poor [95, 96], prognostication remains uncertain [97, 98], ii) patients remain uninformed / unrealistic about their disease and therefore do not participate actively in decision making. Consequently, physicians are often reluctant to discuss palliative care options and, interestingly, when they do so, the reaction of patients involves negative surprise. This might also be attributed to the fact that public understanding of these diseases is not linked to dying, unlike for example cancer [99]. With current advances in the interventional pulmonary medicine, options are available to palliate the most distressing symptoms of advanced lung diseases. Pulmonary physicians may play a big role in providing the education and offering both medical and psychological support to both patients and their families.

CONFLICT OF INTEREST

The authors declare no conflict of interest, financial or otherwise.

ACKNOWLEDGEMENTS

Declared none.

REFERENCES

[1] World Health Organization. WHO definition of palliative care-2005. Available at: http://www.who.int/cancer/palliative/definition/en/print.html

[2] Earle CC, Neville BA, Landrum MB, Ayanian JZ, Block SD, Weeks JC. Trends in the aggressiveness of cancer care near the end of life. J Clin Oncol 2004; 22(2): 315-21. [http://dx.doi.org/10.1200/JCO.2004.08.136] [PMID: 14722041]

[3] National hospice and palliative care organization. National hospice and palliative care organization. Available at: http://www.nhpco.org/

[4] Lim RB. End-of-life care in patients with advanced lung cancer. Ther Adv Respir Dis 2016; 10(5): 455-67. [http://dx.doi.org/10.1177/1753465816660925] [PMID: 27585597]

[5] CDC. Leading causes of death. Available at: http://www.cdc.gov/nchs/fastats/leading-causes-of-death.htm

[6] Siegel RL, Miller KD, Jemal A. Cancer statistics, 2016. CA Cancer J Clin 2016; 66(1): 7-30. [http://dx.doi.org/10.3322/caac.21332] [PMID: 26742998]

[7] Surveillance, epidemiology, and end results program. Available at: http://seer.cancer.gov/

[8] Ellershaw J, Smith C, Overill S, Walker SE, Aldridge J. Care of the dying: setting standards for symptom control in the last 48 hours of life. J Pain Symptom Manage 2001; 21(1): 12-7. [http://dx.doi.org/10.1016/S0885-3924(00)00240-2] [PMID: 11223310]

[9] Stone P, Rees E, Hardy JR. End of life care in patients with malignant disease. Eur J Cancer 2001; 37(9): 1070-5. [http://dx.doi.org/10.1016/S0959-8049(01)00087-9] [PMID: 11378335]

[10] Kvale PA, Selecky PA, Prakash UB, *et al.* Palliative care in lung cancer: ACCP evidence-based clinical practice guidelines (2nd edition). Chest. 2007; 132: pp. 368S-403S.

[11] Disler RT, Currow DC, Phillips JL, Smith T, Johnson MJ, Davidson PM. Interventions to support a palliative care approach in patients with chronic obstructive pulmonary disease: an integrative review. Int J Nurs Stud 2012; 49(11): 1443-58. [http://dx.doi.org/10.1016/j.ijnurstu.2012.02.004] [PMID: 22405402]

[12] Morita T, Ichiki T, Tsunoda J, Inoue S, Chihara S. A prospective study on the dying process in terminally ill cancer patients. Am J Hosp Palliat Care 1998; 15(4): 217-22. [http://dx.doi.org/10.1177/104990919801500407] [PMID: 9729972]

[13] Tsim S, Davidson S. End-of-life care in a general respiratory ward in the United Kingdom. Am J Hosp Palliat Care 2014; 31(2): 172-4. [http://dx.doi.org/10.1177/1049909113481261] [PMID: 23503567]

[14] Brown CE, Engelberg RA, Nielsen EL, Curtis JR. Palliative care for patients dying in the intensive care unit with chronic lung disease compared with metastatic cancer. Ann Am Thorac Soc 2016; 13(5): 684-9. [http://dx.doi.org/10.1513/AnnalsATS.201510-667OC] [PMID: 26784137]

[15] Abernethy AP, Currow DC, Frith P, Fazekas BS, McHugh A, Bui C. Randomised, double blind, placebo controlled crossover trial of sustained release morphine for the management of refractory dyspnoea. BMJ 2003; 327(7414): 523-8. [http://dx.doi.org/10.1136/bmj.327.7414.523] [PMID: 12958109]

[16] Jennings A-L, Davies AN, Higgins JP, Gibbs JS, Broadley KE. A systematic review of the use of opioids in the management of dyspnoea. Thorax 2002; 57(11): 939-44. [http://dx.doi.org/10.1136/thorax.57.11.939] [PMID: 12403875]

[17] Currow D, Johnson M, White P, Abernethy A. Evidence-based intervention for chronic refractory breathlessness: practical therapies that make a difference. Br J Gen Pract 2013; 63(616): 609-10. [http://dx.doi.org/10.3399/bjgp13X674611] [PMID: 24267852]

[18] Simon ST, Higginson IJ, Booth S, Harding R, Bausewein C. Benzodiazepines for the relief of breathlessness in advanced malignant and non-malignant diseases in adults. Cochrane Database Syst Rev 2010; CD007354(1): CD007354. [http://dx.doi.org/10.1002/14651858.CD007354.pub2] [PMID: 20091630]

[19] Mercadante S, Villari P, Ferrera P. Refractory death rattle: deep aspiration facilitates the effects of antisecretory agents. J Pain Symptom Manage 2011; 41(3): 637-9. [http://dx.doi.org/10.1016/j.jpainsymman.2010.06.012] [PMID: 21131169]

[20] Lilly EJ, Senderovich H. Palliative care in chronic obstructive pulmonary disease. J Crit Care 2016; 35: 150-4. [http://dx.doi.org/10.1016/j.jcrc.2016.05.019] [PMID: 27481751]

[21] Psallidas I, Kalomenidis I, Porcel JM, Robinson BW, Stathopoulos GT. Malignant pleural effusion: from bench to bedside. Eur Respir Rev 2016; 25(140): 189-98.

[http://dx.doi.org/10.1183/16000617.0019-2016] [PMID: 27246596]

[22] Meyer PC. Metastatic carcinoma of the pleura. Thorax 1966; 21(5): 437-43. [http://dx.doi.org/10.1136/thx.21.5.437] [PMID: 5969243]

[23] Stathopoulos GT, Kalomenidis I. Malignant pleural effusion: tumor-host interactions unleashed. Am J Respir Crit Care Med 2012; 186(6): 487-92. [http://dx.doi.org/10.1164/rccm.201203-0465PP] [PMID: 22652027]

[24] Thomas R, Francis R, Davies HE, Lee YC. Interventional therapies for malignant pleural effusions: the present and the future. Respirology 2014; 19(6): 809-22. [http://dx.doi.org/10.1111/resp.12328] [PMID: 24947955]

[25] Martínez-Moragón E, Aparicio J, Sanchis J, Menéndez R, Cruz Rogado M, Sanchis F. Malignant pleural effusion: prognostic factors for survival and response to chemical pleurodesis in a series of 120 cases. Respiration 1998; 65(2): 108-13. [http://dx.doi.org/10.1159/000029240] [PMID: 9580921]

[26] Mongardon N, Pinton-Gonnet C, Szekely B, Michel-Cherqui M, Dreyfus JF, Fischler M. Assessment of chronic pain after thoracotomy: a 1-year prevalence study. Clin J Pain 2011; 27(8): 677-81. [http://dx.doi.org/10.1097/AJP.0b013e31821981a3] [PMID: 21705876]

[27] Heffner JE, Nietert PJ, Barbieri C. Pleural fluid pH as a predictor of pleurodesis failure: analysis of primary data. Chest 2000; 117(1): 87-95. [http://dx.doi.org/10.1378/chest.117.1.87] [PMID: 10631204]

[28] Vogelzang NJ, Rusthoven JJ, Symanowski J, *et al.* Phase III study of pemetrexed in combination with cisplatin *versus* cisplatin alone in patients with malignant pleural mesothelioma. J Clin Oncol 2003; 21(14): 2636-44. [http://dx.doi.org/10.1200/JCO.2003.11.136] [PMID: 12860938]

[29] Clive AO, Bhatnagar R, Psallidas I, Maskell NA. Individualised management of malignant pleural effusion. Lancet Respir Med 2015; 3(7): 505-6. [http://dx.doi.org/10.1016/S2213-2600(15)00183-6] [PMID: 26170072]

[30] Bugalho A, Ferreira D, Dias SS, *et al.* The diagnostic value of transthoracic ultrasonographic features in predicting malignancy in undiagnosed pleural effusions: a prospective observational study. Respiration 2014; 87(4): 270-8. [http://dx.doi.org/10.1159/000357266] [PMID: 24480900]

[31] Qureshi NR, Rahman NM, Gleeson FV. Thoracic ultrasound in the diagnosis of malignant pleural effusion. Thorax 2009; 64(2): 139-43. [http://dx.doi.org/10.1136/thx.2008.100545] [PMID: 18852159]

[32] Leung AN, Müller NL, Miller RR. CT in differential diagnosis of diffuse pleural disease. AJR Am J Roentgenol 1990; 154(3): 487-92. [http://dx.doi.org/10.2214/ajr.154.3.2106209] [PMID: 2106209]

[33] Porcel JM, Hernández P, Martínez-Alonso M, Bielsa S, Salud A. Accuracy of fluorodeoxyglucose-PET imaging for differentiating benign from malignant pleural effusions: a meta-analysis. Chest 2015; 147(2): 502-12. [http://dx.doi.org/10.1378/chest.14-0820] [PMID: 25188411]

[34] Jones PW, Moyers JP, Rogers JT, Rodriguez RM, Lee YC, Light RW. Ultrasound-guided thoracentesis: is it a safer method? Chest 2003; 123(2): 418-23. [http://dx.doi.org/10.1378/chest.123.2.418] [PMID: 12576360]

[35] Mercaldi CJ, Lanes SF. Ultrasound guidance decreases complications and improves the cost of care among patients undergoing thoracentesis and paracentesis. Chest 2013; 143(2): 532-8. [http://dx.doi.org/10.1378/chest.12-0447] [PMID: 23381318]

[36] Hooper C, Lee YCG, Maskell N. Investigation of a unilateral pleural effusion in adults: British Thoracic Society Pleural Disease Guideline 2010. Thorax 2010; 65(Suppl 2): ii4-17.

[37] Folch E, Mahajan A, Majid A. Pleural manometry: ready for prime time. J Bronchology Interv Pulmonol 2013; 20(4): 297-8. [http://dx.doi.org/10.1097/LBR.0000000000000019] [PMID: 24162110]

[38] Maldonado F, Mullon JJ. Counterpoint: should pleural manometry be performed routinely during thoracentesis? No. Chest 2012; 141(4): 846-8. [http://dx.doi.org/10.1378/chest.11-3233] [PMID: 22474146]

[39] Henderson DW, Reid G, Kao SC, van Zandwijk N, Klebe S. Challenges and controversies in the diagnosis of mesothelioma: Part 1. Cytology-only diagnosis, biopsies, immunohistochemistry, discrimination between mesothelioma and reactive mesothelial hyperplasia, and biomarkers. J Clin Pathol 2013; 66(10): 847-53. [http://dx.doi.org/10.1136/jclinpath-2012-201303] [PMID: 23814259]

[40] Menzies R, Charbonneau M. Thoracoscopy for the diagnosis of pleural disease. Ann Intern Med 1991; 114(4): 271-6. [http://dx.doi.org/10.7326/0003-4819-114-4-271] [PMID: 1987873]

[41] Rahman NM, Ali NJ, Brown G, *et al.* British Thoracic Society Pleural Disease Guideline Group. Local anaesthetic thoracoscopy: British Thoracic Society Pleural Disease Guideline 2010. Thorax 2010; 65 (Suppl. 2): ii54-60. [http://dx.doi.org/10.1136/thx.2010.137018] [PMID: 20696694]

[42] Hallifax RJ, Corcoran JP, Ahmed A, *et al.* Physician-based ultrasound-guided biopsy for diagnosing pleural disease. Chest 2014; 146(4): 1001-6. [http://dx.doi.org/10.1378/chest.14-0299] [PMID: 24832701]

[43] Roberts ME, Neville E, Berrisford RG, Antunes G, Ali NJ. BTS Pleural Disease Guideline Group. Management of a malignant pleural effusion: British Thoracic Society Pleural Disease Guideline 2010. Thorax 2010; 65 (Suppl. 2): ii32-40. [http://dx.doi.org/10.1136/thx.2010.136994] [PMID: 20696691]

[44] Putnam J. Lung, chest wall, pleura, and mediastinum. Sabiston Textbook of Surgery. Philadelphia, PA: Elsevier Saunders 2012. [http://dx.doi.org/10.1016/B978-1-4377-1560-6.00058-5]

[45] Furrer M, Rechsteiner R, Eigenmann V, Signer C, Althaus U, Ris HB. Thoracotomy and thoracoscopy: postoperative pulmonary function, pain and chest wall complaints. Eur J Cardiothorac Surg 1997; 12(1): 82-7. [http://dx.doi.org/10.1016/S1010-7940(97)00105-X] [PMID: 9262085]

[46] Dajczman E, Gordon A, Kreisman H, Wolkove N. Long-term postthoracotomy pain. Chest 1991; 99(2): 270-4. [http://dx.doi.org/10.1378/chest.99.2.270] [PMID: 1989781]

[47] Rodriguez-Panadero F, Antony VB. Pleurodesis: state of the art. Eur Respir J 1997; 10(7): 1648-54. [http://dx.doi.org/10.1183/09031936.97.10071648] [PMID: 9230261]

[48] Simoff MJ, Lally B, Slade MG, *et al.* Symptom management in patients with lung cancer: Diagnosis and management of lung cancer, 3rd ed: American College of Chest Physicians evidence-based clinical practice guidelines. Chest. 2013; 143: pp. e455S-97S.

[49] Van Meter ME, McKee KY, Kohlwes RJ. Efficacy and safety of tunneled pleural catheters in adults with malignant pleural effusions: a systematic review. J Gen Intern Med 2011; 26(1): 70-6. [http://dx.doi.org/10.1007/s11606-010-1472-0] [PMID: 20697963]

[50] Davies HE, Mishra EK, Kahan BC, *et al.* Effect of an indwelling pleural catheter vs chest tube and talc pleurodesis for relieving dyspnea in patients with malignant pleural effusion: the TIME2 randomized controlled trial. JAMA 2012; 307(22): 2383-9. [http://dx.doi.org/10.1001/jama.2012.5535] [PMID: 22610520]

[51] Walker S, Zubrinic M, Massey C, Shargall Y, Bédard E, Darling G. A prospective study of patient-

centred outcomes in the management of malignant pleural effusions. Int J Palliat Nurs 2016; 22(7): 351-8.
[http://dx.doi.org/10.12968/ijpn.2016.22.7.351] [PMID: 27444164]

[52] Puri V, Pyrdeck TL, Crabtree TD, *et al.* Treatment of malignant pleural effusion: a cost-effectiveness analysis. Ann Thorac Surg 2012; 94(2): 374-9.
[http://dx.doi.org/10.1016/j.athoracsur.2012.02.100] [PMID: 22579398]

[53] Olden AM, Holloway R. Treatment of malignant pleural effusion: PleuRx catheter or talc pleurodesis? A cost-effectiveness analysis. J Palliat Med 2010; 13(1): 59-65.
[http://dx.doi.org/10.1089/jpm.2009.0220] [PMID: 19839739]

[54] Lee YC, Fysh ET, Thomas R, *et al.* Australasian Malignant Pleural Effusion (AMPLE) Trial: A Multicentre Randomised Study Comparing Indwelling Pleural Catheter versus Talc Pleurodesis.Leural Disease: Clinical Studies. 2016.

[55] Fysh ET, Tremblay A, Feller-Kopman D, *et al.* Clinical outcomes of indwelling pleural catheter-related pleural infections: an international multicenter study. Chest 2013; 144(5): 1597-602.
[http://dx.doi.org/10.1378/chest.12-3103] [PMID: 23828305]

[56] Lui MM, Thomas R, Lee YC. Complications of indwelling pleural catheter use and their management. BMJ Open Respir Res 2016; 3(1): e000123.
[http://dx.doi.org/10.1136/bmjresp-2015-000123] [PMID: 26870384]

[57] Thomas R, Piccolo F, Miller D, *et al.* Intrapleural Fibrinolysis for the Treatment of Indwelling Pleural Catheter-Related Symptomatic Loculations: A Multicenter Observational Study. Chest 2015; 148(3): 746-51.
[http://dx.doi.org/10.1378/chest.14-2401] [PMID: 25742001]

[58] Dresler CM, Olak J, Herndon JE II, *et al.* Cooperative Groups Cancer and Leukemia Group B; Eastern Cooperative Oncology Group; North Central Cooperative Oncology Group; Radiation Therapy Oncology Group. Phase III intergroup study of talc poudrage vs talc slurry sclerosis for malignant pleural effusion. Chest 2005; 127(3): 909-15.
[http://dx.doi.org/10.1378/chest.127.3.909] [PMID: 15764775]

[59] Tan C, Sedrakyan A, Browne J, Swift S, Treasure T. The evidence on the effectiveness of management for malignant pleural effusion: a systematic review. Eur J Cardiothorac Surg 2006; 29(5): 829-38.
[http://dx.doi.org/10.1016/j.ejcts.2005.12.025] [PMID: 16626967]

[60] Yim AP, Chan AT, Lee TW, Wan IY, Ho JK. Thoracoscopic talc insufflation *versus* talc slurry for symptomatic malignant pleural effusion. Ann Thorac Surg 1996; 62(6): 1655-8.
[http://dx.doi.org/10.1016/S0003-4975(96)00808-9] [PMID: 8957368]

[61] Bethune N. Pleural poudrage: a new technique for deliberate production of pleural adhesions as a preliminary to lobectomy. J Thorac Surg 1935; 4: 251-61.

[62] Agarwal R, Paul AS, Aggarwal AN, Gupta D, Jindal SK. A randomized controlled trial of the efficacy of cosmetic talc compared with iodopovidone for chemical pleurodesis. Respirology 2011; 16(7): 1064-9.
[http://dx.doi.org/10.1111/j.1440-1843.2011.01999.x] [PMID: 21605278]

[63] Kishi K, Homma S, Sakamoto S, *et al.* Efficacious pleurodesis with OK-432 and doxorubicin against malignant pleural effusions. Eur Respir J 2004; 24(2): 263-6.
[http://dx.doi.org/10.1183/09031936.04.00137403] [PMID: 15332395]

[64] Ren S, Terman DS, Bohach G, *et al.* Intrapleural staphylococcal superantigen induces resolution of malignant pleural effusions and a survival benefit in non-small cell lung cancer. Chest 2004; 126(5): 1529-39.
[http://dx.doi.org/10.1378/chest.126.5.1529] [PMID: 15539723]

[65] Hamed H, Fentiman IS, Chaudary MA, Rubens RD. Comparison of intracavitary bleomycin and talc

for control of pleural effusions secondary to carcinoma of the breast. Br J Surg 1989; 76(12): 1266-7. [http://dx.doi.org/10.1002/bjs.1800761214] [PMID: 2481558]

[66] Diacon AH, Wyser C, Bolliger CT, *et al.* Prospective randomized comparison of thoracoscopic talc poudrage under local anesthesia *versus* bleomycin instillation for pleurodesis in malignant pleural effusions. Am J Respir Crit Care Med 2000; 162(4 Pt 1): 1445-9. [http://dx.doi.org/10.1164/ajrccm.162.4.2002030] [PMID: 11029359]

[67] Zimmer PW, Hill M, Casey K, Harvey E, Low DE. Prospective randomized trial of talc slurry vs bleomycin in pleurodesis for symptomatic malignant pleural effusions. Chest 1997; 112(2): 430-4. [http://dx.doi.org/10.1378/chest.112.2.430] [PMID: 9266880]

[68] Ong KC, Indumathi V, Raghuram J, Ong YY. A comparative study of pleurodesis using talc slurry and bleomycin in the management of malignant pleural effusions. Respirology 2000; 5(2): 99-103. [http://dx.doi.org/10.1046/j.1440-1843.2000.00235.x] [PMID: 10894097]

[69] Fentiman IS, Rubens RD, Hayward JL. A comparison of intracavitary talc and tetracycline for the control of pleural effusions secondary to breast cancer. Eur J Cancer Clin Oncol 1986; 22(9): 1079-81. [http://dx.doi.org/10.1016/0277-5379(86)90009-X] [PMID: 3536525]

[70] Kuzdzał J, Sładek K, Wasowski D, *et al.* Talc powder vs doxycycline in the control of malignant pleural effusion: a prospective, randomized trial. Med Sci Monit 2003; 9(6): PI54-9. [PMID: 12824959]

[71] Parulekar W, Di Primio G, Matzinger F, Dennie C, Bociek G. Use of small-bore vs large-bore chest tubes for treatment of malignant pleural effusions. Chest 2001; 120(1): 19-25. [http://dx.doi.org/10.1378/chest.120.1.19] [PMID: 11451810]

[72] Caglayan B, Torun E, Turan D, *et al.* Efficacy of iodopovidone pleurodesis and comparison of small-bore catheter *versus* large-bore chest tube. Ann Surg Oncol 2008; 15(9): 2594-9. [http://dx.doi.org/10.1245/s10434-008-0004-1] [PMID: 18594928]

[73] Ferrer J, Montes JF, Villarino MA, Light RW, García-Valero J. Influence of particle size on extrapleural talc dissemination after talc slurry pleurodesis. Chest 2002; 122(3): 1018-27. [http://dx.doi.org/10.1378/chest.122.3.1018] [PMID: 12226049]

[74] Werebe EC, Pazetti R, Milanez de Campos JR, *et al.* Systemic distribution of talc after intrapleural administration in rats. Chest 1999; 115(1): 190-3. [http://dx.doi.org/10.1378/chest.115.1.190] [PMID: 9925083]

[75] Masuda E, Sista AK, Pua BB, Madoff DC. Palliative procedures in lung cancer. Semin Intervent Radiol 2013; 30(2): 199-205. [http://dx.doi.org/10.1055/s-0033-1342962] [PMID: 24436537]

[76] Ibrahim WH. Massive haemoptysis: the definition should be revised. Eur Respir J 2008; 32(4): 1131-2. [http://dx.doi.org/10.1183/09031936.00080108] [PMID: 18827169]

[77] Cohen E. Con: right-sided double-lumen endotracheal tubes should not be routinely used in thoracic surgery. J Cardiothorac Vasc Anesth 2002; 16(2): 249-52. [http://dx.doi.org/10.1053/jcan.2002.31092] [PMID: 11957180]

[78] Conlan AA, Hurwitz SS. Management of massive haemoptysis with the rigid bronchoscope and cold saline lavage. Thorax 1980; 35(12): 901-4. [http://dx.doi.org/10.1136/thx.35.12.901] [PMID: 7268664]

[79] Valipour A, Kreuzer A, Koller H, Koessler W, Burghuber OC. Bronchoscopy-guided topical hemostatic tamponade therapy for the management of life-threatening hemoptysis. Chest 2005; 127(6): 2113-8. [http://dx.doi.org/10.1378/chest.127.6.2113] [PMID: 15947328]

[80] Crosta C, Spaggiari L, De Stefano A, Fiori G, Ravizza D, Pastorino U. Endoscopic argon plasma coagulation for palliative treatment of malignant airway obstructions: early results in 47 cases. Lung

Cancer 2001; 33(1): 75-80.
[http://dx.doi.org/10.1016/S0169-5002(00)00245-2] [PMID: 11429198]

[81] Morice RC, Ece T, Ece F, Keus L. Endobronchial argon plasma coagulation for treatment of hemoptysis and neoplastic airway obstruction. Chest 2001; 119(3): 781-7.
[http://dx.doi.org/10.1378/chest.119.3.781] [PMID: 11243957]

[82] Mal H, Rullon I, Mellot F, *et al.* Immediate and long-term results of bronchial artery embolization for life-threatening hemoptysis. Chest 1999; 115(4): 996-1001.
[http://dx.doi.org/10.1378/chest.115.4.996] [PMID: 10208199]

[83] Santos RS, Raftopoulos Y, Keenan RJ, Halal A, Maley RH, Landreneau RJ. Bronchoscopic palliation of primary lung cancer: single or multimodality therapy? Surg Endosc 2004; 18(6): 931-6.
[http://dx.doi.org/10.1007/s00464-003-9202-x] [PMID: 15108108]

[84] Kazi AA, Flowers WJ, Barrett JM, O'Rourke AK, Postma GN, Weinberger PM. Ethical issues in laryngology: tracheal stenting as palliative care. Laryngoscope 2014; 124(7): 1663-7.
[http://dx.doi.org/10.1002/lary.24531] [PMID: 24254967]

[85] Mahmood K, Wahidi MM. Ablative therapies for central airway obstruction. Semin Respir Crit Care Med 2014; 35(6): 681-92.
[http://dx.doi.org/10.1055/s-0034-1395501] [PMID: 25463159]

[86] Hooper RG, Jackson FN. Endobronchial electrocautery. Chest 1985; 87(6): 712-4.
[http://dx.doi.org/10.1378/chest.87.6.712] [PMID: 3996055]

[87] Boxem TV, Muller M, Venmans B, *et al.* Nd-YAG laser vs bronchoscopic electrocautery for palliation of symptomatic airway obstruction: a cost-effectiveness study. Chest 1999; 116: 1108-12.

[88] Raben A, Mychalczak B. Brachytherapy for non-small cell lung cancer and selected neoplasms of the chest. Chest 1997; 112(4) (Suppl.): 276S-86S.
[http://dx.doi.org/10.1378/chest.112.4_Supplement.276S] [PMID: 9337304]

[89] Hilaris BS, Mastoras DA. Contemporary brachytherapy approaches in non-small-cell lung cancer. J Surg Oncol 1998; 69(4): 258-64.
[http://dx.doi.org/10.1002/(SICI)1096-9098(199812)69:4<258::AID-JSO11>3.0.CO;2-A] [PMID: 9881944]

[90] Ung YC, Yu E, Falkson C, Haynes AE, Stys-Norman D, Evans WK. Lung Cancer Disease Site Group Of Cancer Care Ontario's Program In Evidence-Based Care. The role of high-dose-rate brachytherapy in the palliation of symptoms in patients with non-small-cell lung cancer: a systematic review. Brachytherapy 2006; 5(3): 189-202.
[http://dx.doi.org/10.1016/j.brachy.2006.05.001] [PMID: 16864071]

[91] Hosni A, Bezjak A, Rink A, *et al.* High dose rate brachytherapy as a treatment option in endobronchial tumors. Lung Cancer Int 2016; 2016: 3086148.
[http://dx.doi.org/10.1155/2016/3086148] [PMID: 27493804]

[92] Huret B, Perez T, Dhalluin X, Dewavrin F, Ramon PP, Fournier C. Treatment of malignant central airways obstruction by rigid bronchoscopy. Rev Mal Respir 2015; 32(5): 477-84.
[http://dx.doi.org/10.1016/j.rmr.2013.09.018] [PMID: 26072007]

[93] Furukawa K, Ishida J, Yamaguchi G, *et al.* The role of airway stent placement in the management of tracheobronchial stenosis caused by inoperable advanced lung cancer. Surg Today 2010; 40(4): 315-20.
[http://dx.doi.org/10.1007/s00595-008-4058-2] [PMID: 20339985]

[94] Gaafar AH, Shaaban AY, Elhadidi MS. The use of metallic expandable tracheal stents in the management of inoperable malignant tracheal obstruction. Eur Arch Otorhinolaryngol 2012; 269(1): 247-53.
[http://dx.doi.org/10.1007/s00405-011-1569-z] [PMID: 21431955]

[95] Mosterd A, Hoes AW. Clinical epidemiology of heart failure. Heart 2007; 93(9): 1137-46.

[http://dx.doi.org/10.1136/hrt.2003.025270] [PMID: 17699180]

[96] Pauwels RA, Rabe KF. Burden and clinical features of chronic obstructive pulmonary disease (COPD). Lancet 2004; 364(9434): 613-20.
[http://dx.doi.org/10.1016/S0140-6736(04)16855-4] [PMID: 15313363]

[97] Lunney JR, Lynn J, Foley DJ, Lipson S, Guralnik JM. Patterns of functional decline at the end of life. JAMA 2003; 289(18): 2387-92.
[http://dx.doi.org/10.1001/jama.289.18.2387] [PMID: 12746362]

[98] Curtis JR. Palliative and end-of-life care for patients with severe COPD. Eur Respir J 2008; 32(3): 796-803.
[http://dx.doi.org/10.1183/09031936.00126107] [PMID: 17989116]

[99] Coventry PA, Grande GE, Richards DA, Todd CJ. Prediction of appropriate timing of palliative care for older adults with non-malignant life-threatening disease: a systematic review. Age Ageing 2005; 34(3): 218-27.
[http://dx.doi.org/10.1093/ageing/afi054] [PMID: 15863407]

CHAPTER 17

Whole Lung Lavage for Pulmonary Alveolar Proteinosis

Suhaib Khan and **Ahmed Awab***

University of Oklahoma Health Sciences Center, Oklahoma City, Oklahoma, USA

Abstract: Pulmonary Alveolar Proteinosis (PAP) is a rare disease characterized by the accumulation of proteinaceous material in the alveoli, resulting in progressive hypoxemia and functional limitation. Whole lung lavage under general anesthesia with normal saline has become established as a safe and effective treatment for PAP. The technique varies slightly from institution to institution, but essentially involves the instillation and removal of 500-1000ml aliquots of normal saline from one lung at a time, which removes the offending material from the alveoli. There is often significant functional improvement within weeks that can persist for months or years. Repeat lavage can be done when symptoms return.

Keywords: Alveolar proteinosis, Lung Lavage, Pulmonary alveolar proteinosis, Whole lung lavage.

INTRODUCTION

Pulmonary Alveolar Proteinosis (PAP), also called alveolar proteinosis, alveolar lipoproteinois, alveolar phospholipidosis, pulmonary alveolar lipoproteinsosis and pulmonary alveolar phospholipoproteinosis, is a rare disorder that is characterized by abnormal intraalveolar surfactant accumulation. The estimated annual incidence and prevalence of PAP has been reported as 0.36 and 3.70 cases per million population, respectively [1]. Due to rarity of the disease there are no randomized trials to date for treatment and most of the guidelines are based on small cases series and case reports.

This book chapter aims to provide an understanding of various whole lung lavage techniques reported in the literature for treatment of this rare conditions. This chapter will initially discuss the pathophysiology briefly, followed by whole lung lavage techniques.

* **Corresponding author Ahmed Awab:** 920 S.L. Young Blvd, WP1310,, Oklahoma City, OK 73104, USA; Tel: 405-271-6173; Fax: 405-271-5982; E-mail: aawab@ouhsc.edu

PATHOPHYSIOLOGY

Novel insight over the last two decades has led to a greater understanding of the spectrum of disease processes that may lead to PAP. Abnormalities of surfactant remain central to the pathogenesis of PAP. Surfactant consists of a mixture of proteins and lipids secreted by type II pneumocytes and is cleared by type II pneumocytes and alveolar macrophages. Mutations in surfactant proteins lead to qualitative and quantitative alterations of secreted surfactants, thus leading to ineffective surfactant and abnormal clearance [2]. Granulocyte monocyte colony stimulating factor (GM-CSF) is a key cytokine in PAP pathophysiology [3, 4]. *In vitro,* GM-CSF, stimulates differentiation, proliferation and survival of myeloid cells [3, 4]. GM-CSF knockout mice show isolated lung lesions reminiscent of PAP seen in humans [3]. In humans, the GM-CSF receptor has two subunits, alpha and beta. The CSF2RA and CSF2RB are the two genes which code for alpha and beta subunits and mutations in either of these two genes, prevent GM-CSF signaling and induce PAP with intra-alveolar surfactant accumulation without interstitial infiltrates [2].

It is now thought that PAP can be divided into two categories:

1. **Autoimmune PAP**, consisting approximately up to 90% cases of PAP, and associated with the presence of circulating GM-CSF autoantibodies.
2. **Non-autoimmune PAP**, which is further subdivided into, congenital (caused by mutations in genes coding for surfactant proteins –B or C, ABCA3, and alpha chain of granulocyte-macrophage colony-stimulating factor receptor, GM-CSF-Rα), and secondary PAP (in the settings of hematologic malignancies, opportunistic infections, inhalation of toxic substances, chemotherapy treatments and lysinuric protein intolerance) [5, 6].

WHOLE LUNG LAVAGE

History

After the identification of the first case of PAP by Dr. Benjamin Castleman of the Massachusetts General Hospital in July 1953, various empirical therapies were proposed. These included antibiotics, corticosteroids and attempts at physical dissolution through administration of potassium iodide, streptokinase, trypsin, heparin and acetylcysteine [7, 8]. In November 1960, Dr. Jose Ramirez-Rivera at Veterans' Administration Hospital in Baltimore applied repeated "segmental flooding", as a means of physically removing the accumulated material [9 - 12]. His technique consisted of "blind" placement of a percutaneous transtracheal endobronchial catheter. Through this catheter, aliquots of 100 ml of warmed saline were instilled at a rate of 50-60 drops per minute. This usually triggered

45-70 minutes of vigorous coughing spells which typically produced "30-40 ml of white viscid material". This process was repeated four times a day for 2-3 weeks, using physical positioning to direct saline to a different lung segment every time [13]. This procedure even though prolonged and distressing for the patient, provided the first therapy with reproducible and functionally significant improvements in symptoms and pulmonary functions [1]. Even though the "segmental flooding" provided proof that physical removal of adequate amounts of the material provided functional improvement, the technique was imperfect and denounced by many colleagues at that time [13].

In July 1964, Ramirez-Rivera proceeded with a trial of whole-lung lavage, using up to 3L saline added with heparin or acetylcysteine, initially under local anesthesia [14]. This human trial provided further evidence that such a procedure was potentially safe and feasible. Over next four decades, further advancements were made and the procedure was further refined using general anesthesia, increased lavage volumes [15, 16], use of saline alone [17 - 19] and successful treatment of bilateral sequential whole lung lavage in the same treatment session [20]. In case of severe hypoxia, utilization of extracorporeal membrane oxygenation has been reported [21].

Indications for Whole Lung Lavage

The main indication for whole lung lavage (WLL) is the limitation of daily activities due to dyspnea [20]. Therefore an individual whose work requires more physical exertion like a laborer should have lower threshold for undergoing WLL as compared to someone who has a sedentary life style. Some authors have suggested that patients with $PaO2$ of less than 70mm Hg (9.3kPa) or a P (A-a) O2 of more than 40 mm Hg (5.3 KPa) are more likely to progress and hence require WLL [20].

Technical Aspects of Whole Lung Lavage

Due to lack of randomized trials, there are no specific guidelines for the technique of performing WLL and each institute has built up their own protocol with slight variations. The technique discussed in this section is similar to practice at other centers.

Following induction of general anesthesia, a double lumen endotracheal tube is introduced by an experienced anesthetist. A fiberoptic bronchoscopy is performed to confirm the placement of double lumen endotracheal tube. The seal of the balloons in tested by increasing peak airway pressure to 50cm of water pressure transiently and immersing the non-ventilated lumen of the tube in a water basin to look for a leak. Both lungs are ventilated with 100% oxygen for at least 20 minutes to eliminate nitrogen from alveolar gas. The target lung is than isolated at the end of expiration. The lung volume of that lung at the end of expiration is estimated from preoperative measurements of functional residual capacity (FRC). The volume of gas is gradually absorbed from the non-ventilated lung at a rate of approximately 100ml/min (estimated oxygen consumption at rest from one lung). Warm normal saline is introduced into the lung through a closed system at the same rate as oxygen is absorbed, until estimated FRC value has been reached. At this point the lung is completely de-gassed and full of saline. In incremental fashion of tidal volume (500ml-1000ml), saline is flowed into the lung under gravitational force-that is a saline column of not more than 50cm-and then out again *via* the closed system into a measuring cylinder. The volume and temperature (approximately 37°C) of instilled saline are closely controlled and monitored. The initial returns are typically milky or turbid. The process of filling and washing the lungs is continued until the effluent becomes clear. The total volumes of saline required can range from 20 to 40L. At the termination of procedure, the residual saline is drained and aspirated from the lung and ventilation with 100% oxygen is resumed. The double lumen endotracheal tube is replaced by single lumen endotracheal tube and the patient is monitored in recovery unit for an hour on mechanical ventilation. At the end of recovery time the patient is awakened and extubated. The patient is further monitored and can usually be discharged on same day.

Role of Body Position in Drainage

The role of chest percussion and body positioning was investigated by Perez *et al.* in 2004. In this study five patient underwent whole lung lavage [22]. The lung lavage was performed in three sequential stages. In stage 1, the patient was placed in supine position, during which time there was instillation and removal of fluid until the effluent fluid became clear. During stage 2, manual percussion of chest wall was done in order to assist clearance. Percussion was administered during both instillation and removal of fluid. The patient was placed in prone position during stage 3 for positional drainage, while continuing the percussion. The results of this limited study demonstrated that application of different maneuvers is superior to single maneuver in clearing the solid material from the lungs of PAP patient. It is hypothesized that prone positioning potentially facilitates drainage from posterior segments of the lungs [22]. The main side effect of prone positioning was potential danger of dislodging of endotracheal tube from its position [22]. There are reports in literature which describe a 30 degree lateral decubitus position in order to preserve the ratio of ventilation/perfusion of the dependent ventilated lung [23]. One report described the use of dorsal decubitus position, with a reverse Trendelenburg as well Trendelenburg positioning to facilitate the gravitational instillation and removal of warm saline from the lungs

[24]. In one study the patient was placed in lateral decubitus position, with the lavage of non-dependent lung and ventilation of dependent lung [30]. The rationale behind this technique was to improve ventilation perfusion mismatch as the blood flow will increase towards the nondependent lung. In one report intraoperative diuresis with Furosemide at a dosage of 115 mg/H was used.

Role of Percussion

The role of manual percussion *versus* mechanical percussion has been investigated in study that demonstrated that optical density of recovered lavage fluid was greater from patients who received manual percussion than those who received percussion using mechanical devices or no percussion [25]. Another study revealed that the use of manual percussion of manual percussion as an adjunct to lavage was very effective in removing proteinaceous material [22].

Bilateral sequential lung lavage has been reported in the literature. In one case series, six bilateral whole lung lavages were performed without any major complications and were associated with clinical and functional improvement of PAP patients submitted to this procedure [24]. Another study from China reported bilateral sequential whole lung lavage in same treatment session for 12 patients with significant improvement in symptoms, chest radiograph and difference in alveolar to arterial tension. However, no significant improvement in immediate pulmonary function test was noted [26].

Safety of Whole Lung Lavage

The major side effect from whole lung lavage is hypoxemia which can be improved by ventilation with high inspired oxygen concentration [27, 28]. During the filling phase arterial oxygenation improves due to increase in airway pressure and shunting of blood to the contralateral ventilated lung [20]. Emptying of the lung causes a decrease in airway pressure and perfusion of the surfactant filled alveoli creates a shunt in the lung undergoing treatment and hence a fall in $PaO2$ [20]. The utilization of hyperbaric oxygen, partial cardiopulmonary bypass and temporary veno-venous extracorporeal gas exchange for patients with severe hypoxemia and in children undergoing whole lung lavage has been reported in the literature [1].

Mal-positioning of double lumen endobronchial tube with overspill of lavage fluid into ventilated lung is also a potential adverse event [20]. Barotrauma can also occur with rapid instillation of large volumes of fluid. Other reported complications include hydropnemothorax, surgical emphysema and pleural collections [28, 29]. The risk of hypothermia can be minimized by close monitoring of patient's body temperature and keeping the body warm using heating pads.

Timing of Whole Lung Lavage

The time from diagnosis of PAP to performing WLL is variable ranging between immediate lavage to lavage done at 210 months with a median of 2 months [1]. The majority of patients (79%) underwent WLL within 12 months of diagnosis [1].

The timing of repeat WLL is also variable and tailored according to the patient's symptoms, in patients with severe symptoms requiring early repeat procedure. It has been reported that the number of repeat procedures performed was proportional to the duration of follow-up, such that 66% patient, who followed for more than 1 year, underwent more than one lavage [2]. In one study, the median symptom free time period after first WLL was 3 years, with 70% patient followed beyond 3 years remaining free of recurrent PAP symptoms [30]. In another report, a much shorter median duration of benefit of 15 months was reported, after which patient required a repeat lavage [1].

Follow-up on Change in Lung Mechanics and Outcomes after WLL

Due to lack of randomized clinical trials, the true therapeutic impact of WLL cannot be determined. Based on available date the patient who underwent WLL showed better survival as compared to patients who did not underwent WLL, with 5-year actuarial survival rate from diagnosis of 94% ± 2% compared to 85% ± 5% for those not receiving WLL therapy [1].

From clinical stand-point WLL has been associated with improvement in dyspnea symptoms [30]. A report of 47 patients with paired pre-lavage and post-lavage data demonstrates that there was 85% improvement in PaO2 [A-a] gradient, FEV1, vital capacity, DLCO [27]. More recently, a study following long term effect of WLL reported a significant improvement in FVC immediately following WLL, with the effect persisting up to 1-year of the procedure [30]. The DLCO did not improve 1 week following WLL, but showed improvement in 6 months. There was also significant improvement in mean distance walked in meters at 6 months following WLL [30].

FUTURE DIRECTIONS

With the implication of anti GM-CSF antibody in the pathogenesis of autoimmune alveolar proteinosis, human recombinant GM-CSF has been tried as a therapeutic agent. There are some reports of complete remission, and many instances of clinical response. Both inhaled and subcutaneous route have been tried. One meta-analysis of observational studies of both inhaled and injected GM-FSG showed a pooled response rate of 59%, with a relapse rate of nearly 30% [31]. In the absence of large trials, GM-SCF therapy remains an off-label indication for the treatment of alveolar proteinosis. Other treatments with limited data include rituximab and exchange transfusion [32, 33]. Lung transplant has been attempted with reports of recurrence of disease in the transplanted lung [34]. Multiple clinical trials are accruing patients for one or more of the above described therapies. More information can be obtained at http://clinicaltrials.gov.

CONFLICT OF INTEREST

The authors declare no conflict of interest, financial or otherwise.

ACKNOWLEDGEMENTS

Declared none.

REFERENCES

[1] Seymour JF, Presneill JJ. Pulmonary alveolar proteinosis: progress in the first 44 years. Am J Respir Crit Care Med 2002; 166(2): 215-35. [http://dx.doi.org/10.1164/rccm.2109105] [PMID: 12119235]

[2] Borie R, Danel C, Debray MP, *et al.* Pulmonary alveolar proteinosis. Eur Respir Rev 2011; 20(120): 98-107. [http://dx.doi.org/10.1183/09059180.00001311] [PMID: 21632797]

[3] Stanley E, Lieschke GJ, Grail D, *et al.* Granulocyte/macrophage colony-stimulating factor-deficient mice show no major perturbation of hematopoiesis but develop a characteristic pulmonary pathology. Proc Natl Acad Sci USA 1994; 91(12): 5592-6. [http://dx.doi.org/10.1073/pnas.91.12.5592] [PMID: 8202532]

[4] Dranoff G, Crawford AD, Sadelain M, *et al.* Involvement of granulocyte-macrophage colony-stimulating factor in pulmonary homeostasis. Science 1994; 264(5159): 713-6. [http://dx.doi.org/10.1126/science.8171324] [PMID: 8171324]

[5] Inoue Y, Trapnell BC, Tazawa R, *et al.* Japanese center of the rare lung diseases consortium. Characteristics of a large cohort of patients with autoimmune pulmonary alveolar proteinosis in Japan. Am J Respir Crit Care Med 2008; 177(7): 752-62. [http://dx.doi.org/10.1164/rccm.200708-1271OC] [PMID: 18202348]

[6] Trapnell BC, Whitsett JA, Nakata K. Pulmonary alveolar proteinosis. N Engl J Med 2003; 349(26): 2527-39. [http://dx.doi.org/10.1056/NEJMra023226] [PMID: 14695413]

[7] Davidson JM, Macleod WM. Pulmonary alveolar proteinosis. Br J Dis Chest 1969; 63(1): 13-28. [http://dx.doi.org/10.1016/S0007-0971(69)80040-9] [PMID: 4886263]

[8] De Sanctis PN. Pulmonary alveolar proteinosis. A review of the findings and theories to date, with a digression on Pneumocystis carinii pneumonia. BMQ 1962; 13: 19-35. [PMID: 13884520]

[9] Moertel CG, Woolner LB, Bernatz PE. Pulmonary alveolar proteinosis; report of case. Proc Staff Meet Mayo Clin 1959; 34(6): 152-7.

[PMID: 13658247]

[10] Ramirez J, Campbell GD. Pulmonary alveolar proteinosis. Endobronchial treatment. Ann Intern Med 1965; 63: 429-41. [http://dx.doi.org/10.7326/0003-4819-63-3-429] [PMID: 14330592]

[11] Ramirez J, Nyka W, McLAUGHLIN J. Pulmonary alveolar proteinosis. Diagnostic technics and observations. N Engl J Med 1963; 268: 165-71. [http://dx.doi.org/10.1056/NEJM196301242680401] [PMID: 13990655]

[12] Ramirez J, Schultz RB, Dutton RE. Pulmonary alveolar proteinosis: A new technique and rationale for treatment. Arch Intern Med 1963; 112: 419-31. [http://dx.doi.org/10.1001/archinte.1963.03860030173021] [PMID: 14045290]

[13] Ramírez-Rivera J. The strange beginnings of diagnostic and therapeutic bronchoalveolar lavage. P R Health Sci J 1992; 11(1): 27-32. [PMID: 1603932]

[14] Ramirez J, Kieffer RF Jr, Ball WC Jr. Bronchopulmonary lavage in man. Ann Intern Med 1965; 63(5): 819-28. [http://dx.doi.org/10.7326/0003-4819-63-5-819] [PMID: 5848630]

[15] Wasserman K, Blank N, Fletcher G. Lung lavage (alveolar washing) in alveolar proteinosis. Am J Med 1968; 44(4): 611-7. [http://dx.doi.org/10.1016/0002-9343(68)90062-4] [PMID: 5642718]

[16] Ramirez J. Pulmonary alveolar proteinosis. Treatment by massive bronchopulmonary lavage. Arch Intern Med 1967; 119(2): 147-56. [http://dx.doi.org/10.1001/archinte.1967.00290200071003] [PMID: 6017123]

[17] Wasserman K. Evaluation of solutions used for lung lavage in alveolar proteinosis. Rounds of the Teaching Staff of Wadsworth Hospital Centre 1968; 11: 217-22.

[18] Kao D, Wasserman K, Costley D, Benfield JR. Advances in the treatment of pulmonary alveolar proteinosis. Am Rev Respir Dis 1975; 111(3): 361-3. [PMID: 1119744]

[19] Sunderland WA, Klein RL. Heparin absorption during heparin-saline lung lavage in a patient with pulmonary alveolar proteinosis. Chest 1973; 63(6): 1033-4. [http://dx.doi.org/10.1378/chest.63.6.1033] [PMID: 4711851]

[20] Shah PL, Hansell D, Lawson PR, Reid KB, Morgan C. Pulmonary alveolar proteinosis: clinical aspects and current concepts on pathogenesis. Thorax 2000; 55(1): 67-77. [http://dx.doi.org/10.1136/thorax.55.1.67] [PMID: 10607805]

[21] Cohen ES, Elpern E, Silver MR. Pulmonary alveolar proteinosis causing severe hypoxemic respiratory failure treated with sequential whole-lung lavage utilizing venovenous extracorporeal membrane oxygenation: a case report and review. Chest 2001; 120(3): 1024-6. [http://dx.doi.org/10.1378/chest.120.3.1024] [PMID: 11555544]

[22] Perez A IV, Rogers RM. Enhanced alveolar clearance with chest percussion therapy and positional changes during whole-lung lavage for alveolar proteinosis. Chest 2004; 125(6): 2351-6. [http://dx.doi.org/10.1378/chest.125.6.2351] [PMID: 15189962]

[23] Campo I, Kadija Z, Mariani F, *et al.* Pulmonary alveolar proteinosis: diagnostic and therapeutic challenges. Multidiscip Respir Med 2012; 7(1): 4. [http://dx.doi.org/10.1186/2049-6958-7-4]

[24] Silva A, Moreto A, Pinho C, Magalhães A, Morais A, Fiuza C. Bilateral whole lung lavage in pulmonary alveolar proteinosis--a retrospective study. Rev Port Pneumol 2014; 20(5): 254-9. [http://dx.doi.org/10.1016/j.rppneu.2014.04.004] [PMID: 25042291]

[25] Hammon WE, McCaffree DR, Cucchiara AJ. A comparison of manual to mechanical chest percussion

for clearance of alveolar material in patients with pulmonary alveolar proteinosis (phospholipidosis). Chest 1993; 103(5): 1409-12.
[http://dx.doi.org/10.1378/chest.103.5.1409] [PMID: 8486019]

[26] Xie SG, Cai BQ, Zhang H, Liu YJ, Liu T. Bilateral sequential whole lung lavage in the same treatment session for pulmonary alveolar proteinosis. Zhonghua Nei Ke Za Zhi 2007; 46(2): 118-22.
[PMID: 17445437]

[27] Rogers RM, Levin DC, Gray BA, Moseley LW Jr. Physiologic effects of bronchopulmonary lavage in alveolar proteinosis. Am Rev Respir Dis 1978; 118(2): 255-64.
[PMID: 697176]

[28] Prakash UB, Barham SS, Carpenter HA, Dines DE, Marsh HM. Pulmonary alveolar phospholipoproteinosis: experience with 34 cases and a review. Mayo Clin Proc 1987; 62(6): 499-518.
[http://dx.doi.org/10.1016/S0025-6196(12)65477-9] [PMID: 3553760]

[29] Kariman K, Kylstra JA, Spock A. Pulmonary alveolar proteinosis: prospective clinical experience in 23 patients for 15 years. Lung 1984; 162(4): 223-31.
[http://dx.doi.org/10.1007/BF02715650] [PMID: 6492867]

[30] Beccaria M, Luisetti M, Rodi G, *et al.* Long-term durable benefit after whole lung lavage in pulmonary alveolar proteinosis. Eur Respir J 2004; 23(4): 526-31.
[http://dx.doi.org/10.1183/09031936.04.00102704] [PMID: 15083749]

[31] Khan A, Agarwal R, Aggarwal AN. Effectiveness of granulocyte-macrophage colony-stimulating factor therapy in autoimmune pulmonary alveolar proteinosis: a meta-analysis of observational studies. Chest 2012; 141(5): 1273-83.
[http://dx.doi.org/10.1378/chest.11-0951] [PMID: 22016491]

[32] Kavuru MS, Malur A, Marshall I, *et al.* An open-label trial of rituximab therapy in pulmonary alveolar proteinosis. Eur Respir J 2011; 38(6): 1361-7.
[http://dx.doi.org/10.1183/09031936.00197710] [PMID: 21478218]

[33] Garber B, Albores J, Wang T, Neville TH. A plasmapheresis protocol for refractory pulmonary alveolar proteinosis. Lung 2015; 193(2): 209-11.
[http://dx.doi.org/10.1007/s00408-014-9678-2] [PMID: 25557091]

[34] Parker LA, Novotny DB. Recurrent alveolar proteinosis following double lung transplantation. Chest 1997; 111(5): 1457-8.
[http://dx.doi.org/10.1378/chest.111.5.1457] [PMID: 9149615]

CHAPTER 18

Bronchial Thermoplasty

Steven J. Campbell and **Shaheen Islam***

Section of Interventional Pulmonology, Division of Pulmonary, Allergy, Critical Care and Sleep Medicine, Ohio State University Wexner Medical Center, Columbus, Ohio, USA

Abstract: Treatment of severe asthma refractory to standard therapies such as inhaled corticosteroids or bronchodilators is limited. Newer pharmacologic agents focus on the allergic subset of asthmatics limiting their use to a smaller subgroup. Bronchial thermoplasty is a novel procedure developed over the past decade where airway smooth muscles are ablated using radiofrequency thermal energy during bronchoscopy to prevent bronchoconstriction. Current data suggest that the procedure is relatively safe with a potential for transient and mild worsening of respiratory symptoms. Bronchial thermoplasty has shown a significant decrease in the number of exacerbations and emergency department visits during the year following therapy. While FDA approved since 2010 for refractory asthma not responding to conventional therapies, some individual health plans are yet to approve it for reimbursement limiting its wide use. Current guidelines endorse cautionary use until further data is available regarding the efficacy of the procedure.

Keywords: Allergic subset, Asthma refractory, Bronchial thermoplasty, Bronchoconstriction, Bronchodilators, Exacerbations, Inhaled corticosteroids.

INTRODUCTION

Asthma affects more than 334 million people worldwide and more than 24 million people in the United States alone [1, 2]. It is estimated that asthma is directly responsible for $56 billion dollars per year in health care costs [3]. The disease is caused by chronic inflammation of the large and small airways resulting in airway hyper-responsiveness and excessive mucous secretion [4]. Asthma treatment involves four main tenets: using objective measures of lung function to monitor severity and assess symptoms; instituting environmental control measures to reduce asthma symptoms and exacerbations; having a collaborative patient-doctor model with sufficient patient education; and effectively prescribing therapy that reduces inflammation and exacerbations [5]. The backbone of asthma therapy is

* **Corresponding author Shaheen Islam:** Section of Interventional Pulmonology, Division of Pulmonary, Allergy, Critical Care and Sleep Medicine, Ohio State University Wexner Medical Center, Columbus, Ohio, USA; Tel: (614) 292-6563; Fax: (614)-293-4799; E-mail: shaheen.islam@osumc.edu

Ali I. Musani (Ed.)

inhaled corticosteroids (ICS) that aim to reduce inflammation along with inhaled short- and long-acting β2 receptor agonists that relax airway smooth muscle (ASM).

Unfortunately, 5-10% of asthmatics will not achieve control even with large doses of ICS. Not surprisingly these patients end up utilizing a disproportionate share of healthcare resources [6 - 8]. Therapies for severe asthma are limited. A subset of patients with poorly controlled asthma along with allergic sensitization and elevated Immunoglobulin E (IgE) levels may benefit from subcutaneous omalizumab. This drug is a humanized monoclonal antibody targeting IgE and has been shown to reduce asthma exacerbations in patients refractory to ICS [9 - 11]. Many patients with severe asthma remain symptomatic despite the addition of omalizumab to their regimen. The leukotriene receptor antagonists have had mixed results in clinical trials [12, 13]. Several new therapies have emerged that target the cascade of inflammatory mediators. For example, mepolizumab targets IL-5 which modulates eosinophil function and recruitment. Clinical trials have shown fewer exacerbations and reduced oral glucocorticoid requirements [14, 15]. While these immunotherapies are promising, they are in the early stages of development and only are applicable for the subpopulation of allergic asthmatics. Recently bronchial thermoplasty has emerged as a potential therapeutic option in the hopes of improving poorly controlled asthma for a broader subset of asthmatics.

Overview

Bronchial thermoplasty (BT) is the procedure of applying radio frequency (RF) thermal energy to the airways *via* a bronchoscope with the goal of ablating airway smooth muscle (ASM). BT reduces airway smooth muscle mass through application of controlled heat to the airway mucosa. Frictional heat is generated at tissue interfaces where the flow of current meets resistance. BT is currently being utilized in approximately 41 countries with over 4500 patients who have undergone the procedure (data courtesy of Boston Scientific). BT was approved in April 2010 by the US Food and Drug Administration (FDA) for adult patients (age >18 years) "whose severe and persistent asthma is not well-controlled with inhaled corticosteroids and long acting β-agonist medications" [16]. The contra-indications to BT listed by the FDA include: presence of an implanted electronic device (*e.g.* pacemaker or defibrillator), sensitivities to any of the medications used for bronchoscopy, or patients previously treated with BT. Additionally, BT should be deferred for the following reasons: active respiratory infection, asthma exacerbation within the past 2 weeks, coagulopathy, or inability to temporarily withhold anticoagulant medications.

ASM is an attractive target for several reasons. Contraction of ASM cells causes bronchoconstriction [17]. Hypertrophy and hyperplasia of ASM are responsible for airway remodeling [18]. Finally, ASM cells play a role in the inflammatory response through their interaction with mast cells and T lymphocytes [19]. While BT would seem to have a benefit in asthma based solely on the reduction of ASM mass, there is speculation that a more complex interaction is involved. For example, BT may alter airway function by reducing the contractility of airway smooth muscle [20]. Of note, BT does not treat the smaller, more distal airways which in asthmatics may be the predominant sites of airflow limitation, increased resistance, and airway hyper-responsiveness [21].

BT reduces airway smooth muscle mass through application of controlled heat to the airway mucosa. Frictional heat is generated at tissue interfaces where the flow of current meets resistance.

Technique

The device currently used is the Alair Bronchial Thermoplasty system (Boston Scientific, Natick, MA). The system consists of an RF controller (Alair model ATS 200, Fig. **1**) and a single-use catheter (Alair ATS 2-5) with an expandable wire array (Fig. **2**) that is connected to the RF controller. The distal 4-electrode array can be expanded by squeezing the handle located at the proximal end of the catheter so all four of them are in contact with mucosa (Fig. **3**). The catheter is serially deployed in the airways to sequentially treat all visible bronchial segments in a distal to proximal fashion without overlap [22]. There is a foot paddle connected to RF controller to activate the RF energy application. A grounding pad is placed on the patient and is also connected to the RF controller to complete the electric circuit during activation. The fraction of inspired oxygen is kept below 40% to prevent airway fire. When the wires come in contact the airway wall, monopolar RF energy is applied and is converted to heat targeting a tissue temperature of 65°C for 10 seconds. The RF controller has a 25 watt generator but a maximum of 18 watts of energy at 460 MHz is applied during the activation. Patients generally require 50-80 activations during each bronchoscopy.

The procedure can be done under moderate sedation or general anesthesia. We prefer general anesthesia as it minimizes cough reflex. An ultrathin bronchoscope allows access to the smaller distal airways and is our preference. After adequate sedation is obtained, the bronchoscope is introduced to inspect the airways and clean the airways of any mucus secretion. Additionally, glycopyrrolate can be used to control secretions.

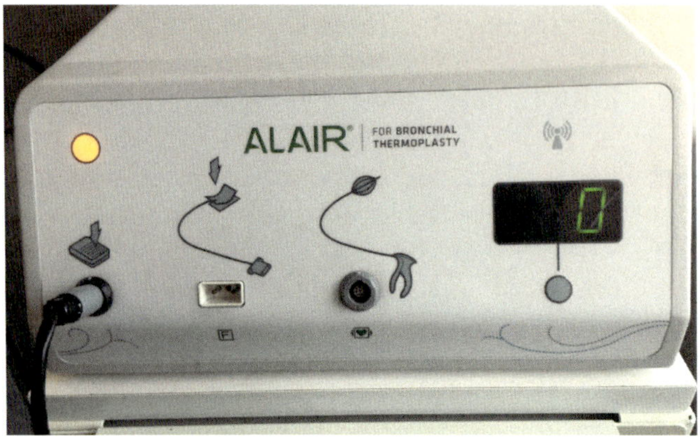

Fig. (1). Alair RF controller Model ATS 200. The display on the right side of the front panel shows the total number of activations.

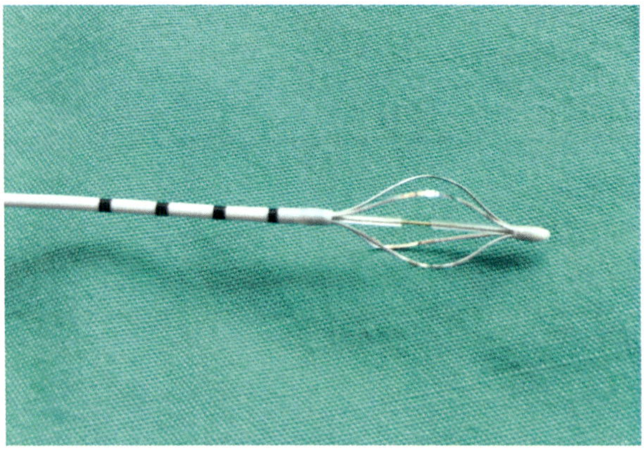

Fig. (2). Single-use Alair catheter with 4 electrode wire array (expanded in picture). The four black marks on the catheter are placed 5mm apart.

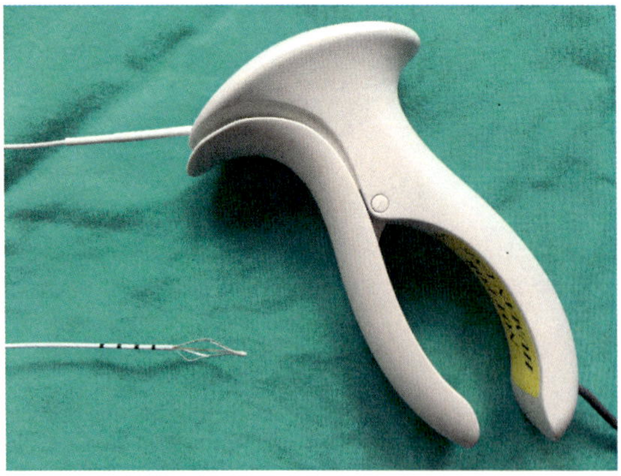

Fig. (3). Handle of the Alair catheter partially squeezed with the distal end of the wired array. Please note the attached cord at the lower end of the handle that is connected to the RF controller.

Once in the target lobe, a general inspection of the airways is done first to identify all the sub-segments and to formulate a plan to sequentially treat all of the sub-segments. Then the thermoplasty probe is inserted through the working channel of the flexible bronchoscope. The probe has four markings every 5mm to indicate the location of the distal end of the probe in the airways when the wire array cannot be seen in the bronchi (Fig. **4**). After the catheter is placed in appropriate position the distal wire array is then expanded by squeezing the handle. Once the foot paddle is pressed and released, the controller is programmed to apply RF energy for 10 seconds. There is an audible sound on the controller indicating the duration of RF energy application.

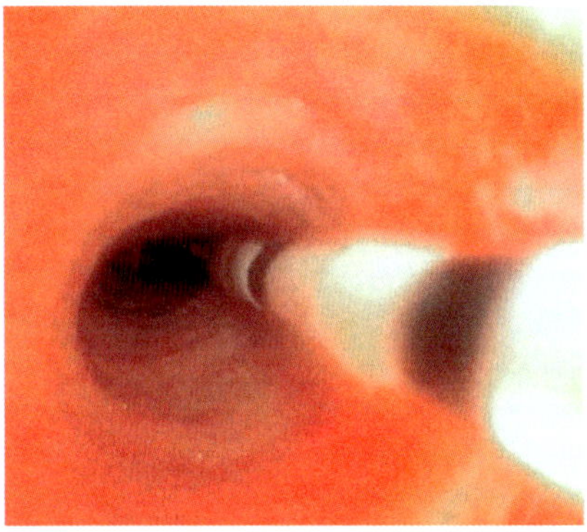

Fig. (4). The wired array is about 1.5cm distally in the bronchus Note the two black markers on the catheter.

After the energy is applied, the probe is then pulled proximally about 5 mm and the whole process is repeated until the wire arrays are outside the bronchus (Fig. **5**). The treatment is then continued on the next target bronchus. The total number of activations and the segments treated are recorded.

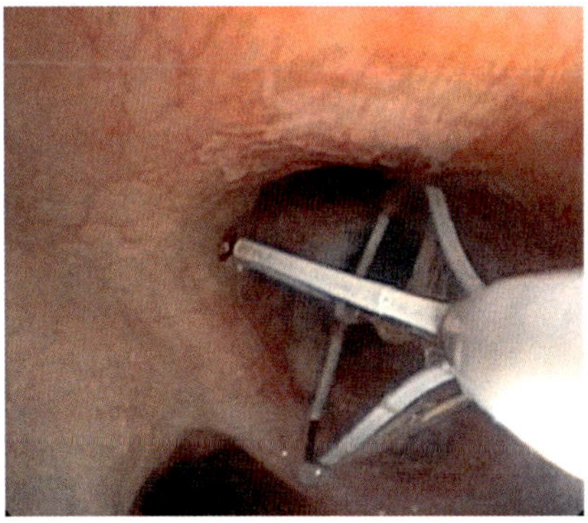

Fig. (5). The expanded catheter at the proximal end of a small bronchus. Note all 4 wires are in contact with the mucosa.

BT is performed in three sequential bronchoscopies spaced three weeks apart each. The target areas are the right lower lobe, left lower lobe, and bilateral upper lobes respectively [23]. By convention the right middle lobe is excluded from treatment. The reason for this omission is that the right middle lobe bronchus is typically a smaller diameter and there are concerns that BT may cause stenosis [24]. The treatment takes place over three separate sessions to give shorter procedure times (each bronchoscopy takes 45-60 minutes) and to mitigate the potential risk of inducing an asthma exacerbation in a susceptible population. Additionally, patients are given oral corticosteroids, usually prednisone (50mg), for 5 days starting 2 to 3 days prior to the first BT to minimize post-procedure airway inflammation [25].

Evidence

Initial studies were performed in canines where the airways of healthy dogs received thermal energy *via* an RF catheter. There was a significant decrease in airway responsiveness to methacholine when thermal energy at 65°C and 75°C was used. Histologic evaluation of canine airways showed persistent ASM reduction and no evidence of smooth muscle regeneration up to 3 years following treatment [26]. A follow up study examined high resolution CT scans and for the dogs whom had underwent BT the investigators found increased airway luminal areas at any dose of inhaled methacholine [27]. The preliminary animal data suggested that by targeting ASM with BT there was the potential to reduce bronchial hyper-responsiveness and airflow obstruction in asthmatics [4].

The first data from a human population was a feasibility study of nine patients who were planning to undergo a lobectomy or pneumonectomy for known or suspected lung cancer [28]. Of note is that the study population did not carry a diagnosis of asthma, and only eight patients ended up receiving treatment. BT was given 2-3 weeks prior to surgery and limited to segmental bronchi that were within the lobe(s) planned for resection. No adverse effects were observed in this small population, including no new symptoms or unscheduled visits for medical care. On repeat bronchoscopic evaluation at the time of surgery the majority of airways appeared normal. All airways treated at 55°C appeared normal, whereas in some of the patients treated at 65°C the authors observed erythema, edema, blanching, and airway narrowing with mucous retention. The authors postulated that these changes would have resolved if longer follow-up been available based on animal data. Histologically, at 65°C there was a reduction in ASM on average of approximately 50% compared to a 5% reduction in the 55°C group. The treatment effect was confined to the airway wall and the immediate peribronchial region. With evidence of tolerability and reduction of ASM in humans the way was set for further clinical trials.

Cox and colleagues conducted a nonrandomized, prospective study involving 16 adult patients with stable mild to moderate asthma [29]. All subjects tolerated BT well and were discharged at the end of a 6-hour observation period. No patients required post-procedure admission. The majority of side effects related to the procedure were related to airway irritation and included cough, dyspnea, wheeze, and bronchospasm. In the study these events tended to be mild, occurring within a few days of the procedure and resolving within a week. Long-term safety data was extrapolated from there being no significant change in FEV1 and no new findings on computed tomography (CT) scan (*e.g.* bronchiectasis or other parenchymal abnormality) at two years. The study was not powered to evaluate efficacy, however there was a significant reduction in airway hyper-responsiveness as measured by an increase in the provocative concentration of methacholine causing a 20% decline in FEV1 (PC_{20}). In addition, at 12 weeks post BT the study participants reported a significant increase in symptom-free days.

The next breakthrough for BT was the Asthma Intervention Research (AIR) trial, a multicenter randomized controlled study which enrolled 112 adult patients with moderate to severe asthma [30]. The study noted significantly more symptom-free days (86 additional symptom-free days per subject per year) and better scores on the asthma quality of life questionnaire (AQLQ) in the treatment group. These patients also had a significant reduction in mild exacerbations (10 fewer per subject per year). The benefits persisted after 1 year in the study. Notably there were no significant differences in pre-bronchodilator FEV1 or airway hyper-responsiveness measured by PC_{20}. Adverse events in this study were primarily related to worsening of asthma symptoms within the first week following treatment and tended to be mild. A notable shortcoming in this study was that it was unblinded and there was no sham group. The AIR trial was followed by the Research in Severe Asthma (RISA) trial which involved 32 patients with severe asthma [31]. While this was a smaller study, the findings were similar to the AIR trial in that there was a significant improvement in asthma symptoms and quality of life despite unimpressive improvements in pulmonary function. BT was again well tolerated in the study group.

As any invasive procedure is likely to produce a strong placebo response in patients with asthma, the efficacy of BT was in doubt given that prior trials did not include a sham group [32]. Thus the AIR-2 trial was designed as a randomized, double-blind, sham-controlled study [33]. 288 adult patients classified as severe asthma were randomized. The AQLQ score improved by 1.16 ± 1.23 in the sham group and by 1.35 ± 1.10 in the thermoplasty group. While an AQLQ score increase of 1 (range, 0.77-1.51) is considered a moderate improvement, the absolute difference between the two groups was only 0.19 (non-significant). This might suggest that there was not a meaningful improved quality of life in patients who received BT compared to those who received a sham procedure. There was a significant decrease in the number of exacerbations (32% risk reduction), emergency department visits (84% risk reduction) and days lost from school or work (66% risk reduction) during the year following BT. However, these outcomes are all tied to each other and there was an outlier in the sham group with 9 hospitalizations whom may have skewed the results towards BT [21]. AIR-2 showed no statistically significant difference in important endpoints such as FEV1, total symptom scores, morning peak flow measurements, and rescue medication use. Following the results of the AIR-2 trial the use of BT was FDA approved.

Safety and Complications

To address long-term outcomes and safety, cohorts from the aforementioned studies were followed for several additional years. Five-year follow up data from the first thermoplasty study (AIR) showed no difference in exacerbation rates, ED visits, hospitalizations, or oral corticosteroid use between the BT and control groups [34]. There were no declines in pulmonary function tests or new abnormalities visualized on chest radiograph. The improvements in airway hyper-responsiveness measured by PC_{20} persisted out to 3 years that suggested long-term efficacy. In regards to the RISA trial only the BT arm was followed out to 5 years, and they exhibited a decreased rate of hospitalizations and emergency department visits compared to before therapy [35]. Again, there was no noticeable decline in pulmonary function tests. Finally, most of the AIR-2 patients who had received BT were followed for 5 years [36]. Similar to the follow up RISA study, the control patients of AIR-2 were not followed due to ethical considerations of withholding a potentially beneficial therapy from these patients for several additional years. Compared to before BT, patients in AIR-2 had fewer exacerbations and emergency department visits. Pulmonary function tests remained stable and no changes were seen on serial CT scans. While the safety data is encouraging, without follow up data in the sham control arm the persistent effectiveness of BT cannot be adequately assessed.

Common side effects from the procedure are coughing, wheezing, exacerbation of asthma, and respiratory infections in the treated airways. Data from AIR-2 showed a small risk (3.4%) of requiring hospital admission post procedure for worsening dyspnea. While in general 5 year safety data from the aforementioned trials is reassuring, a larger cohort is needed to help understand the full spectrum of potential adverse events that may arise. Notably in the AIR trial among the 45 BT treated patients one went on to develop a lung abscess 14 months post treatment [34]. At that time it was felt that the abscess was not secondary to treatment given the time delay and the histologic characteristics of the resected tissue specimen. However, a recent case report showed a woman whom developed a lung abscess three days following her second BT session [37]. The authors were unsure why this ensued but they postulated it might have been related to transient localized airway obstruction. Also worth noting is that in AIR-2 one patient presented with significant hemoptysis from the right upper lobe 1 month after the last BT session and required bronchial artery embolization. Slight bleeding had been observed during the treatment of this lobe thus it was presumed to be a procedural complication [33]. Another recent case report described recurrent lung atelectasis secondary to fibrin plugs as an early complication of BT, which again highlights the need for more robust monitoring data [38].

Procedural Costs and Cost-effectiveness

Effective January 2014, the Centers for Medicare and Medicaid Services (CMS) approved two Current Procedural Terminology (CPT) codes for reimbursement of BT procedures. The CPT for a single lobe treatment is (*e.g.* lower lobes) 31660, and for 2 or more lobes is 31661. The Relative Value Index (RVU) associated with 31660 and 31661 are 4.25 and 4.50 respectively. The average physician professional fees reimbursed by CMS in Ohio in 2016 for 31660 and 31661 are $212.22 and $222.84 respectively while the facility fee is about $2980.56. Even though BT is approved by the CMS, some individual health plans have yet to approve BT for reimbursement. The list price for the generator from Boston Scientific is $89,900 with each disposable catheter costing about $2500. Usually, each patient is scheduled for three procedures.

A recent study examined the cost-effectiveness of omalizumab, BT, and standard therapy (*i.e.* inhaled corticosteroids with or without long-acting beta-agonists) over a predicted five year period in patients with moderate-to-severe asthma in the US [39]. In terms of quality-adjusted life years (QALYs) gained omalizumab was the most effective (3.08 for standard therapy, 3.24 for BT, and 3.26 for omalizumab), however it was also the most expensive over 5-years ($15,400 for standard therapy, $28,100 for BT, and $117,000 for omalizumab). BT could be cost-effective if policy makers were willing to pay over $80,000 per QALY. However, the authors caution that there is significant uncertainty over BT as the chance of this new therapy being cost-effective compared to omalizumab and standard therapy was only 67%.

Limitations

Patients with very severe airflow obstruction were excluded in the aforementioned major clinical trials. Patients with an FEV_1 of less than 60% of predicted were not enrolled in AIR and AIR-2. A small case series of 8 patients with very severe asthma showed no serious adverse events with BT and suggested that it could be of utility in this population, but more data are needed [40]. In addition, AIR-2 did not include phenotypic data on the study participants, thus it is not clear which asthma groupings may benefit more or less from BT.

Current criticism states that the definitive AIR-2 trial did not show any clinically significant benefit when compared to the sham group. Critics argue that what may seem like promising results are perhaps entwined with a placebo effect [21]. In addition, the follow up data from AIR-2 did not include patients from the sham group thus putting into question the knowledge gleaned regarding the risks and benefits of thermoplasty. These criticisms along with the expensive and invasive nature of BT have kept it from being more widely adopted into clinical practice. Current American Thoracic / European Respiratory Societal guidelines endorse cautionary use of BT and an overall sense of low confidence for benefiting patients with severe asthma [41].

CONCLUSIONS

Bronchial thermoplasty is a novel therapy that targets the ASM in the hopes of providing a rescue option for refractory asthmatics. Current data suggest that aside from the potential for transient and mild worsening of respiratory symptoms the procedure is relatively safe, although recent case reports emphasize vigilant monitoring for complications. Selected patients with moderate to severe asthma refractory to conventional pharmacologic therapies are the intended population, although the ideal phenotype is unknown. Controversy remains over the actual benefits given the significant placebo effect observed with the AIR-2 trial. Data from trials preceeding AIR-2 may be unreliable given the lack of a sham thermoplasty arm [21]. More studies are underway to help assess the long-term effectiveness of BT such as the Bronchial Thermoplasty in Severe Persistent Asthma (PAS2) trial. Current societal guidelines do not strongly endorse BT citing the need for more data [41].

CONFLICT OF INTEREST

The authors declare no conflict of interest, financial or otherwise.

ACKNOWLEDGEMENTS

Declared none.

REFERENCES

[1] Network TG. The Global Asthma Report 2014. Available at: http://www.globalasthmareport.org/index.php

[2] CDC. National Current Asthma Prevalance 2014. Available at: http://www.cdc.gov/asthma/most_recent_data.htm

[3] Barnett SB, Nurmagambetov TA. Costs of asthma in the United States: 2002-2007. J Allergy Clin Immunol 2011; 127(1): 145-52. [http://dx.doi.org/10.1016/j.jaci.2010.10.020] [PMID: 21211649]

[4] Laxmanan B, Hogarth DK. Bronchial thermoplasty in asthma: current perspectives. J Asthma Allergy 2015; 8: 39-49. [http://dx.doi.org/10.2147/JAA.S49306] [PMID: 26028976]

[5] Program NAEaP. Guidelines for the diagnosis and management of asthma 1991. Available at: http://www.nhlbi.nih.gov/health-pro/guidelines/current/asthma-guidelines/full-report

[6] Godard P, Chanez P, Siraudin L, Nicoloyannis N, Duru G. Costs of asthma are correlated with severity: a 1-yr prospective study. Eur Respir J 2002; 19(1): 61-7. [http://dx.doi.org/10.1183/09031936.02.00232001] [PMID: 11843329]

[7] Ivanova JI, Bergman R, Birnbaum HG, Colice GL, Silverman RA, McLaurin K. Effect of asthma exacerbations on health care costs among asthmatic patients with moderate and severe persistent asthma. J Allergy Clin Immunol 2012; 129(5): 1229-35. [http://dx.doi.org/10.1016/j.jaci.2012.01.039] [PMID: 22326484]

[8] Moore WC, Bleecker ER, Curran-Everett D, *et al.* National Heart, Lung, Blood Institute's Severe Asthma Research Program. Characterization of the severe asthma phenotype by the National Heart, Lung, and Blood Institute's Severe Asthma Research Program. J Allergy Clin Immunol 2007; 119(2): 405-13. [http://dx.doi.org/10.1016/j.jaci.2006.11.639] [PMID: 17291857]

[9] Busse WW. Anti-immunoglobulin E (omalizumab) therapy in allergic asthma. Am J Respir Crit Care Med 2001; 164(8 Pt 2): S12-7. [http://dx.doi.org/10.1164/ajrccm.164.supplement_1.2103026] [PMID: 11704612]

[10] Hanania NA, Alpan O, Hamilos DL, *et al.* Omalizumab in severe allergic asthma inadequately controlled with standard therapy: a randomized trial. Ann Intern Med 2011; 154(9): 573-82. [http://dx.doi.org/10.7326/0003-4819-154-9-201105030-00002] [PMID: 21536936]

[11] Solèr M, Matz J, Townley R, *et al.* The anti-IgE antibody omalizumab reduces exacerbations and steroid requirement in allergic asthmatics. Eur Respir J 2001; 18(2): 254-61. [http://dx.doi.org/10.1183/09031936.01.00092101] [PMID: 11529281]

[12] Robinson DS, Campbell D, Barnes PJ. Addition of leukotriene antagonists to therapy in chronic persistent asthma: a randomised double-blind placebo-controlled trial. Lancet 2001; 357(9273): 2007-11. [http://dx.doi.org/10.1016/S0140-6736(00)05113-8] [PMID: 11438132]

[13] Virchow JC Jr, Prasse A, Naya I, Summerton L, Harris A. Zafirlukast improves asthma control in patients receiving high-dose inhaled corticosteroids. Am J Respir Crit Care Med 2000; 162(2 Pt 1): 578-85. [http://dx.doi.org/10.1164/ajrccm.162.2.9905041] [PMID: 10934090]

[14] Bel EH, Wenzel SE, Thompson PJ, *et al.* SIRIUS Investigators. Oral glucocorticoid-sparing effect of mepolizumab in eosinophilic asthma. N Engl J Med 2014; 371(13): 1189-97. [http://dx.doi.org/10.1056/NEJMoa1403291] [PMID: 25199060]

[15] Ortega HG, Liu MC, Pavord ID, *et al.* MENSA Investigators. Mepolizumab treatment in patients with severe eosinophilic asthma. N Engl J Med 2014; 371(13): 1198-207. [http://dx.doi.org/10.1056/NEJMoa1403290] [PMID: 25199059]

[16] Administration FaD. FDA approves new device for adults with severe and persistent asthma 2010.

[17] Doeing DC, Solway J. Airway smooth muscle in the pathophysiology and treatment of asthma. J Appl Physiol 2013; 114(7): 834-43. [http://dx.doi.org/10.1152/japplphysiol.00950.2012] [PMID: 23305987]

[18] Siddiqui S, Martin JG. Structural aspects of airway remodeling in asthma. Curr Allergy Asthma Rep 2008; 8(6): 540-7.
[http://dx.doi.org/10.1007/s11882-008-0098-3] [PMID: 18940147]

[19] Black JL, Panettieri RA Jr, Banerjee A, Berger P. Airway smooth muscle in asthma: just a target for bronchodilation? Clin Chest Med 2012; 33(3): 543-58.
[http://dx.doi.org/10.1016/j.ccm.2012.05.002] [PMID: 22929101]

[20] Dyrda P, Tazzeo T, DoHarris L, *et al.* Acute response of airway muscle to extreme temperature includes disruption of actin-myosin interaction. Am J Respir Cell Mol Biol 2011; 44(2): 213-21.
[http://dx.doi.org/10.1165/rcmb.2009-0259OC] [PMID: 20395634]

[21] Iyer VN, Lim KG. Bronchial thermoplasty: Where there is smoke, there is fire. Allergy Asthma Proc 2015; 36(4): 251-5.
[http://dx.doi.org/10.2500/aap.2015.36.3857] [PMID: 26108081]

[22] Mayse ML, Laviolette M, Rubin AS, *et al.* Clinical pearls for bronchial thermoplasty. J Bronchology Interv Pulmonol 2007; 14: 115-23.

[23] Laxmanan B, Egressy K, Murgu SD, White SR, Hogarth DK. Recent advances in chest medicine: Advances in bronchial thermoplasty. Chest 2016.
[http://dx.doi.org/10.1016/j.chest.2016.03.012]

[24] Cox PG, Miller J, Mitzner W, Leff AR. Radiofrequency ablation of airway smooth muscle for sustained treatment of asthma: preliminary investigations. Eur Respir J 2004; 24(4): 659-63.
[http://dx.doi.org/10.1183/09031936.04.00054604] [PMID: 15459147]

[25] Kynyk J, Benninger C, Wood KL. Bronchial thermoplasty. Otolaryngol Clin North Am 2014; 47(1): 77-86.
[http://dx.doi.org/10.1016/j.otc.2013.09.007] [PMID: 24286681]

[26] Danek CJ, Lombard CM, Dungworth DL, *et al.* Reduction in airway hyperresponsiveness to methacholine by the application of RF energy in dogs. J Appl Physiol 2004; 97(5): 1946-53.
[http://dx.doi.org/10.1152/japplphysiol.01282.2003] [PMID: 15258133]

[27] Brown RH, Wizeman W, Danek C, Mitzner W. In vivo evaluation of the effectiveness of bronchial thermoplasty with computed tomography. J Appl Physiol 2005; 98(5): 1603-6.
[http://dx.doi.org/10.1152/japplphysiol.01210.2004] [PMID: 15718404]

[28] Miller JD, Cox G, Vincic L, Lombard CM, Loomas BE, Danek CJ. A prospective feasibility study of bronchial thermoplasty in the human airway. Chest 2005; 127(6): 1999-2006.
[http://dx.doi.org/10.1378/chest.127.6.1999] [PMID: 15947312]

[29] Cox G, Miller JD, McWilliams A, Fitzgerald JM, Lam S. Bronchial thermoplasty for asthma. Am J Respir Crit Care Med 2006; 173(9): 965-9.
[http://dx.doi.org/10.1164/rccm.200507-1162OC] [PMID: 16456145]

[30] Cox G, Thomson NC, Rubin AS, *et al.* AIR Trial Study Group. Asthma control during the year after bronchial thermoplasty. N Engl J Med 2007; 356(13): 1327-37.
[http://dx.doi.org/10.1056/NEJMoa064707] [PMID: 17392302]

[31] Pavord ID, Cox G, Thomson NC, *et al.* RISA Trial Study Group. Safety and efficacy of bronchial thermoplasty in symptomatic, severe asthma. Am J Respir Crit Care Med 2007; 176(12): 1185-91.
[http://dx.doi.org/10.1164/rccm.200704-571OC] [PMID: 17901415]

[32] Wechsler ME, Kelley JM, Boyd IO, *et al.* Active albuterol or placebo, sham acupuncture, or no intervention in asthma. N Engl J Med 2011; 365(2): 119-26.
[http://dx.doi.org/10.1056/NEJMoa1103319] [PMID: 21751905]

[33] Castro M, Rubin AS, Laviolette M, *et al.* AIR2 Trial Study Group. Effectiveness and safety of bronchial thermoplasty in the treatment of severe asthma: a multicenter, randomized, double-blind, sham-controlled clinical trial. Am J Respir Crit Care Med 2010; 181(2): 116-24.

[http://dx.doi.org/10.1164/rccm.200903-0354OC] [PMID: 19815809]

[34] Thomson NC, Rubin AS, Niven RM, *et al.* AIR Trial Study Group. Long-term (5 year) safety of bronchial thermoplasty: Asthma Intervention Research (AIR) trial. BMC Pulm Med 2011; 11: 8. [http://dx.doi.org/10.1186/1471-2466-11-8] [PMID: 21314924]

[35] Pavord ID, Thomson NC, Niven RM, *et al.* Research in Severe Asthma Trial Study Group. Safety of bronchial thermoplasty in patients with severe refractory asthma. Ann Allergy Asthma Immunol 2013; 111(5): 402-7. [http://dx.doi.org/10.1016/j.anai.2013.05.002] [PMID: 24125149]

[36] Wechsler ME, Laviolette M, Rubin AS, *et al.* Asthma Intervention Research 2 Trial Study Group. Bronchial thermoplasty: Long-term safety and effectiveness in patients with severe persistent asthma. J Allergy Clin Immunol 2013; 132(6): 1295-302. [http://dx.doi.org/10.1016/j.jaci.2013.08.009] [PMID: 23998657]

[37] Balu A, Ryan D, Niven R. Lung abscess as a complication of bronchial thermoplasty. J Asthma 2015; 52(7): 740-2. [http://dx.doi.org/10.3109/02770903.2015.1005844] [PMID: 25766745]

[38] Facciolongo N, Menzella F, Lusuardi M, *et al.* Recurrent lung atelectasis from fibrin plugs as a very early complication of bronchial thermoplasty: a case report. Multidiscip Respir Med 2015; 10(1): 9. [http://dx.doi.org/10.1186/s40248-015-0002-7] [PMID: 25852934]

[39] Zafari Z, Sadatsafavi M, Marra CA, Chen W, FitzGerald JM. Cost-Effectiveness of Bronchial Thermoplasty, Omalizumab, and Standard Therapy for Moderate-to-Severe Allergic Asthma. PLoS One 2016; 11(1): e0146003. [http://dx.doi.org/10.1371/journal.pone.0146003] [PMID: 26751790]

[40] Doeing DC, Mahajan AK, White SR, Naureckas ET, Krishnan JA, Hogarth DK. Safety and feasibility of bronchial thermoplasty in asthma patients with very severe fixed airflow obstruction: a case series. J Asthma 2013; 50(2): 215-8. [http://dx.doi.org/10.3109/02770903.2012.751997] [PMID: 23252954]

[41] Chung KF, Wenzel SE, Brozek JL, *et al.* International ERS/ATS guidelines on definition, evaluation and treatment of severe asthma. Eur Respir J 2014; 43(2): 343-73. [http://dx.doi.org/10.1183/09031936.00202013] [PMID: 24337046]

CHAPTER 19

Bronchoscopic Lung Volume Reduction

Rabih I. Bechara*

Cancer Treatment Centers of America at Southeastern Regional Medical Center, Newnan, GA 30265, USA

Medical College of Georgia, School of Medicine, Augusta University, GA 30912, USA

Abstract: Emphysema is a form of the chronic obstructive pulmonary disease characterized by destruction of alveolar tissue, abnormal and permanent enlargement of the airspaces distal to the terminal bronchioles. The physiologic consequences of the anatomical changes include loss of elastic recoil, early airway closure during exhalation, and air trapping in the distal air spaces. Alveolar wall destruction with the formation of emphysematous blebs and bullae leads to increased physiologic dead space and loss of gas exchanging surface. Further, air trapping and hyperinflation press the diaphragm into a flat configuration and place all the muscles of respiration at a mechanical overstretch disadvantage. In combination, these mechanisms lead to refractory dyspnea in affected individuals.

Lung volume reduction surgery (LVRS) is a surgical treatment for patients with advanced emphysema whose dyspnea is poorly controlled with the usual therapies. LVRS entails reducing the lung volume by wedge excisions of emphysematous tissue. However, surgical morbidity is high, and non-pulmonary comorbidities may preclude surgery. Minimally invasive techniques have been created, and provide similar benefits to surgical outcomes with significantly less morbidity and mortality. Bronchoscopic Lung Volume Reduction (BLVR) refers to techniques developed to treat hyperinflation due to emphysema, using devices deployed *via* a flexible bronchoscope. The devices and techniques for BLVR will be reviewed in this manuscript.

Keywords: Airway Bypass, Coils, COPD, Emphysema, Endobronchial Valve, Hydrogel, Lung Volume Reduction, Thermal Ablation.

INTRODUCTION

Over the past decade, since the publishing of the original National Emphysema Treatment Trial (NETT) results in the New England Journal of Medicine [1], the concept of a procedural intervention in patients with emphysema has grown. Chronic Obstructive Pulmonary Disease (COPD) remains the third leading

* **Corresponding author Rabih I. Bechara:** Medical College of Georgia, School of Medicine, Augusta University, GA 30912, USA; Tel/Fax: +1404-778-3261; E-mail: Rabih.Bechara@ctca-hope.com

Ali I. Musani (Ed.)

cause of death in the United States (Centers for Disease Control [CDC] and Prevention's National Center for Health Statistics [NCHS], Deaths: Preliminary Data for 2008) [2]. As such, the potential for an intervention that can help control morbidity and improve quality of life could have incredible application throughout the world.

The goal of surgery was the removal of 25-30% of the diseased lung. The reported ninety-day mortality of 7.9% in the surgical group *vs.* the 1.3% mortality in the medical control group was significant. There were also significant post-operative morbidities (air leak greater than seven days, prolonged hospitalization, and readmission to the intensive care unit, *etc.*) in the surgical group *vs.* the medical group. When subgroup analysis was completed, approximately 30% of surgical patients demonstrated clinically significant improvement in exercise capacity and quality of life scoring.

These results were encouraging but underscored the fact that major surgical procedure needed for this procedure was being performed on very poor candidates. Minimally invasive techniques need to be created to allow the opportunity to provide the potential physiologic advantages to both the patients that would be candidates for volume reduction surgery, but more importantly, to that patient with severe morbidities due to their emphysema, who are otherwise not surgical candidates and subsequently may receive the greatest benefits.

The following chapter highlights the work that is currently ongoing in the area of bronchoscopic lung volume reduction. There are tools now clinically available in some locations throughout the world, but no standardized technique exists.

Endobronchial Blockers

The initial attempts at bronchoscopic lung volume reduction were aimed to correct loss of elastic recoil in emphysematous lung, by blocking those airways with the most severe airflow limitation [3 - 5]. This therapy was used for patients with heterogeneous emphysema. The blockage was to induce resorption atelectasis in the more distal lung segments, thereby allowing expansion of healthier lung with resultant improvement in overall elastic recoil. Additionally, reductions of anatomic dead space would translate into a decrease in dynamic air trapping and thus improved exercise inspiratory capacity. Like LVRS, the reduction of hyperinflation would provide further benefits to optimizing chest wall dimensions and the operating length of the diaphragm.

Early endobronchial blockers were comprised of silicone (Fig. **1**), vascular balloons filled with radio-opaque contrast; however, custom built stainless steel stents with occlusive bio-compatible sponges in the center were soon constructed

[5]. Unfortunately, experience with this modality of BLVR revealed that the benefit seen in improvement of dyspnea and exercise tolerance afforded by the blockers was overshadowed by post-procedural complications. These included significant and numerous issues with the migration of the blockers after implantation and subsequent post-obstructive pneumonia due to the accumulation of distal secretions, which necessitated repeated bronchoscopies [3 - 5].

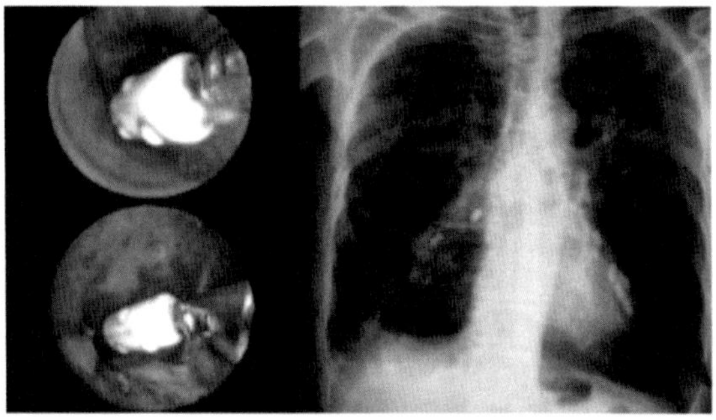

Fig. (1). Watanabe spigot and example of an endobronchial blocker.

Ultimately, further advancements for this route of BLVR were abandoned in favor of other modalities that sought to address the issues of drainage of distal secretions as well as, migration of the implanted devices.

One-way Endobronchial Valves

The experience with endobronchial blockers highlighted what the desired characteristics of an endobronchial device aimed to reduce lung volumes should be [5]. The ideal device should cause distal atelectasis in the target lung units, be able to be implanted *via* flexible bronchoscopy without risk for subsequent migration, removable if required, and should allow drainage of distal secretions while blocking airflow into airways [5].

The intended physiologic basis for this modality is similar to LVRS. Despite that, only a minority of patients achieve complete collapse of the selected area distal to the implanted valves [6 - 11]. In the remaining, majority of patients, the valves divert airflow from the segments of the lung with the most severe disease to airways with less airflow limitation, thereby attempting to reduce the amount of physiologic dead space and improve dynamic airflow trapping. The one-way valve mechanisms seek to permit drainage of secretions distal to the valve in an attempt to reduce the incidence of post-obstructive pneumonia [6 - 11]. Two types of valves have been developed with this goal. Their clinical efficacy at achieving the desired effect has been studied over the last ten years.

Endobronchial Valve (EBV)

The valve with the largest amount of data to date is the Zephyr endobronchial valve (Pulmonx, Redwood City, CA) formerly known as the Emphasys Zephyr EBV. This device is comprised of a central silicone one-way duckbill valve attached to a Nitinol (nickel-titanium alloy) self-expanding retaining frame that is wrapped in a silicone seal [11] (Fig. **2**). After selection of a single target lobe, the Zephyr valves are implanted unilaterally in a three-step process. The valves are removable in the event of improper positioning or complications from the valve. The valve sits flush with the carina of the segmental bifurcation when correctly positioned [6 - 8, 11] (Fig. **3**).

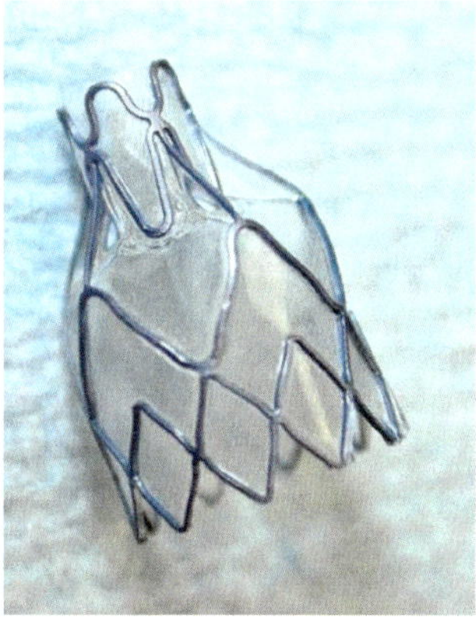

Fig. (2). The Emphasys Endobronchial Valve (EBV) with the central one-way silicone duckbill valve attached to a nitinol self-expanding retaining frame that itself is wrapped in a silicone seal. Used with permission, Pulmonx Inc.

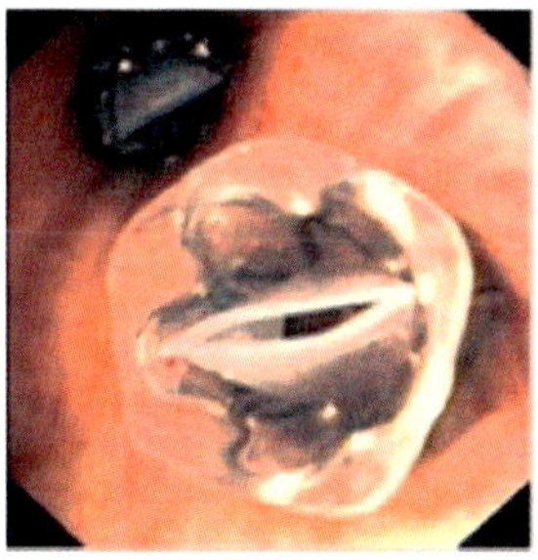

Fig. (3). The Emphasys Endobronchial Valve (EBV) in good position after implantation in the right upper lobe. Used with permission, Pulmonx Inc.

After the initial pilot studies by Toma *et al.* and Yim *et al.* suggested efficacy and relative safety of the procedure, some smaller studies without control arms were conducted [11]. These case series consistently were able to demonstrate improvements in subjective scores of dyspnea but were unable to delineate a clear improvement in traditionally measured physiologic markers such as FEV1 or six-minute walk distances (6MWT) [6 - 8].

The Endobronchial Valve for Emphysema PalliatioN Trial (VENT) study was a multicenter prospective double-blinded trial, which enrolled 321 patients that were randomly assigned in a 2:1 ratio to unilateral therapy with a Zephyr Valve (220 patients) *vs.* standard medical management (101 patients) for their emphysema.8 Eligibility and exclusion criteria mirrored that from the NETT subgroup identified as responders. Namely, patients with heterogeneous emphysema, a forced expiratory volume in one second (FEV1) of 15% to 45% of the predicted value, residual volume of more than 150% of predicted value, a body-mass index (BMI) of 31.1 or less for men or 32.3 or less for women, a partial pressure of carbon dioxide (PaCO2) of less than 50 mm Hg, a partial pressure of oxygen (PaO2) of more than 45 mm Hg on room air, and a post-rehabilitation 6 minute walk distance of at least 1,40 m (459 ft.) were enrolled. Patients were excluded if they had a carbon monoxide diffusing capacity (DLCO) of less than 20% of the predicted value, the presence of giant bullae, alpha-1 anti-trypsin deficiency, previous thoracotomy, excessive sputum, severe pulmonary hypertension, active infection, or unstable cardiac conditions.

The data obtained from the VENT study demonstrated small improvements in their primary efficacy outcomes of FEV1 (4.3%; 95% CI +/- 1.4 to 7.2) and 6MWT (2.5%; 95% CI +/- -1.1 to 6.1) as compared to decreases in the control group at six months with FEV1 (2.5%; 95% CI -5.4 to 0.4) and 6MWT (3.2%; 95% CI -8.9 to 2.4). Modest improvements were demonstrated in secondary efficacy measures of quality of life and dyspnea, such as the St. George's Respiratory Questionnaire (SGRQ), BODE (Body Mass index, Obstructive lung disease, Dyspnea, and Exercise tolerance) index, average daily oxygen use, and maximum workload by cycle ergometry.

A non-statistically significant trend towards a greater rate of major complications (6.1% in the valve implant group *vs.* 1.2% in control groups) was reported. Twelve patients developed post-obstructive pneumonia with half of those requiring removal of their valves. Hemoptysis (6%), pneumothorax (4.2%), and exacerbations of chronic obstructive pulmonary disease (COPD) requiring hospital admission occurred with greater frequency in the EBV group. Six deaths occurred in the intervention arm in contrast to none in the control arm. Mortalities were not felt to be associated with the procedure or the valve implants. At the twelve-month follow-up, a statistically significant difference in survival benefit was not demonstrated on multivariate Cox regression analysis.

In the follow-up phase of the study, valve migration, post-obstructive pneumonia distal to the valve, hemoptysis, and COPD exacerbations occurred, requiring the removal of eighty-five valves in thirty-five patients. The success rate of valve removal was 97.7%. Post completion of the study another eight patients had elective removals of the EBV due to adverse events. The European cohort of 171 patients demonstrated similar results to the US cohort data reported [6]. The FDA review of the study did not result in approval of the device for BLVR due to the lack of clinically significant response seen in FEV1 [3 - 16].

Further subgroup analysis of HRCT data revealed a correlation of clinical success with fissure integrity affording greater improvements in symptoms, measured physiologic markers and reductions in lung volumes resulting in expansion of the less diseased neighboring lung. Small studies with longer-term follow-up have also shown that patients who have atelectasis of the target segments show a survival benefit over other groups receiving BLVR [7, 11].

These results support theories raised in earlier studies and the experience seen with endobronchial blocker use that collateral ventilation may have a role to play in blunting the benefit and lung volume reduction that is achieved with endobronchial airway obstructive techniques. Ventilation through accessory pathways (collateral ventilation) is the likely cause of the high percentage of patients who had lobar exclusion with valve blockade but did not achieve selected atelectasis [7, 14]. The European cohort of the VENT (Euro-VENT), also an RCT, confirmed fissure integrity and lobar occlusion as predictors of successful valve treatment [32]. A reduction in the volume of the treated lobe of the lung (target lobe volume reduction, TLVR) of 80% was demonstrated in patients with a complete fissure and complete lobar occlusion. In a retrospective analysis, 32% of the patients with a complete fissure had TLVR >50%, compared with only 4% of patients with an incomplete fissure [33]. Moreover, decreased the volume of the treated lobe correlated positively with lung function, exercise tolerance, quality of life, and the BODE index (body mass index, airflow obstruction, dyspnea, and exercise capacity index in chronic obstructive pulmonary disease). Thus a radiologically demonstrable uninterrupted fissure of >90% on at least one HRCT plane—axial, sagittal, or frontal—seems to be a surrogate for absent or minimal collateral ventilation. In contrast, the presence of a parenchymal bridge connecting the lobes for ≥ 10% of the fissure is assumed to indicate a high degree of collateral ventilation, leading to retrograde re-aeration of the occluded lobe and nullifying the valve effect. While the interlobar fissure in the left lung is complete in half of the cases, the fissures in the right lung are often incomplete [34]. Evaluation of fissure integrity demands radiological expertise, so in addition to visual quantification dedicated software is used for fissure analysis [35, 36]. A catheter-based pulmonary assessment system enables invasive quantification of collateral ventilation. The lobe to be treated is occluded bronchoscopically using a balloon catheter, and respiratory flow and pressure are measured. A decrease in flow speaks for only minor collateral ventilation, while unchanged flow indicates high collateral ventilation [14] (Fig. **4**).

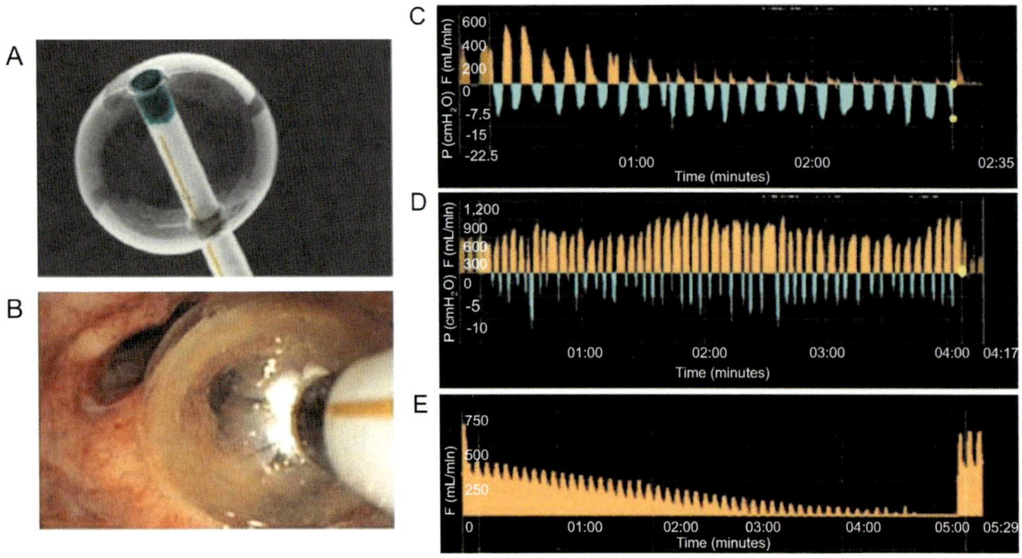

Fig. (4). The Chartis system with attached measurement catheter that is aimed to assess the presence of collateral ventilation to identify patients that will have a more favorable response to treatment. Used with permission, Pulmonx Inc.

Intra-bronchial Valve (IBV)

The Spiration intra-bronchial valve (Olympus, Redmond, WA) is a self-expanding Nitinol frame consisting of a central core with five distal anchors and six proximal curved radial struts [9, 10]. This structure supports a polyurethane membrane, which acts as a one-way umbrella valve when implanted against the bronchial wall [9, 10] (Fig. **5**). Aside from support the central core also serves as a removal rod or if the device needs manipulation after initial deployment [9, 10]. After selection of the target airways, appropriately sized valves are chosen. In a somewhat similar technique to the EBV placement, the IBV is inserted *via* the working channel of a flexible bronchoscope on a catheter loader. Once in position, the valve is deployed so it will sit flush with the carina of the segmental bronchus [10] (Fig. **6**).

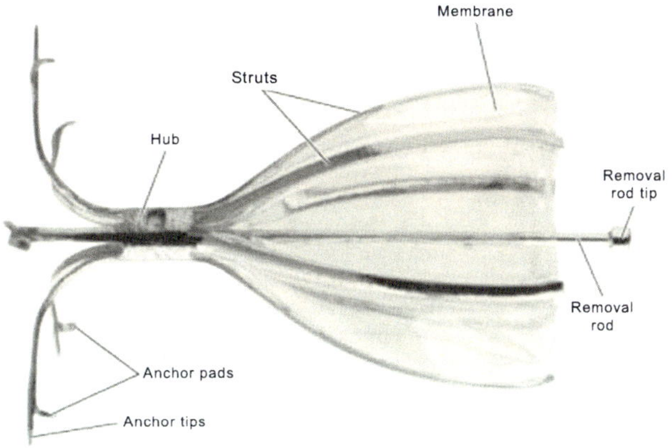

Fig. (5). The Spiration Intra-bronchial Valve (IBV) with nitinol frame mounted silicone umbrella valve and a central core strut use to manipulate or remove the valve once deployed.

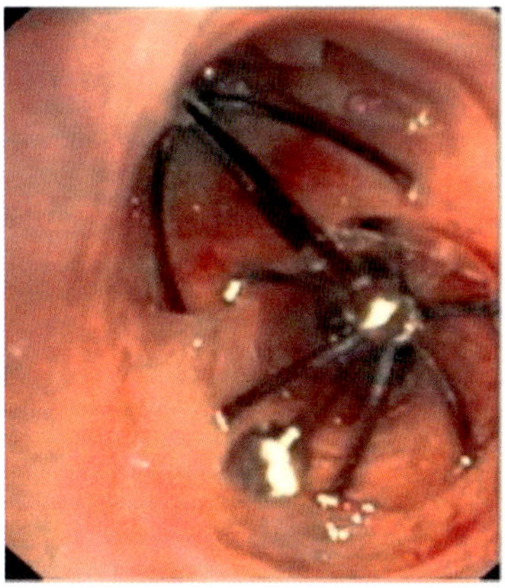

Fig. (6). Diagrams of the Spiration Intra-bronchial Valve (IBV) showing the valve in good position after implantation and function allowing drainage of secretions but blocking entry of air flow.

Two articles on the same set of patients, detailing experience with the placement of these valves have been published [9, 10]. One significant difference from EBV studies is the bilateral targeting and placement of these valves in the upper lobes. Similar to the trials for EBV, these trials used selection criteria that closely mirrored the NETT trial subgroup that demonstrated the greatest benefit. Patients enrolled in both studies had severe heterogeneous predominantly upper lobe emphysema with a FEV1 of 15% to 45% predicted, TLC greater than100% predicted, RV greater than 150% predicted, PaCO2 of less than 50 mmHg, PaO2 greater than 45 mmHg, and a post rehabilitation six minute walk of greater than 140m. Exclusion criteria removed patients with a FEV1 less than 20% predicted, DLCO less than 20% predicted, homogenous emphysema, active infection, a recent COPD exacerbation, giant bullae, pulmonary hypertension, or oxygen requirements greater than 6 liters per minute (LPM).

The two articles share ninety-one subjects at eleven US and international centers. For reasons not explained in either article, seven subjects from two additional centers were included in the initial article, which was not included in the later more comprehensive article. Results of both reports were similar. The pilot study, by Sherman *et al.* [10], was a single-arm, open-label case series using a multi-lobar bilateral treatment approach. Primary outcomes of the study focused on safety based on the incidence of valve migration, erosion, or infection. Efficacy based on FEV1, 6MWT, and SGRQ were the secondary endpoints. Other potential measures of efficacy included change in oxygen supplementation requirements, improvement in Medical Outcome Study Short-Form Health Survey (SF-36) scores, and improvement in the modified Medical Research Council dyspnea score [9, 10].

During the study period, the protocol was changed twice. After the first third of patients were enrolled, the protocol was modified to include, at the discretion of the investigator, valve treatment to the lingula in addition to the left upper lobe with the intention to increase the amount of atelectasis achieved. Then, after enrollment of the second third of patients, the protocol was reverted to excluding the lingula from treatment with the addition of further radiographic measurements for evaluating response to the valve implants. Changes to the protocol for follow-up included cessation of a second bronchoscopy one-month post procedure as it was felt to be of low yield. Quantitative Computer Tomography (QCT) of patients for volumetric analysis of lobar volumes was added to the study protocol during the last third of the investigation as an additional marker for efficacy of treatment [9, 10].

The results of this pilot study were encouraging. No patients were lost to follow-up, although twenty-six patients withdrew from the study related to adverse events associated with the valve implants. The majority of patients with later withdrawals (defined as withdrawal after six months post procedure) were either related to a perceived lack of improvement by the patient or other issues such as a new diagnosis of lung cancer [10].

As the primary endpoint was to evaluate safety data a detailed analysis of all adverse events was performed. None of the deaths were determined to be procedure related. No migration or erosion was noted throughout the study. Dyspnea post procedure day three was seen in eight patients and was felt to be related to implant triggered bronchospasm. Only two of these patients required valve removal to alleviate the symptoms with the remainder improving with bronchodilator treatment. Other procedure-related complications included myocardial infarction, injury to bronchi from deep valve placement, and transient hypercarbia requiring temporary ventilatory overnight support. Across the course of the study, a total of forty-four valves were removed due to persistent bronchospasm, recurrent COPD exacerbations, pneumonia, or pneumothorax [9, 10].

A total of eleven patients developed pneumothorax with six requiring chest tube placements. Subsequent analysis revealed a higher incidence of left-sided pneumothorax in the patients who had received additional valve implants to the lingula. As in prior studies of other modalities of BLVR, a close correlation was noted between the amount of atelectasis achieved and incidence of pneumothorax [9, 10]. The suggested mechanism for this has been related to rapid atelectasis of the lung parenchyma in the presence of adhesions, tension on adjacent tissue, or overexpansion of blebs and bullae that may accompany the lung reduction. Also, there were three deaths associated with pneumothorax in the study population

In comparison to the LVRS patients in the NETT, morbidity and mortality data (49.8%) were more favorable for the IBV data, which demonstrated a 5.5% 30-day morbidity for major cardio-pulmonary complications [9, 10]. Health-related quality of life (HRQL) measures at six months achieving the -4 points clinically significant threshold in the NETT patients was 60% in comparison to 55% for patients with IBV implants [9, 10]. These result comparisons suggest an improved risk/benefit ratio in terms HRQL measures for IBV treatment.

On the evaluation of the secondary endpoints of efficacy, no statistically significant change or improvement was seen in any of the measured physiologic indices such as FEV1, TLC, RV, or 6MWT. Improvement in HRQL measures was noted in the majority of patients as measured by the SGRQ and SF-36. This population of patients with clinically significant improvement in SGRQ increased with time and remained statistically significant. Similar results of discordance between the improvements in HRQL measures and physiologic indices in the population of patients with severe emphysema have been seen in other studies of BLVR and LVRS.

It has been suggested that in this population of patients the traditional physiologic measures of FEV1 and lung volume do not accurately predict effects of changes in regional lung volume when the obstructive defect is known to be fixed. Additionally, issues with the effort dependent variability of FEV1 in severe emphysema due to loss of elastic recoil could limit its utility as an outcome measure [9].

To further investigate these proposed mechanisms, researchers employed a QCT evaluation to assess changes in regional lung volume [9]. Using a previously validated quantitative volumetric CT assessment tool, a statistically significant average upper lobe volume reduction of roughly 300ml was seen six months post-treatment in 93% of patients. This volume reduction increased across all time points in the study period and was accompanied by a respective increase in the volume of the untreated and less severely emphysematous lung. A significant correlation was then noted among patients with improvements in their HRQL responses and QCT assessed volume increases of greater than 10% in the non-treated lung [9].

The above observations lead the investigators of the study to postulate a third mechanism to be contributory to the improvement in HRQL that were observed. In addition to lobar atelectasis causing lung volume reduction and improvements in dynamic hyperinflation, an inter-lobar shift of ventilation was identified [9]. In essence, with increased ventilation to the less severely emphysematous lower lobes and shunting of airflow away from the poorly perfused lobes targeted for treatment, an improvement in the ventilation-perfusion ratio was achieved. This improvement most likely represents an element of the observed improvements in dyspnea and HRLQ after treatment [9]. The investigators acknowledged that the above three mechanisms were most likely interlinked and each plays some role in improvements noted by the patients [9].

Currently, the IBV valves are available for use in the United States with a Federal Drug Administration (FDA) humane use only indication for prolonged surgical air leaks pending further studies that hope to elucidate clinically significant efficacy. A multicenter trial that randomly assigned 277 subjects to IBV treatment *versus* sham bronchoscopy has been completed, but the results are not yet available. The primary outcome measures were an improvement in the SGRQ, and regional lung volume changes on computed tomography at six months [17].

Lung Volume Reduction Coil (LVRC) Implants

Experience with an endobronchial blocker and one-way airway valves for volume reduction have been plagued with lack of response felt to be related to the presence of collateral ventilation [6, 8, 9, 14]. Another approach to BLVR to overcome this challenge is the Lung Volume Reduction Coil (LVRC), an implant that physically compresses target areas in patients with severe heterogeneous emphysema to avoid the issue of collateral ventilation altogether. The RePneu Airway Coil (PenumRx, Inc. Mountain View, CA) is a nitinol wire that is preformed in a shape that compresses the lung parenchyma once deployed in the target airways [13, 16] (Fig. 7). This approach is intended to lead to a genuine reduction in lung volume from the surrounding area.

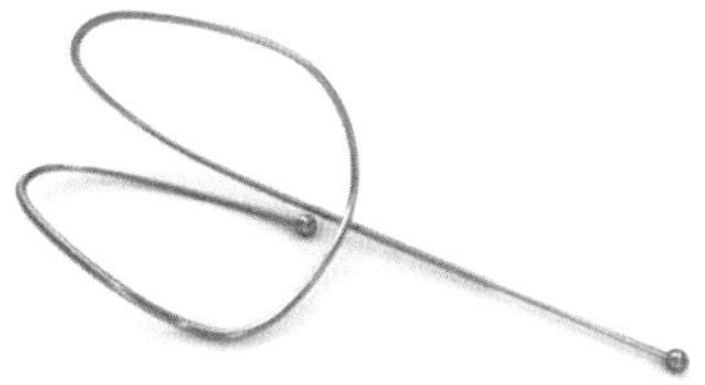

Fig. (7). The nitinol airway coil implant is seen here in its preformed shape. Used with permission, PneumRx Inc.

The airway implants are placed under general anesthesia with flexible bronchoscopy *via* a rigid bronchoscope or large endotracheal tube [13, 16]. A guidewire is advanced into the target segment under fluoroscopic guidance. The length of the airway is then measured using a graduated catheter passed over the guidewire. This allows selection of the appropriate length of the LVRC implant (Fig. **8**). After removal of the guidewire, a straightened LVRC is advanced under fluoroscopic guidance into the airway *via* the catheter using a grasper holding the proximal end of the implant (Fig. **9**). Proper positioning of the implant aligns the distal tip of the LVRC 15mm from the pleura [13, 16] (Fig. **10**). The LVRC assumes its preformed shape once the catheter is removed, thereby bending the airway and compressing the surrounding lung parenchyma. Finally, the proximal end of the LVRC is released from the grasper and the bronchoscope removed. Repositioning or removal of the implant is performed by reversal of the above-described procedure [13, 16].

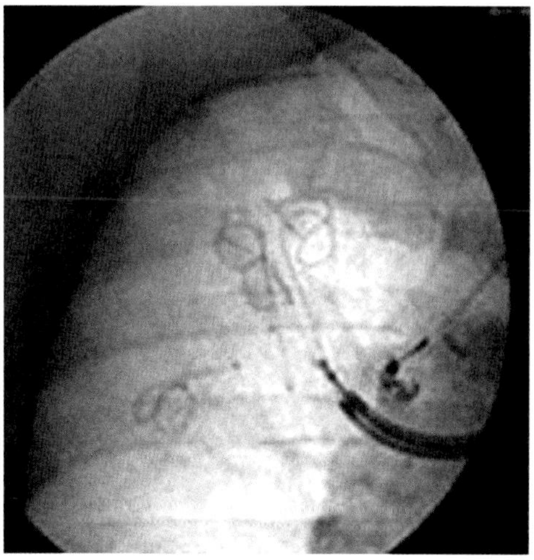

Fig. (8). Once the coil has been advanced into position, the guide catheter is withdrawn with the coil returning to its preformed shape compressing the surrounding lung parenchyma with it. Used with permission, PneumRx Inc.

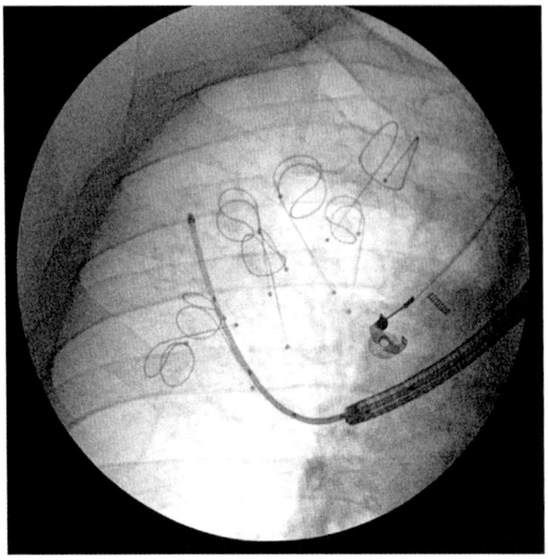

Fig. (9). The fluoroscopic guidance allows optimal positioning of the guide catheter and airway coil. Previously placed implants are also visible. Courtesy G.Deslée.

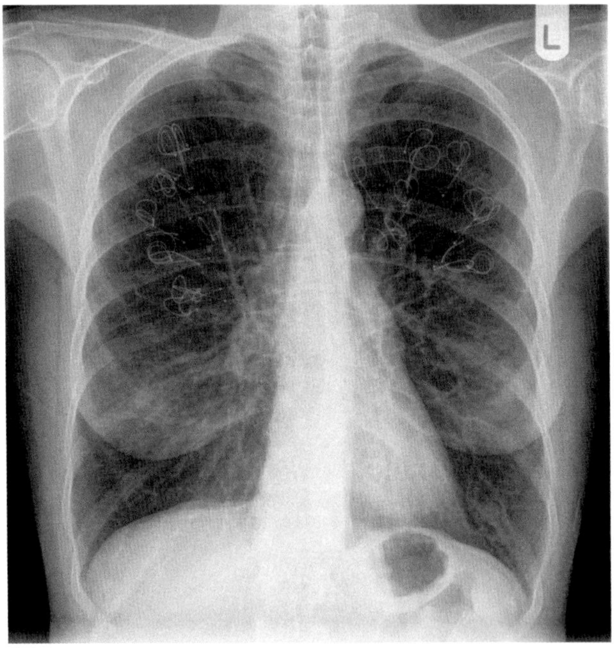

Fig. (10). The implanted airway coils can be seen in bilateral upper lobes on radiographic imaging. Courtesy D.J. Slebos.

After initial animal studies, a pilot study was conducted that enrolled eleven patients (eight with severe homogeneous emphysema and three with a severe heterogeneous disease) [13]. Two procedures were performed on each patient one to three months apart. Three to six LVRC implants were placed during each session. Six patients received LVRC implants bilaterally, four had unilateral treatment, and one patient did not get a second treatment.

The primary endpoint of the pilot study was safety data measured by analysis of adverse events. Heath *et al.* showed in this trail that the procedure was feasible and observed adverse effects were comprised of initial episodes of dyspnea, cough, transient chest pain and exacerbation of COPD that resolved with treatment. No serious adverse events occurred, and none of the LVRC implants required removal during the six-month study period. The data further suggested that in addition to improvements in HRQL there were clinically significant improvements in pulmonary function indices such as FEV1, FVC, and 6 MWT in patients with the heterogeneous disease [13]. The study was not designed with adequate power to detect a statistical difference in efficacy data as this was a secondary endpoint.

The second generation coil was developed and used in the second LVRC study [16]. The trial focused on patients with only upper lobe predominant heterogeneous emphysema. Inclusion and exclusion criteria were almost identical to other BLVR studies [16].

Once patients were identified, an assessment of the degree of emphysema was done using CT imaging. Visual assessment of sagittal reconstructions of full inspiratory thin slice CT scans in addition to digital assessment, were used to select and quantify patients with disease that were suspected to have enough destruction of upper lobe parenchyma to derive benefit from treatment, yet have enough tissue to allow LVRC placement with subsequent compression of surrounding parenchyma [16]. Upon completion of initial evaluations, an additional exclusion criterion was added; patients with greater than 75% destruction of their upper lobes on digital assessment were excluded.

Sixteen patients had twenty-eight sequentially staged LRVC placement procedures. An average of ten coils was placed per procedure. To further standardize the approach, coils were also placed in predetermined segments independent of CT findings. Bilateral implants were placed in twelve patients. Four patients receiving unilateral treatment due to: ineligible targets contralaterally, significant clinical improvement from the initial treatment, or limitations from cardiac comorbidities [16].

No implant migration, erosion of airways, or need to remove any of the implants occurred during the six-month follow-up. One patient developed a pneumothorax one hour after the procedure. This resolved in one day with chest tube decompression. Additionally, 75% of patients had mild (less than 5ml) hemoptysis. Transient self-limited chest pain thought to be related to pleural traction occurred in four patients. The frequency of COPD exacerbations and coughing were the most common issues post-implantation. These events decreased to pre-procedural levels after the first month. Mucosal damage, edema, and bronchoconstriction associated with the placement of the LVRC implants were postulated to be the reason for the respiratory events noted [13, 16]. Yet, undocumented concerns still exist for the development of pulmonary torsion, airway erosion, and infarction due to compression of blood vessels in the target lung.

Six months post procedure, an improvement is HRQL was seen similar to BLVR patients treated by both one-way valves and endobronchial blockers. The almost fifteen point reduction in SGRQ however, was greater than that reported even in the favorable response sub-group of the NETT LRVS study [13]. Unlike the other BLVR device implants, this study showed a 14.9% clinically significant ($p<0.005$) improvement in FEV1, 13.4% improvement in FVC, 11% reduction in RV, and a clinically relevant 84-meter improvement in 6MWT [16]. As efficacy was again a secondary endpoint of this study, these results need to be interpreted with cautious optimism while awaiting further data from more adequately powered studies.

Two trials are currently ongoing to more completely address the clinical efficacy of LVRC in effecting BLVR. The larger US study intended to recruit 315 patients has not yet started enrolling patients at the time of writing of this publication. A smaller study registered in the UK is currently ongoing, and data is not available for interpretation or comment.

Bronchoscopic Thermal Vapor Ablation (BTVA)

Bronchoscopic thermal vapor ablation (BTVA) was developed as another technique to selectively treat portions of the lung which are diseased. Scarring and contraction is produced by inducing an inflammatory response to thermal injury of soft tissue as a means of lung volume reduction [16, 18 - 21]. Animal studies have delineated the effects and extent of varying doses of treatment.

The thermal energy is delivered *via* bronchoscopic introduction of heated water vapor into the lung parenchyma and airways using the InterVapor system (Uptake Medical, Tustin, CA) [18 - 21]. The system is comprised of a device to precisely delivery heated water vapor, a delivery handle (Fig. **11**), and a delivery catheter with an occlusion balloon near the tip. All procedures were performed under general anesthesia with flexible bronchoscopy *via* a large (size nine or ten) endotracheal tube. Two operators are needed to optimally carry out this procedure, the first performing the bronchoscopy and the second manipulating the catheter system and delivery handle for the vapor therapy. Once the target segment is identified, the vapor delivery catheter was advanced into the airway with subsequent inflation of the occlusion balloon at the tip of the catheter. (Fig. **12**) The desired dose of thermal energy, using steam, is delivered to the airway. A five-minute period between treatments is required to prevent accumulative thermal energy causing a more significant injury.

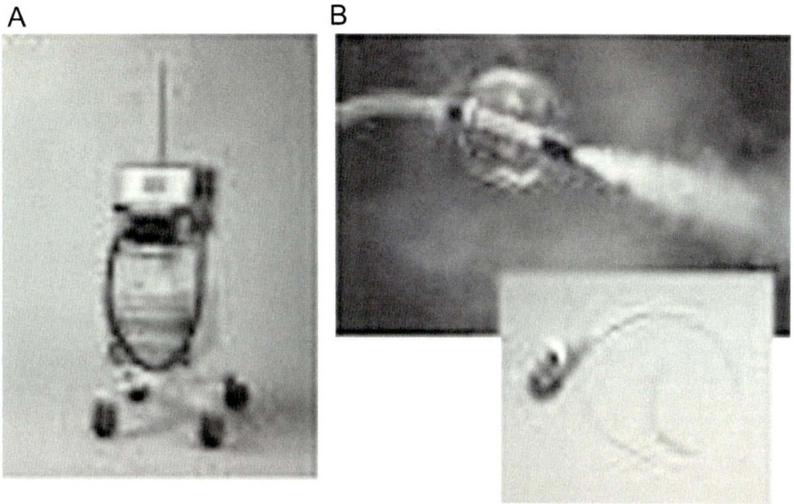

Fig. (11). The InterVapor system used to generate the steam to deliver thermal energy to the target segments. The single patient use disposable catheter is also seen. Used with permission, Uptake Medical.

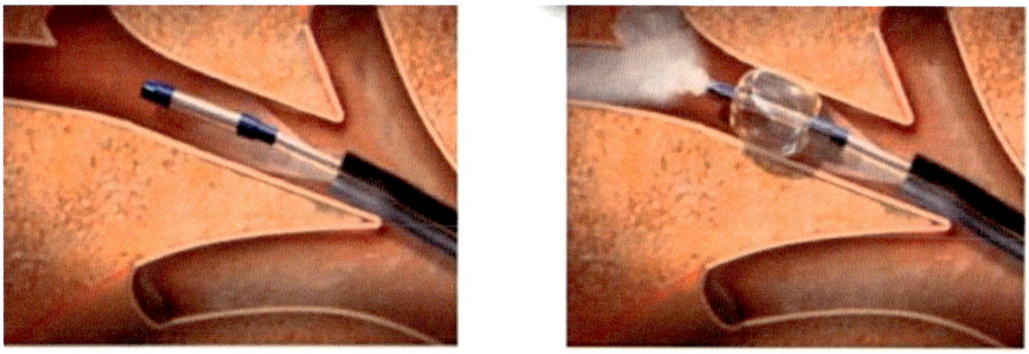

Fig. (12). The tip of the delivery catheter with an inflated occlusive balloon that avoids unintended proximal delivery of steam. Used with permission, Uptake Medical.

Extrapolating from the animal studies on BTVA a unilateral dose of five calories/gram of lung tissue treated was selected for the first pilot study in humans done by Snell *et al.* [21]. Patients with heterogeneous upper lobe emphysema who had a FEV1 between 15% and 45% predicted, TLC at least 100% predicted, RV greater than 150% predicted a post-rehabilitation 6MWT of more than 140m,

PaCO2 less than 50 mmHg, and a PaO2 greater than 45 mmHg were enrolled. In summary, the criteria were similar to studies done to evaluate other BLVR modalities.

All of the eleven patients enrolled in the pilot study received unilateral treatment to the lobe thought to have the most severe disease by the investigators [21]. No procedural complications were reported. Symptoms of nausea, cough, transient fatigue, and mild to moderate hemoptysis were noted post-procedurally. Almost 64% of patients had subsequent exacerbations of their COPD with roughly half of these felt to be related to infection by the authors. Two of the seven patients with COPD exacerbations required hospitalization. Two additional patients developed pneumonitis, one requiring hospital admission and treatment. Atrial tachycardia and anxiety in one patient also required inpatient treatment. Overall, BTVR was felt to be relatively safe and thus a feasible procedure [21].

Secondary endpoint evaluations in this pilot study included quantitative volumetric CT assessment [21]. A 16% volume reduction of the treated lobe was seen on chest CT analysis. The amount of volume loss noted appeared to correlate with improvements seen on SGRQ ($r = 0.83$). In conjunction with the observed target lobe volume loss, a comparable increase in the ipsilateral non-treated lobe volume of 24% was observed [21]. Total lung volume was not changed. Of the thirty-three segments treated with BTVA, thirty-one of the segmental airways showed narrowing or occlusion. Bronchoscopy repeated six months after the treatment did not reveal granulation tissue or airway inflammation. Improvements were seen in HRLQ with an increase of 15.3 points on the SGRQ [21]. Pulmonary function testing, however, did not reveal any significant changes from baseline measurements of FEV1, FVC, TLC, or RV [21]. Additionally no change was seen in 6 MWT at the end of the six-month study period [21].

This pilot study was critical in elucidating the favorable procedural safety data observed. A similar inflammatory response seen in animal studies was also noted in humans. Initially, there is a blanching of the airways and an immediate chest x-ray change that likely represents alveolar edema [21]. This is followed by mild non-specific airway symptoms seen for seven to fourteen days post-procedure [21]. At six months, 94% of the treated airways are at least partially occluded on CT imaging due to fibrosis of the targeted areas [21]. The increased incidence of COPD exacerbations and cough symptoms are probably related to above-described induced inflammatory changes [21].

Further studies assessing the dosimetry of thermal energy delivered have been completed. Most patients evaluated demonstrated improvement in physiologic parameters in addition to HRQL. Volumetric assessments were also improved as compared to previous studies. Similar post-procedure complications were noted, particularly COPD exacerbations due to the inflammatory modified response [18 - 20].

Larger trails evaluating BTVA are currently underway and should be able to address any concerns of safety of the treatment. It appears the increased thermal energy delivered in the latter studies was more effective; however, further dosimetric studies may be required to strike a balance between adverse events and efficacy [18 - 21]. The lack of a control arm will also need to be addressed in future studies.

Biological Lung Volume Reduction

Biological lung volume reduction (BiLVR) is based on the bronchoscopic application of a fibrin hydrogel into the airways of hyperinflated areas of emphysematous lungs to cause scar tissue formation, which will lead to a reduction of the overall lung volumes and air trapping. The first studies were performed by Ingenito *et al.* [22, 23] in sheep models of emphysema with promising results. The hydrogel contains biodegradable complexes of poly--lysine and chondroitin sulfate that initiate a localized inflammatory reaction that collapses, remodels, and reduces the volume of emphysematous lung over three to six weeks.

The procedure consists on instilling fibrinogen suspension and thrombin solution into the selected subsegmental airway through a dual lumen catheter over ten to fifteen seconds to ensure rapid polymerization of the hydrogel, followed immediately by injection of air to push the reagents peripherally [24, 25]. Most recently, with the introduction of AeriSeal (Aeris Therapeutics, Woburn, Mass., USA) as a foam sealant that is prepared at the bedside right before the procedure, the instillation is performed through a single lumen catheter [26] (Fig. **12**).

The use of BLVR has shown to be useful in the treatment of severe upper lobe predominant emphysema [24] as well as homogeneous emphysema [25], with significant improvement in physiological (FEV1 and FVC), functional (6-minute walk test) and symptomatic (dyspnea index) parameters at six months. The degree of response was dose dependent and more durable with 20mL per site dosing compared to the only 10mL. Patients with heterogeneous emphysema with Global Initiative for Chronic Obstructive Lung Disease (GOLD) stage III have shown the best response from this procedure [26]. All studies have also proved BiLVR to be very safe, with no mortality associated with the procedure [24 - 26]. Self-limited side effects like dyspnea, fever, radiographic infiltrate and chest pain right after the procedure have been reported [26].

Contrary to other bronchoscopic techniques of lung volume reduction, like endobronchial valves, the effect of silver in patients with upper lobe predominant emphysema is not related to interlobar fissure integrity [27].

Recently, in a randomized trial, 57 patients were randomly assigned to ELS (two subsegments in each upper lobe) plus medical therapy or medical therapy alone and followed for six months. Significant improvements from baseline were noted in lung function, dyspnea, and quality of life at three months when compared to control, and the benefits persisted for six months [37]. However, clinically significant adverse events requiring hospitalization occurred in 44 percent of the treatment group in addition to two deaths. The study was terminated early due to financial problems.

Airway Bypass

Van Allen and colleagues described "collateral ventilation" for the first time in 1930 [28] by describing the passage of gases between different lung lobules without the existence of anatomical passageways. Later on, Hogg *et al.* [29] demonstrated that collateral ventilation is substantially increased in emphysema and that in emphysematous lungs there is lower resistance through some of the collateral channels than through the airways themselves.

Based on the results of multiple studies showing the benefits from decreasing dynamic hyperinflation in emphysematous patients by lung volume reduction surgery [30], Lausberg *et al.* [31] hypothesized that creation of new exit pathways from the lung parenchyma into the airways (airway bypass) would allow the trapped gas to escape during exhalation. Lausberg's study, performed in homogeneous emphysematous lungs removed at the time of lung transplantation, demonstrated a significant improvement in FEV1 after the bronchoscopic creation of three to five extra-anatomic bronchopulmonary passages compared to baseline.

The Exhale Emphysema Treatment System (Bronchus Technologies, Inc, Mountain View, Calif) has been used to create airway bypass in all the studies since Lausberg's trial. This system comes with a Doppler transducer catheter (Exhale Doppler Probe); a Doppler processing unit to amplify the sounds of the Doppler probe; a transbronchial dilatation needle for passage creation and dilatation; and the Exhale Drug-Eluting Stent, which is composed of stainless steel, paclitaxel, and silicone.

The creation of a passage requires three steps: first, bronchoscopic identification of a location (segmental bronchi) that is free of blood vessels by using the Doppler probe; second, fenestration of the bronchial wall using the transbronchial needle and dilating balloon; and third, placement of the drug-eluting stent to hold the passage open [12] (Fig. **13**). The average of implanted stents has varied from six to eight per person [12], placed on a single bronchoscopic session performed under general anesthesia and orotracheal intubation (Fig. **14**). Serious but rare complications related to the procedure include major hemoptysis, pneumothorax with chest tube insertion and respiratory failure. More common complications were related to COPD exacerbations or pulmonary infections that needed hospitalization for more than seven days [15].

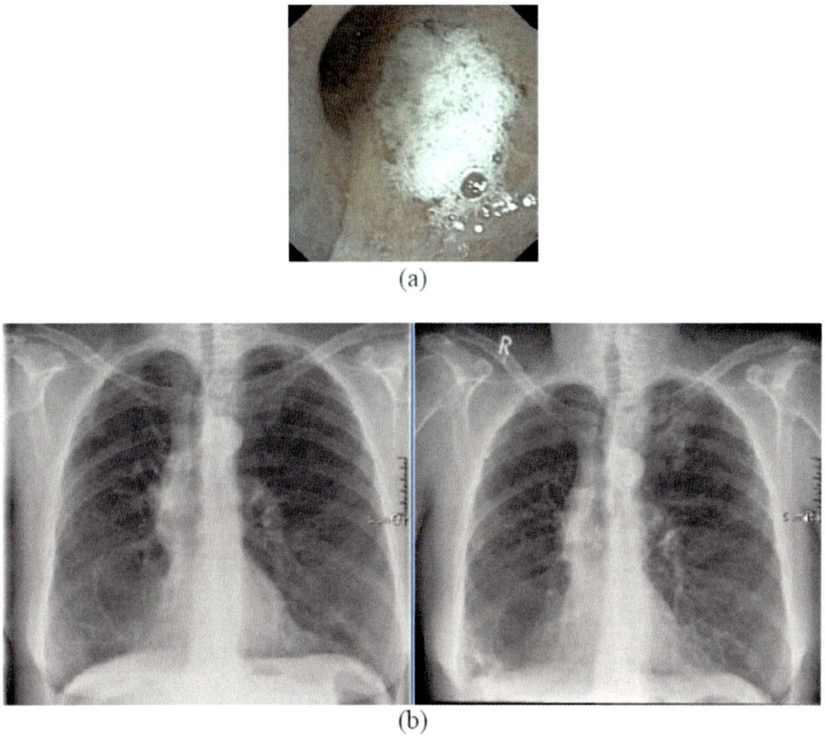

Fig. (13). Bronchoscopic instillation of the biological foam into the segmental airway (a) will create an inflammatory reaction leading to collapse (b) and formation of scar tissue.
(Courtesy of Aeris Therapeutics, Woburn, Mass.)

Early results from studies were promising and revealed significant improvement in different parameters at one month compared to baseline, although the only improvement in residual volume and dyspnea scores remained significant at six months [12]. These results prompted the development of a multicenter, double-blind, randomized, sham-controlled trial (Exhale airway stents for emphysema-EASE trial) [15]. The study recruited 315 patients with homogeneous emphysema. Even though significant improvement in pulmonary function and dyspnea scores was found at day one after the procedure in the airway bypass group, these changes were not different from those found in the sham control group at 3, 6 and 12 months follow-up. This technology is not being pursued any further.

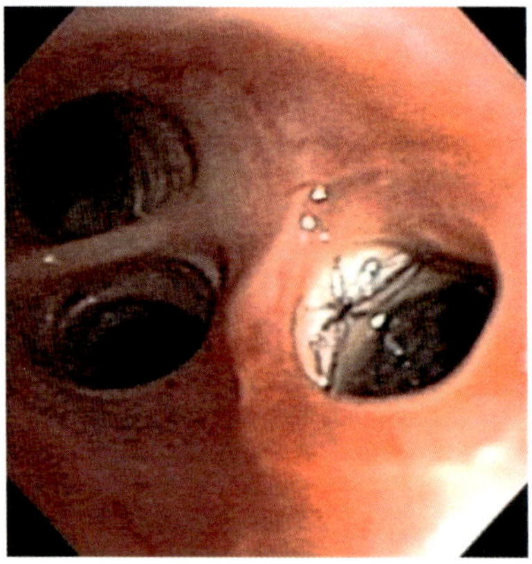

Fig. (14). Image of an implanted stent after six months.
(From Cardoso PFG, *et al*. Clinical application of airway bypass with paclitaxel-eluting stents: early results. J Thorac Cardiovasc Surg 2007; 134:974-81).

CONCLUSION

COPD is a widespread disease associated with significant morbidity and mortality. Initial therapeutic approach to patients should include strict weaning off tobacco, vaccination against influenza and pneumococci, improvement of physical fitness, and pharmacotherapy. From the original concept of surgical lung volume reduction to the multiple options discussed above, it is evident that the endoscopic management of COPD is actively being pursued. Identifying a bronchoscopic approach that has an actual impact on this patient population will be a major accomplishment in the management of patients with COPD.

The use of more traditional markers of improvement (*i.e.*, increases in FEV1and FVC) may be the incorrect approach to evaluating the success of BLVR procedures. The resurgence in work on the physiologic improvements in patients successfully treated with these techniques should identify better parameters that can be used in addition to the quality of life scores to mark successful interventions.

The successful use of bronchoscopic lung volume reduction may allow for better bridging for lung transplant patients as well as overall improvement in severe emphysematous patients functionality. Currently, in the United States, no technique is FDA approved. Also, collateral ventilation influences some procedures, and others are not. As such, identifying the most appropriate bronchoscopic approach that has an actual impact on this patient population, and plays a great impact on the success or failure of the intervention. It is important for all physicians involved in the management of these patients to be aware of any clinical trials available and recommend patients to them as this is a significant step for the advancement of these technologies.

CONFLICT OF INTEREST

The authors declare no conflict of interest, financial or otherwise.

ACKNOWLEDGEMENTS

Declared none.

REFERENCES

[1] Fishman A, Martinez F, Naunheim K, *et al.* National Emphysema Treatment Trial Research Group. A randomized trial comparing lung-volume-reduction surgery with medical therapy for severe emphysema. N Engl J Med 2003; 348(21): 2059-73. [http://dx.doi.org/10.1056/NEJMoa030287] [PMID: 12759479]

[2] Control CfD. Centers for Disease control and preventions's national center for health statistics, deaths: Preliminary data for 2008 2008.

[3] Ernst A, Anantham D. Endoscopic management of emphysema. Clin Chest Med 2010; 31(1): 117-26. [Table of Contents]. [http://dx.doi.org/10.1016/j.ccm.2009.08.001] [PMID: 20172437]

[4] Ernst A, Anantham D. Bronchoscopic lung volume reduction. Pulm Med 2011; 2011: 610802. [http://dx.doi.org/10.1155/2011/610802]

[5] Hwong TM, Yim AP. New treatment modalities for end-stage emphysema. Chest Surg Clin N Am 2003; 13(4): 739-53. [http://dx.doi.org/10.1016/S1052-3359(03)00093-0] [PMID: 14682606]

[6] Herth FJ, Noppen M, Valipour A, *et al.* International VENT Study Group. Efficacy predictors of lung volume reduction with Zephyr valves in a European cohort. Eur Respir J 2012; 39(6): 1334-42. [http://dx.doi.org/10.1183/09031936.00161611] [PMID: 22282552]

[7] Hopkinson NS, Kemp SV, Toma TP, *et al.* Atelectasis and survival after bronchoscopic lung volume reduction for COPD. Eur Respir J 2011; 37(6): 1346-51. [http://dx.doi.org/10.1183/09031936.00100110] [PMID: 20947683]

[8] Sciurba FC, Ernst A, Herth FJ, *et al.* VENT Study Research Group. A randomized study of endobronchial valves for advanced emphysema. N Engl J Med 2010; 363(13): 1233-44. [http://dx.doi.org/10.1056/NEJMoa0900928] [PMID: 20860505]

[9] Springmeyer SC, Bolliger CT, Waddell TK, Gonzalez X, Wood DE. IBV Valve Pilot Trials Research Teams. Treatment of heterogeneous emphysema using the spiration IBV valves. Thorac Surg Clin 2009; 19(2): 247-253, ix-x. [ix-x]. [http://dx.doi.org/10.1016/j.thorsurg.2009.02.005] [PMID: 19662968]

[10] Sterman DH, Mehta AC, Wood DE, *et al.* IBV Valve US Pilot Trial Research Team. A multicenter pilot study of a bronchial valve for the treatment of severe emphysema. Respiration 2010; 79(3): 222-33. [http://dx.doi.org/10.1159/000259318] [PMID: 19923790]

[11] Toma TP, Hopkinson NS, Hillier J, *et al.* Bronchoscopic volume reduction with valve implants in patients with severe emphysema. Lancet 2003; 361(9361): 931-3. [http://dx.doi.org/10.1016/S0140-6736(03)12762-6] [PMID: 12648974]

[12] Cardoso PF, Snell GI, Hopkins P, *et al.* Clinical application of airway bypass with paclitaxel-eluting stents: early results. J Thorac Cardiovasc Surg 2007; 134(4): 974-81. [http://dx.doi.org/10.1016/j.jtcvs.2007.05.040] [PMID: 17903516]

[13] Herth FJ, Eberhard R, Gompelmann D, Slebos DJ, Ernst A. Bronchoscopic lung volume reduction with a dedicated coil: a clinical pilot study. Ther Adv Respir Dis 2010; 4(4): 225-31. [http://dx.doi.org/10.1177/1753465810368553] [PMID: 20538661]

[14] Herth FJ, Eberhardt R, Gompelmann D, *et al.* Radiological and clinical outcomes of using Chartis™ to plan endobronchial valve treatment. Eur Respir J 2013; 41(2): 302-8. [http://dx.doi.org/10.1183/09031936.00015312] [PMID: 22556025]

[15] Shah PL, Slebos DJ, Cardoso PF, *et al.* EASE trial study group. Bronchoscopic lung-volume reduction with Exhale airway stents for emphysema (EASE trial): randomised, sham-controlled, multicentre trial. Lancet 2011; 378(9795): 997-1005. [http://dx.doi.org/10.1016/S0140-6736(11)61050-7] [PMID: 21907863]

[16] Slebos DJ, Klooster K, Ernst A, Herth FJ, Kerstjens HA. Bronchoscopic lung volume reduction coil treatment of patients with severe heterogeneous emphysema. Chest 2012; 142(3): 574-82. [http://dx.doi.org/10.1378/chest.11-0730] [PMID: 22116796]

[17] Health NIo. Implantation of endobronchial valves versus intrabronchial valves in patients with severe heterogeneous emphysema 2011.

[18] Emery MJ, Eveland RL, Eveland K, Couetil LL, Hildebrandt J, Swenson ER. Lung volume reduction by bronchoscopic administration of steam. Am J Respir Crit Care Med 2010; 182(10): 1282-91. [http://dx.doi.org/10.1164/rccm.201001-0102OC] [PMID: 20622035]

[19] Gompelmann D, Heussel CP, Eberhardt R, *et al.* Efficacy of bronchoscopic thermal vapor ablation and lobar fissure completeness in patients with heterogeneous emphysema. Respiration 2012; 83(5): 400-6. [http://dx.doi.org/10.1159/000336239] [PMID: 22377613]

[20] Snell G, Herth FJ, Hopkins P, *et al.* Bronchoscopic thermal vapour ablation therapy in the management of heterogeneous emphysema. Eur Respir J 2012; 39(6): 1326-33. [http://dx.doi.org/10.1183/09031936.00092411] [PMID: 22075481]

[21] Snell GI, Hopkins P, Westall G, Holsworth L, Carle A, Williams TJ. A feasibility and safety study of bronchoscopic thermal vapor ablation: a novel emphysema therapy. Ann Thorac Surg 2009; 88(6): 1993-8. [http://dx.doi.org/10.1016/j.athoracsur.2009.06.038] [PMID: 19932274]

[22] Ingenito EP, Reilly JJ, Mentzer SJ, *et al.* Bronchoscopic volume reduction: a safe and effective alternative to surgical therapy for emphysema. Am J Respir Crit Care Med 2001; 164(2): 295-301. [http://dx.doi.org/10.1164/ajrccm.164.2.2011085] [PMID: 11463604]

[23] Ingenito EP, Berger RL, Henderson AC, Reilly JJ, Tsai L, Hoffman A. Bronchoscopic lung volume reduction using tissue engineering principles. Am J Respir Crit Care Med 2003; 167(5): 771-8. [http://dx.doi.org/10.1164/rccm.200208-842OC] [PMID: 12406835]

[24] Criner GJ, Pinto-Plata V, Strange C, *et al.* Biologic lung volume reduction in advanced upper lobe emphysema: phase 2 results. Am J Respir Crit Care Med 2009; 179(9): 791-8. [http://dx.doi.org/10.1164/rccm.200810-1639OC] [PMID: 19179484]

[25] Refaely Y, Dransfield M, Kramer MR, *et al.* Biologic lung volume reduction therapy for advanced homogeneous emphysema. Eur Respir J 2010; 36(1): 20-7. [http://dx.doi.org/10.1183/09031936.00106009] [PMID: 19926742]

[26] Herth FJ, Gompelmann D, Stanzel F, *et al.* Treatment of advanced emphysema with emphysematous lung sealant (AeriSeal®). Respiration 2011; 82(1): 36-45. [http://dx.doi.org/10.1159/000322649] [PMID: 21228545]

[27] Magnussen H, Kramer MR, Kirsten AM, *et al.* Effect of fissure integrity on lung volume reduction

using a polymer sealant in advanced emphysema. Thorax 2012; 67(4): 302-8.
[http://dx.doi.org/10.1136/thoraxjnl-2011-201038] [PMID: 22374920]

[28] Van Allen CM, Lindskog GE, Richter HG. Gaseous Interchange Between Adjacent Lung Lobules. Yale J Biol Med 1930; 2(4): 297-300.
[PMID: 21433459]

[29] Hogg JC, Macklem PT, Thurlbeck WM. The resistance of collateral channels in excised human lungs. J Clin Invest 1969; 48(3): 421-31.
[http://dx.doi.org/10.1172/JCI105999] [PMID: 5773080]

[30] Sciurba FC, Rogers RM, Keenan RJ, *et al.* Improvement in pulmonary function and elastic recoil after lung-reduction surgery for diffuse emphysema. N Engl J Med 1996; 334(17): 1095-9.
[http://dx.doi.org/10.1056/NEJM199604253341704] [PMID: 8598868]

[31] Lausberg HF, Chino K, Patterson GA, Meyers BF, Toeniskoetter PD, Cooper JD. Bronchial fenestration improves expiratory flow in emphysematous human lungs. Ann Thorac Surg 2003; 75(2): 393-7.
[http://dx.doi.org/10.1016/S0003-4975(02)04553-8] [PMID: 12607646]

[32] Herth FJ, Noppen M, Valipour A, *et al.* International VENT Study Group. Efficacy predictors of lung volume reduction with Zephyr valves in a European cohort. Eur Respir J 2012; 39(6): 1334-42.
[http://dx.doi.org/10.1183/09031936.00161611] [PMID: 22282552]

[33] Valipour A, Herth FJ, Burghuber OC, *et al.* VENT Study Group. Target lobe volume reduction and COPD outcome measures after endobronchial valve therapy. Eur Respir J 2014; 43(2): 387-96.
[http://dx.doi.org/10.1183/09031936.00133012] [PMID: 23845721]

[34] Koenigkam-Santos M, de Paula WD, Owsijewitsch M, *et al.* Incomplete pulmonary fissures evaluated by volumetric thin-section CT: semi-quantitative evaluation for small fissure gaps identification, description of prevalence and severity of fissural defects. Eur J Radiol 2013; 82(12): 2365-70.
[http://dx.doi.org/10.1016/j.ejrad.2013.08.029] [PMID: 24016827]

[35] Koenigkam-Santos M, Puderbach M, Gompelmann D, *et al.* Incomplete fissures in severe emphysematous patients evaluated with MDCT: incidence and interobserver agreement among radiologists and pneumologists. Eur J Radiol 2012; 81(12): 4161-6.
[http://dx.doi.org/10.1016/j.ejrad.2012.06.006] [PMID: 22770581]

[36] van Rikxoort EM, Goldin JG, Galperin-Aizenberg M, *et al.* A method for the automatic quantification of the completeness of pulmonary fissures: evaluation in a database of subjects with severe emphysema. Eur Radiol 2012; 22(2): 302-9.
[http://dx.doi.org/10.1007/s00330-011-2278-0] [PMID: 21984417]

[37] Come CE, Kramer MR, Dransfield MT, *et al.* A randomised trial of lung sealant *versus* medical therapy for advanced emphysema. Eur Respir J 2015; 46(3): 651-62.
[http://dx.doi.org/10.1183/09031936.00205614] [PMID: 25837041]

CHAPTER 20

Foreign Body Retrieval

Javier Flandes[1], Juan A. Cascón[2], Rosa Cordovilla[2] and **Javier Alfayate[1,*]**

[1] *Bronchoscopy and Interventional Pulmonology. IIS - Fundación Jiménez Díaz University Hospital –CIBERES, Madrid, Spain*

[2] *Bronchoscopy and Interventional Pulmonology Unit - Hospital Universitario de Salamanca, Salamanca, Spain*

Abstract: The presence of foreign bodies in the airways may be a life-threatening emergency that requires quick and decisive action. Sometimes the foreign body aspiration may go unnoticed by the patient and the doctors, as may manifest in many ways, such as asthma-like symptoms, recurrent infections or even pulmonary abnormalities (*e.g.* bronchiectasis or areas of air-trapping).

Therefore, the diagnosis of these situations can be complex and requires a high degree of clinical suspicion. Among the complementary tests, chest x-ray may provide us with important information on those radiopaque foreign bodies. However, in other instances a computerized tomography (CT) is necessary to confirm the diagnosis and to determine the physical characteristics and exact location of the foreign body.

Since Gustav Killian extracted the first foreign body in 1897 using an esophagoscope, various techniques have been used for this purpose. Due to its larger working channel, rigid bronchoscopy allows an easier handling, removal and treatment of possible complications. Following the invention of the flexible bronchoscope by Shigeto Ikeda, and its subsequent development, this technique has emerged as a less invasive alternative to traditional procedures with encouraging results in selected cases and requiring fewer resources.

Keywords: Aspiration, Basket, Bronchology, CT scan, Chest, Cryoextraction, Flexible bronchoscopy, Fogarty catheter, Forceps, Foreign body, Interventional Pulmonology, Nd-YAG Laser, Rigid Bronchoscopy, X-Ray.

* **Corresponding author Javier Flandes:** Bronchoscopy and Interventional Pulmonology, IIS - Fundación Jiménez Díaz University Hospital - CIBERES, Avenida de los Reyes Católicos, 2, Madrid 28040, Spain; Tel: +34 91 550 48 13; E-mails: jflandes@fjd.es, flandes@fjd.es

Ali I. Musani (Ed.)

INTRODUCTION

Foreign body aspiration represents an urgent condition and requires a quick and decisive action in many cases, as it is potentially life-threatening. Since Gustav Killian in 1897 removed a pork bone from a farmer's airway, using an esophagoscope [1, 2], there have been numerous publications. A wide range of different foreign bodies, clinical presentations and removal procedures have been reported.

Rigid bronchoscopy has been the most commonly used technique for this purpose, as it provides a great number of possibilities regarding both handling of instruments, extraction technique and treatment of complications associated with the procedure.

Following the introduction of flexible bronchoscopy by Shigeto Ikeda in 1967 [3] and its further development, the number of indications of this technique is constantly growing. In the same way, techniques and devices that can be used through the channel of the bronchoscope are also rapidly increasing.

In this chapter, we will discuss the main aspects related to the foreign body retrieval, including the majority of the available techniques, assuming that innovations are constantly emerging in this field in order to achieve the highest success rate and lowest risk for the patient.

EPIDEMIOLOGY

Foreign Bodies in Children

Aspiration of foreign bodies has a higher incidence during childhood; nearly 80% of episodes take place in patients younger than 15 years. It is seen in all age groups but, according to some case series as described by Baharloo *et al.* a peak of incidence is observed around two years old, with a drop in incidence from the third year of life [4]. As for sex, the literature seems to show a predominance of males [5].

As for regarding the nature of the foreign body, they are mainly organic objects (peanuts, beans, seeds); 60-95% depending on the series (Fig. **1**). In terms of location, in pediatric patients, foreign bodies usually lodge in the proximal airways (larynx, vocal cords, trachea and bronchi). In addition, it seems to be a trend towards the right bronchial tree, although this is not as important as in adults, because of the change of position of the main bronchi with child development.

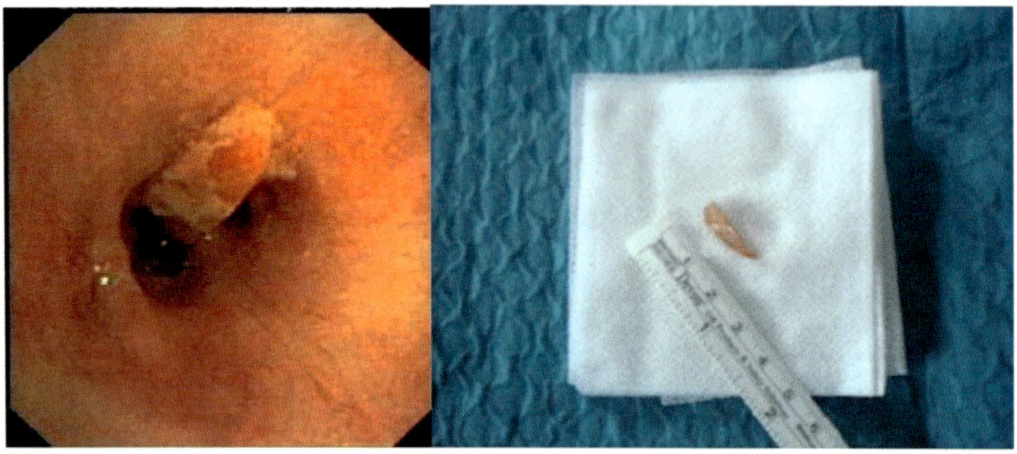

Fig. (1). Sunflower seed shell removed from the right lower lobe of a children.
Source: Interventional Pulmonology Unit. Salamanca University Hospital.

Foreign Bodies in Adults

Adults have a lower incidence of foreign body aspiration than children. Several predisposing factors have been postulated: Altered level of consciousness [6] (*e.g.* head trauma, use of central nervous system depressants such as alcohol or other drugs of abuse), swallowing dysfunction associated with some neurological disorders (*e.g.* Parkinson disease), mental retardation, dental procedures or even tracheostomy care.

There seems to be a male predominance [7, 8], and in terms of age, the published series does not show a peak in incidence, however, it seems logical to think that there is a progressively increased risk in the elderly.

Most often, as described in children, aspirated foreign bodies are organic (nuts, bones) [4], (Fig. **2**) but in other case series inorganic objects are reported (tracheostomy brush, pins, *etc.*) [7] (Fig. **3**). There is enough evidence about the most common location of aspirated foreign bodies. The right bronchial tree is affected in most cases, due to its more vertical course, wider diameter, the airflow and the fact that the carina lies to the left of the midline of the trachea.

DIAGNOSIS

Clinical Findings

Foreign body aspiration can be a life-threatening emergency with a high rate of morbidity and mortality, or conversely go unnoticed in the clinical practice. Despite this fact, symptoms may suddenly worsen and so several centers have set up protocols for the removal of airway foreign bodies as soon as possible [9]. A delayed diagnosis increases the rate of complications (atelectasis, bleeding, granuloma formation, *etc.*) [10].

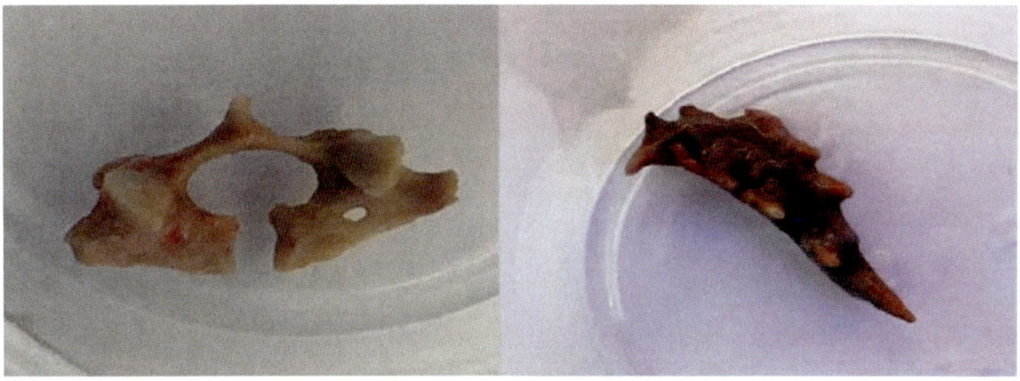

Fig. (2). Left: Chicken vertebrae removed from the left lower lobe of a 76-year-old man.
Right: Lobster shell removed from the intermediary bronchus of a 63-year-old man.
Source: Interventional Pulmonology Unit. Fundación Jiménez Díaz University Hospital.

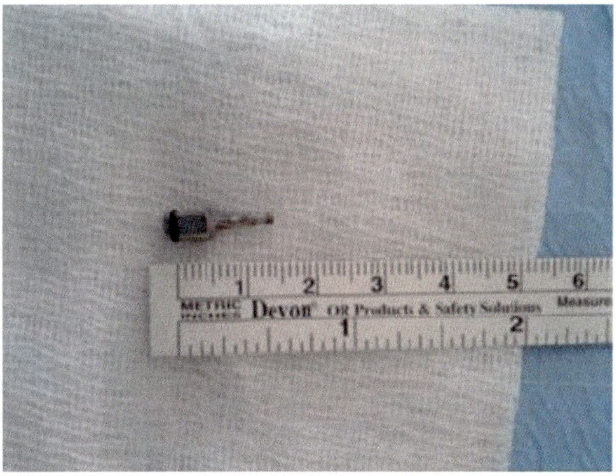

Fig. (3). Dental implant screw removed from right lower lobe.
Source: Interventional Pulmonology Unit. Salamanca University Hospital.

The classic clinical presentation of a foreign body aspiration is choking, later associated with persistent cough and respiratory distress [11]. Other symptoms may appear depending on the location: stridor if it is placed in the subglottic space, wheezing in case of a partial obstruction of the trachea or bronchi. Symptoms may persist, but occasionally are followed by intermittent cough or an asymptomatic period.

Up to 25% of cases, the clinical presentation is not so obvious and many patients do not recall any aspiration episode. It is common to find this insidious clinical presentation, with a wide differential diagnosis, which can hinder the work of the doctor, running several years from the time of aspiration at the time of diagnosis. In some cases, a history of repeated respiratory infections, recurrent pneumonia involving the same lobe accompanied by other radiological findings such as bronchiectasis or loss of lung volume [12] is seen. These symptoms and radiological abnormalities usually resolve after removal of the foreign body and the adequate medical treatment.

Clinical manifestations may mimic other diseases. As dyspnea, coughing and wheezing are frequently present; patients are most commonly misdiagnosed with asthma or recurrent bronchitis [13]. There have also been reported cases where the suspected diagnosis of endobronchial lesion is either benign origin (*e.g.* Carcinoid tumor) or malignant endobronchial component [14, 15].

Likewise, if it occurs in a patient with underline respiratory disease, it may further complicate the diagnosis [16].

Although rare, cases may occur through penetrating wounds (*e.g* firearm shots) resulting in a foreign body lodged in the bronchial tree, which can be accessible endoscopically [17].

In any case, in the diagnosis of foreign body aspiration, a high clinical index of suspicion is necessary [14].

Imaging

Once the clinical evaluation is completed, including a careful history and physical examination, appropriate diagnostic tests are required to reach the diagnosis in a simple and accurate way, minimizing the risks to the patient.

Chest X-ray

In the diagnostic evaluation of patients with a foreign body in the airway, plain radiography in two projections is the first test to be performed because of its wide availability, the important information provided in radiopaque objects and low risk to the patient.

On the one hand, up to 90% of foreign bodies are radiolucent; indirect findings such as atelectasis or air trapping are not always present and 30-50% of pediatric patients with an endobronchial foreign body have normal x-ray [18].

On the other hand, in a series of 31 patients, Pinto *et al.* observed that in 21 cases (67.7%) plain chest radiography showed the presence of foreign-body aspiration and/or pleuroparenchymal abnormalities [19]. Therefore, despite its limitations, simple radiology continues to play a key role in the diagnostic evaluation (Fig. **4**).

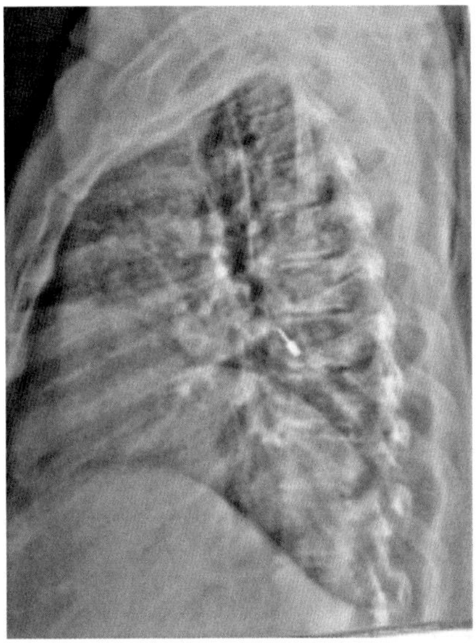

Fig. (4). Chest x-ray showing a radiopaque foreign body (dental implant screw).
Source: Interventional Pulmonology Unit. Salamanca University Hospital.

Computed Tomography (CT)

A contrast-enhanced chest CT scan is the most accurate test to locate the foreign body in the airways as well as to diagnose all secondary findings.

Given the amount of radiation the patient receives, it is important to weigh the risks and benefits of the test, especially in children. Therefore, chest CT scan should be restricted to those patients with a high suspicion of foreign body and a chest x-ray that shows no significant findings.

The most common findings on chest CT scan are [18]:

- Radiopaque foreign bodies: do not pose a significant diagnostic challenge and are mostly metallic objects (except aluminum which does not present sufficient radiopacity to be displayed in plain film).
- Radiolucent foreign bodies: can be both organic and inorganic. We noted that the organic ones produce a more intense tissue reaction and are more often associated with complications.
- Indirect radiological findings:

- Hyperinflation: It is common to find unilateral air trapping caused by a valve mechanism.
- Atelectasis: seen in up to 25% of cases, the incidence increases with delayed diagnosis. A post-obstructive pneumonia may be associated.
- Bronchiectasis: irreversible bronchial dilation, they are more common the longer the foreign body is lodged in the airways.
- Pneumothorax / pneumomediastinum: although rare, they can occur in cases of perforation of the airway.

Moreover, these findings may not be so clear and raise confusion with other entities such as mucus plugging, airway stenosis or endobronchial tumors.

Despite this wide range of findings, the absence of radiological findings suggesting a foreign body in the airways does not rule out the diagnosis [20].

Recent techniques such as virtual bronchoscopy are being used for diagnosis. In a series of 60 cases that included organic and non-metallic foreign bodies, an excellent correlation between the findings of the virtual bronchoscopy and those of rigid bronchoscopy were observed, reaching a positive predictive value of 98.3% [21].

TREATMENT

As a general rule, in the presence of any foreign body in the airway, removal should be considered, either by positional, endoscopic or surgical techniques.

Endoscopic Techniques

Endoscopic retrieval is the technique of choice for a suspected foreign body lodged in the airways. Its wide use, the greater safety of the procedure and the continuous development of therapeutic possibilities allow its implementation.

The debate between rigid and flexible bronchoscopy in pediatric and adult patients, has been widely discussed in the available literature.

Preferences or the routine of the medical team that performs the procedure is an important criterion to consider. Moreover, the patient's condition can force the decision to use one technique or another. In cases of respiratory failure, or procedures that are considered of high risk, seems more appropriate the use of the rigid bronchoscope in the operating room environment and control by anesthesia.

When clinical situation allows it, the best initial approach would be using flexible bronchoscopy as it let us a general look of the anatomical variants, the presence of granulation tissue, the position and characteristics of the object. Even, flexible bronchoscopy can result in definitive treatment with all the guarantees.

Rigid Bronchoscopy

With the emergence of flexible bronchoscopy, the role of the rigid bronchoscopy seemed relegated to the background. However, with the gradual increase in Interventional Pulmonology techniques that can be applied, its use become more common [24].

When compared to the flexible endoscope, the rigid bronchoscope have some advantages thanks to its larger working channel, through which you can use numerous devices and sensors that allow not only the removal of the foreign but also to prevent, control and treat complications that may arise during the procedure.

In pediatric patients, it is the most frequently chosen technique. In a series of 105 cases Divisi *et al.* reported a success rate of 97.2% [25] when using the rigid bronchoscope. In those cases where rigid bronchoscopy was ineffective, surgical removal was performed.

Among the tools we can use through the working channel of the endoscope, the most important are [26]:

- Forceps: many types of forceps are available. They can be classified based upon grasping surface (coarse serration, finer serrations, toothed forceps or broader surface) or jaw movement (two mobile jaws, one moveable jaw and a stationary jaw). The selection of the type of forceps depends on the localization and the nature of the foreign body (Figs. **5** and **6**).
- Cryoextraction: This technique can be applied both with flexible rigid bronchoscopy. Not only can be used for those objects with high water content, but also for the granulation tissue formed.
- Embolectomy: Catheters: by passing the catheter distally to the object and inflating the balloon with air or serum (more rigid) it helps with the mobilization to more accessible areas, where they can be collected with forceps. It is also a good alternative in case of sharp objects that are fixed and wrapped by bronchial mucosa [27]. Caution should be exercised to prevent an over-inflation or a puncture by a sharp object [28].
- Nd:Yag Laser: its role in the retrieval of foreign bodies is somewhat limited. It has been used for treatment of granulation tissue, especially when it affects a large obstruction of the bronchial lumen [29] or to cut metallic objects.
- Flexible bronchoscope: You can introduce the flexible bronchoscope through the working channel in situations with and inadequate view of the object and use the same devices.

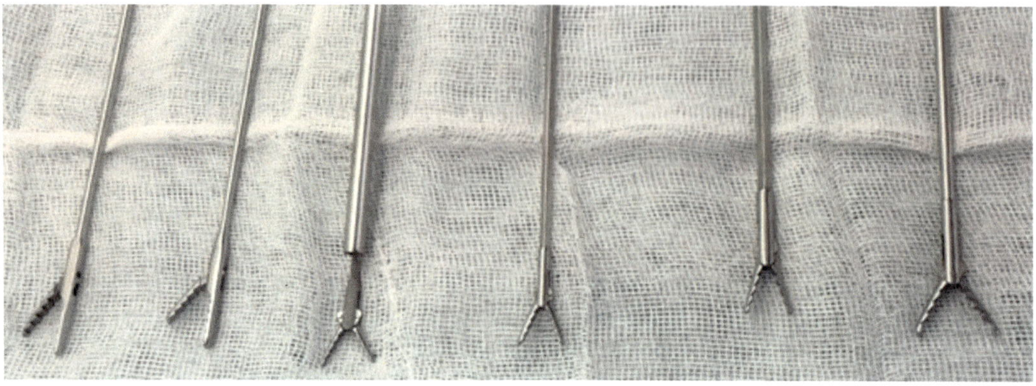

Fig. (5). Different models of forceps for foreign body extraction through the rigid bronchoscope. Source: Interventional Pulmonology Unit. Fundación Jiménez Díaz University Hospital.

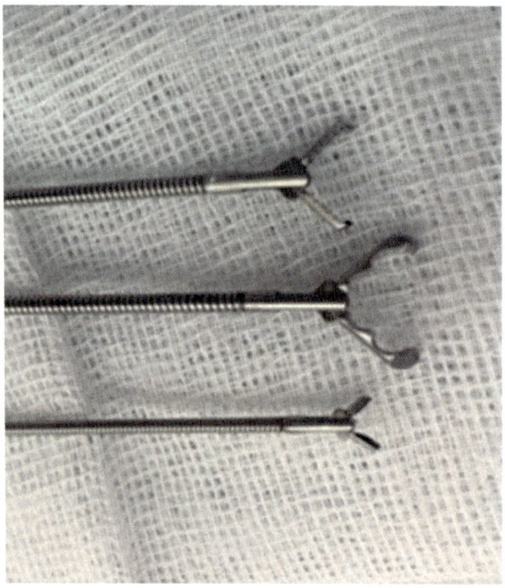

Fig. (6). Rigid forceps for removal of foreign bodies through a rigid bronchoscope.
From top to bottom: Alligator jaw grasping forceps, W-shaped forceps and flat-tip forceps.
Source: Interventional Pulmonology Unit. Fundación Jiménez Díaz University Hospital.

Besides handling the foreign body, the rigid bronchoscope is useful for managing patient ventilation. Recently, Hall *et al.* have proposed a technique that could be applied in patients with a limited respiratory reserve, so that the endoscopist has more time for the extraction. The technique involves placing a modified endotracheal tube (with a cut in its proximal area) on the bronchoscope. The inflation of the balloon of the tube prevents the air to get out and increases positive end expiratory pressure (PEEP) [30].

Like any surgical procedure, after the completion of a rigid bronchoscopy, it should be a period of recovery. In a report publish by Chung *et al.* the average recovery time was about a week, although as noted by the authors, there are several factors that can predict and extended time: preoperative inflammatory findings by radiologic study, a prolonged procedure over 50 minutes, and aggravation of the immediate postoperative radiologic findings [31].

Flexible Bronchoscopy

Ever since the 70's flexible bronchoscopy was found to be a safe technique for the removal of foreign bodies with a decreased morbidity and mortality [32]. The growing number of techniques and devices that can be applied through its working channel increases significantly the therapeutic possibilities.

In children, the rigid bronchoscope was traditionally used as a first choice, since the narrow working channel of the ultrathin bronchoscope had been a limitation when removing foreign bodies. However, Swanson *et al.* showed that, having the appropriate extraction instruments to use through the working channel and placing an endotracheal tube or laryngeal mask, flexible bronchoscopy has proven to be a safe and effective method [33].

In adults, available literature supports the use of the flexible bronchoscope as an adequate technique for foreign body removal. In a series of 33 cases Lan *et al.* described that, after grouping patients, according to the length of time that the foreign body was in the lung, flexible bronchoscopy was effective and safe in most patients [34].

Through the working channel of the flexible bronchoscope can be used [26]:

- Forceps: conventional biopsy forceps may be useful for removal of foreign bodies. As in the rigid bronchoscope, specific forceps with different features (serrated, toothed, spoon) are used according to the location and characteristics of the foreign body (Fig. **7**).
- Cryoprobe: flexible cryoprobe is described as useful and safety in several published cases. It is said to be more effective in mucus plugs, clots and those foreign bodies (both organic and inorganic ones) with high water content [35, 36] (Fig. **8**).
- Snares: consist in a metal loop. Rotation is allowed for a better orientation. The foreign body is wrapped with the snare and pressed against the catheter to allow extraction [37].
- Baskets: can be defined as the most complex version of the loops (snares). They are retractable baskets with about 4-6 rods that allow wrapping the foreign body (Figs. **9** and **10**).

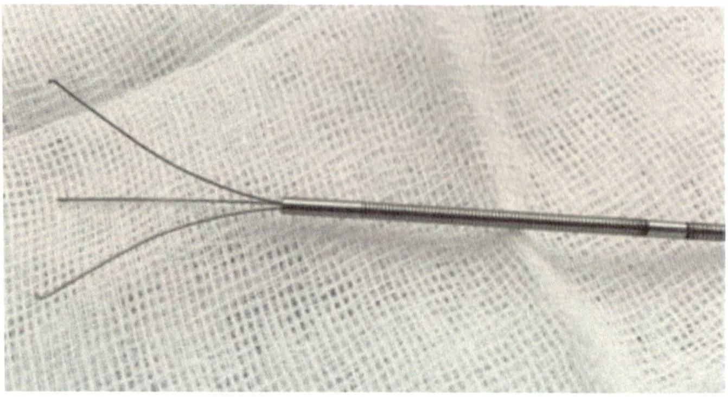

Fig. (7). Tripod forceps for flexible bronchoscope.
Source: Interventional Pulmonology Unit. Fundación Jiménez Díaz University Hospital.

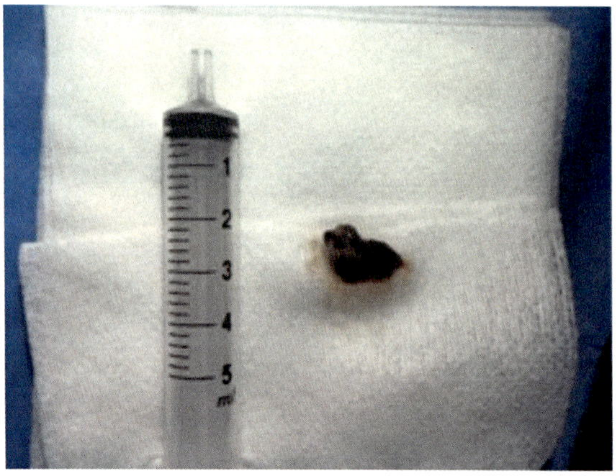

Fig. (8). Blood clot removed using a cryoprobe.
Source: Interventional Pulmonology Unit. Salamanca University Hospital.

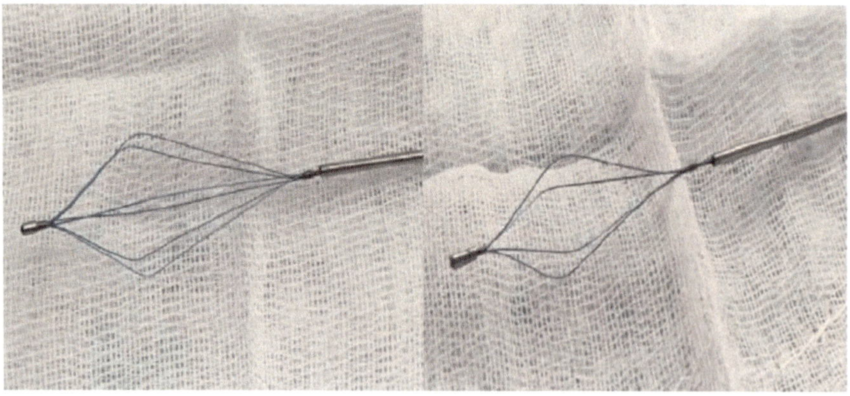

Fig. (9). 6-wire and 4-wire baskets for the extraction of foreign bodies through flexible bronchoscopy.
Source: Interventional Pulmonology Unit. Fundación Jiménez Díaz University Hospital.

In conclusion and in view of the evidence presented in the literature, flexible bronchoscopy can be considered as the initial procedure of choice in adult patients, with a success rate close to 90% [8].

Non-endoscopic Techniques

Positional maneuvers often consist of alternating lateral decubitus and Trendelenburg position depending on the location of the object. In pediatric patients nebulized bronchodilators are also combined with percussion maneuvers [22]. The use of systemic corticosteroids as a useful measure to reduce inflammation in the airways and facilitate the expulsion of the foreign body was also proposed [23].

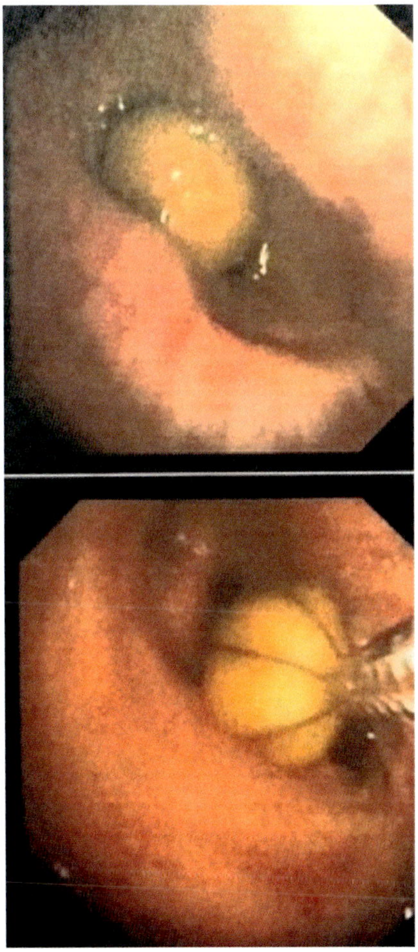

Fig. (10). Endoscopic extraction of a chickpea from the intermediate bronchus using a basket. Source: Interventional Pulmonology Unit. Fundación Jiménez Díaz University Hospital.

These techniques are now obsolete because of the increasing in safety and the new therapeutic possibilities of endoscopic procedures and used only in highly selected cases (very small foreign bodies, young and healthy adults) or in areas with limited resources. Due to the fact the delay in intervention increases the risk of complications; these maneuvers should be stopped if they do not success in a short period of time.

Surgical Resection

Currently, surgical treatment remains the last resort in the removal of foreign bodies. Basically consist of cases with a significant diagnostic delay and major changes in bronchi and lung parenchyma after failed endoscopy. Interventions range from bronchotomy to even pneumonectomy and the complication rate is high.

With a high index of clinical suspicion and the endoscopic techniques available today, surgery remains for highly selected cases [38].

COMPLICATIONS

The number and nature of complications vary with the type of procedure. Below are the most common complications [39]:

- Foreign body fragmentation and distal migration: friable foreign bodies can be broken into small fragments during handling. In some cases, small fragments can be spontaneously expectorated with positional maneuvers. If not, surgical treatment is necessary before the appearance of complications.
- Hemorrhage: This situation is more common in foreign bodies that produce an important inflammatory component, the friable granulation tissue that bleeds during handling. Sharp-edged objects can also damage the bronchial wall during the extraction. The best tool for the management of bleeding is the rigid bronchoscope because it allows the cauterization of the bleeding area by the application of laser.

The risk of bleeding can be reduced by the instillation of cold saline or epinephrine, if the hemodynamic status of the patient allows it safely.

- Bronchial obstruction: caused by an increased inflammatory component secondary to handling or by bleeding.
- Loss of foreign body during its removal: can migrate to the contralateral lung or the upper airway leading to choking.
- Granulation tissue (Fig. **11**).

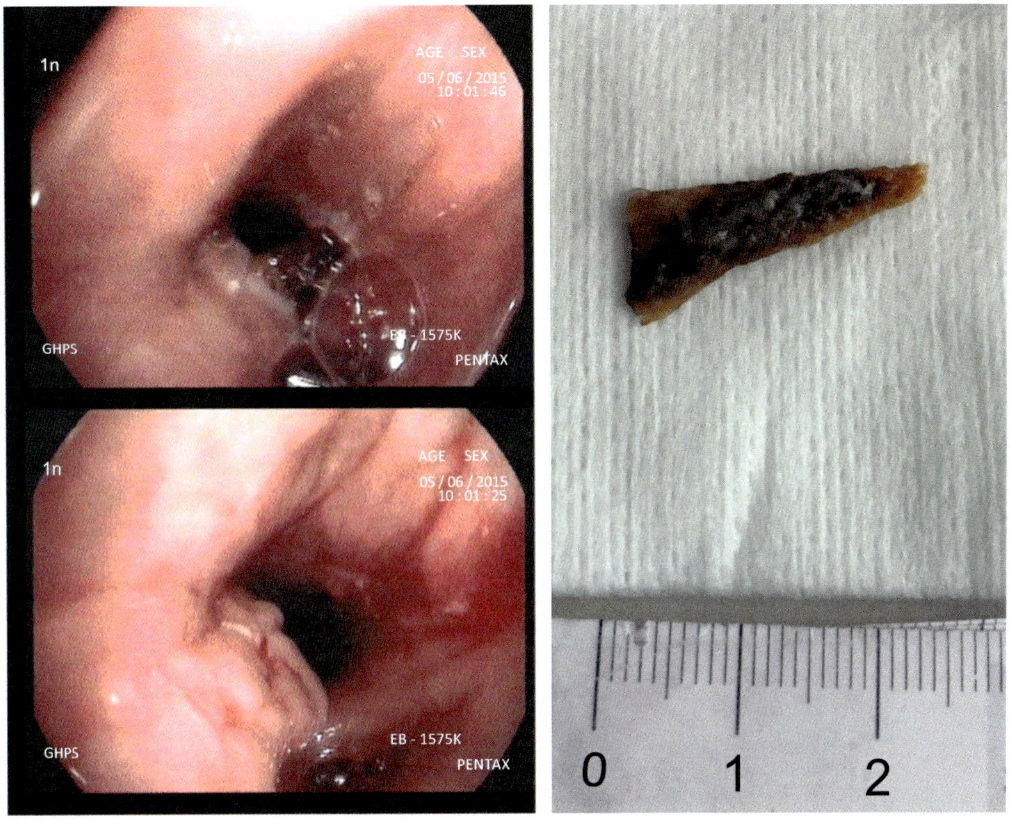

Fig. (11). Left: Aspect before (top) and after endoscopic removal. Foreign body wedged for at least one month, causing intense granulation tissue.
Right: Foreign body removed from the right lower lobe of a 65 year-old-woman, showing inflammatory changes.
Courtesy of Trosini-Désert V. Bronchoscopy Unit. Pitié-Salpêtrière Hospital. Paris. France.

CONCLUSION

Aspiration of foreign bodies is an event that can endanger the lives of patients, especially in children, where the caliber of the airways is smaller and obstruction occurs at the higher levels of the airways. Mortality is much higher in pediatric patients than in adults where barely reaches 0.8 deaths per 100,000 population.

It is important to provide families with the appropriate information to prevent children to handle potentially dangerous objects, to monitor the symptoms and to know what steps to take.

In adults, it should be applied the above to primary caregivers of patients with dementia or neurological disorders who have an increased risk of aspiration.

Dental procedures or tracheostomy care are other high-risk situations.

In patients with suspected foreign body aspiration, both diagnostic and therapeutic decisions should be as fast as possible in order to reduce and prevent life-threatening complications.

CONFLICT OF INTEREST

The authors declare no conflict of interest, financial or otherwise.

ACKNOWLEDGEMENTS

Declared none.

REFERENCES

[1] Killian G. Removal of a bone splinter from the right main bronchus by direct laryngoscopy. Munch Med Wsch 1897; 44: 86.

[2] Panchabhai TS, Mehta AC. Historical perspectives of bronchoscopy. Connecting the dots. Ann Am Thorac Soc 2015; 12(5): 631-41. [http://dx.doi.org/10.1513/AnnalsATS.201502-089PS] [PMID: 25965540]

[3] Ikeda S, Tsuboi E, Ono R, Ishikawa S. Flexible bronchofiberscope. Jpn J Clin Oncol 2010; 40(9): e55-64. [http://dx.doi.org/10.1093/jjco/hyq114] [PMID: 20736215]

[4] Baharloo F, Veyckemans F, Francis C, Biettlot MP, Rodenstein DO. Tracheobronchial foreign bodies: presentation and management in children and adults. Chest 1999; 115(5): 1357-62. [PMID: 10334153]

[5] Ramírez-Figueroa JL, Gochicoa-Rangel LG, Ramírez-San Juan DH, Vargas MH. Foreign body removal by flexible fiberoptic bronchoscopy in infants and children. Pediatr Pulmonol 2005; 40(5): 392-7. [http://dx.doi.org/10.1002/ppul.20242] [PMID: 16130115]

[6] Limper AH, Prakash UB. Tracheobronchial foreign bodies in adults. Ann Intern Med 1990; 112(8): 604-9. [http://dx.doi.org/10.7326/0003-4819-112-8-604] [PMID: 2327678]

[7] Ramos MB, Fernández-Villar A, Rivo JE, *et al.* Extraction of airway foreign bodies in adults: experience from 1987-2008. Interact Cardiovasc Thorac Surg 2009; 9(3): 402-5. [http://dx.doi.org/10.1510/icvts.2009.207332] [PMID: 19491125]

[8] Sehgal IS, Dhooria S, Ram B, *et al.* Foreign body inhalation in the adult population: Experience of 25,998 bronchoscopies and systematic review of the literature. Respir Care 2015; 60(10): 1438-48. [http://dx.doi.org/10.4187/respcare.03976] [PMID: 25969517]

[9] Casalini AG, Majori M, Anghinolfi M, *et al.* Foreign body aspiration in adults and in children: advantages and consequences of a dedicated protocol in our 30-year experience. J Bronchology Interv Pulmonol 2013; 20(4): 313-21. [http://dx.doi.org/10.1097/LBR.0000000000000024] [PMID: 24162114]

[10] Reilly J, Thompson J, MacArthur C, *et al.* Pediatric aerodigestive foreign body injuries are complications related to timeliness of diagnosis. Laryngoscope 1997; 107(1): 17-20. [http://dx.doi.org/10.1097/00005537-199701000-00006] [PMID: 9001259]

[11] Goyal R, Nayar S, Gogia P, Garg M. Extraction of tracheobronchial foreign bodies in children and

adults with rigid and flexible bronchoscopy. J Bronchology Interv Pulmonol 2012; 19(1): 35-43. [http://dx.doi.org/10.1097/LBR.0b013e318244e591] [PMID: 23207261]

[12] Bertolani MF, Marotti F, Bergamini BM, Pellegrino M, Balli R, Calandra Buonaura PL. Extraction of a rubber bullet from a bronchus after 1 year: complete resolution of chronic pulmonary damage. Chest 1999; 115(4): 1210-3.
[http://dx.doi.org/10.1378/chest.115.4.1210] [PMID: 10208235]

[13] Colavita L, Gelli C, Pecorari L, *et al.* A history of recurrent wheezing can delay the diagnosis of foreign body aspiration in a paediatric emergency department 2015.
[http://dx.doi.org/10.1136/bcr-2015-211946]

[14] Lan RS. Non-asphyxiating tracheobronchial foreign bodies in adults. Eur Respir J 1994; 7(3): 510-4.
[http://dx.doi.org/10.1183/09031936.94.07030510] [PMID: 8013610]

[15] Alharthi BJ, Masoodi I, Almourgi MA, Alzahrani S. Occult foreign body in the lung mimicking bronchogenic carcinoma. BMJ Case Rep 2014; 2014: bcr2014207438.
[http://dx.doi.org/10.1136/bcr-2014-207438] [PMID: 25519864]

[16] Møller J, Rasmussen F, Hilberg O, Løkke A. Airway foreign body aspiration: common, yet easily overlooked! Two interesting cases. BMJ Case Rep 2015; 2015: bcr2014209240.
[http://dx.doi.org/10.1136/bcr-2014-209240] [PMID: 26002666]

[17] Lax EA, Kiran SH, Lee MW. Bronchoscopic retrieval of a bullet using a Dormia basket: a case report. J Med Case Reports 2014; 8: 358.
[http://dx.doi.org/10.1186/1752-1947-8-358] [PMID: 25362866]

[18] Hegde SV, Hui PK, Lee EY. Tracheobronchial foreign bodies in children: imaging assessment. Semin Ultrasound CT MR 2015; 36(1): 8-20.
[http://dx.doi.org/10.1053/j.sult.2014.10.001] [PMID: 25639173]

[19] Pinto A, Scaglione M, Pinto F, *et al.* Tracheobronchial aspiration of foreign bodies: current indications for emergency plain chest radiography. Radiol Med (Torino) 2006; 111(4): 497-506.
[http://dx.doi.org/10.1007/s11547-006-0045-0] [PMID: 16779536]

[20] Wunsch R, Wunsch C, Darge K. Foreign body aspiration. Radiologe 1999; 39(6): 467-71.
[http://dx.doi.org/10.1007/s001170050536] [PMID: 10422108]

[21] Behera G, Tripathy N, Maru YK, Mundra RK, Gupta Y, Lodha M. Role of virtual bronchoscopy in children with a vegetable foreign body in the tracheobronchial tree. J Laryngol Otol 2014; 128(12): 1078-83.
[http://dx.doi.org/10.1017/S0022215114002837] [PMID: 25388230]

[22] Cotton EK, Abrams G, Vanhoutte J, Burrington J. Removal of aspirated foreign bodies by inhalation and postural drainage. A survey of 24 cases. Clin Pediatr (Phila) 1973; 12(5): 270-6.
[http://dx.doi.org/10.1177/000992287301200506] [PMID: 4700726]

[23] Pagán Rivera BL, Anselmi FJ, Torres MdelM, Segarra A, Rivera JR. Usefulness Of Glucocorticoids In The Management Of Foreign Body Aspiration. Bol Asoc Med P R 2015; 107(3): 24-7.
[PMID: 26742192]

[24] Alraiyes AH, Machuzak MS. Rigid bronchoscopy. Semin Respir Crit Care Med 2014; 35(6): 671-80.
[http://dx.doi.org/10.1055/s-0034-1395500] [PMID: 25463158]

[25] Divisi D, Di Tommaso S, Garramone M, *et al.* Foreign bodies aspirated in children: role of bronchoscopy. Thorac Cardiovasc Surg 2007; 55(4): 249-52.
[http://dx.doi.org/10.1055/s-2006-924714] [PMID: 17516556]

[26] Ernst A, Herth FJ, Eds. Principles and Practice of Interventional Pulmonology. Springer Science+Business Media New York . 2013.
[http://dx.doi.org/10.1007/978-1-4614-4292-9]

[27] Thornton CS, Yunker WK. Rigid bronchoscopy and balloon dilation for removal of aspirated

thumbtacks: case series and literature review. Int J Pediatr Otorhinolaryngol 2015; 79(9): 1541-3. [http://dx.doi.org/10.1016/j.ijporl.2015.07.007] [PMID: 26209351]

[28] Ross MN, Haase GM, Haase G. An alternative approach to management of Fogarty catheter disruption associated with endobronchial foreign body extraction. Chest 1988; 94(4): 882-4. [http://dx.doi.org/10.1378/chest.94.4.882] [PMID: 3168588]

[29] Hayashi AH, Gillis DA, Bethune D, Hughes D, O'Neil M. Management of foreign-body bronchial obstruction using endoscopic laser therapy. J Pediatr Surg 1990; 25(11): 1174-6. [http://dx.doi.org/10.1016/0022-3468(90)90757-Z] [PMID: 2273434]

[30] Hall MB, Johnston DR, Barth P. Positive pressure bronchoscopy technique: Case report. Ann Otol Rhinol Laryngol 2016; 125(2): 165-8. [http://dx.doi.org/10.1177/0003489415602265] [PMID: 26307070]

[31] Chung MK, Jeong HS, Ahn KM, *et al.* Pulmonary recovery after rigid bronchoscopic retrieval of airway foreign body. Laryngoscope 2007; 117(2): 303-7. [http://dx.doi.org/10.1097/01.mlg.0000250788.93900.ef] [PMID: 17277626]

[32] Cunanan OS. The flexible fiberopticbronchoscope in foreign body removal: experience in 300 cases. Chest 1978.

[33] Swanson KL, Prakash UB, Midthun DE, *et al.* Flexible bronchoscopic management of airway foreign bodies in children. Chest 2002; 121(5): 1695-700. [http://dx.doi.org/10.1378/chest.121.5.1695] [PMID: 12006464]

[34] Lan RS, Lee CH, Chiang YC, Wang WJ. Use of fiberoptic bronchoscopy to retrieve bronchial foreign bodies in adults. Am Rev Respir Dis 1989; 140(6): 1734-7. [http://dx.doi.org/10.1164/ajrccm/140.6.1734] [PMID: 2604299]

[35] Sriratanaviriyakul N, Lam F, Morrissey BM, Stollenwerk N, Schivo M, Yoneda KY. Safety and clinical utility of flexible bronchoscopic cryoextraction in patients with non-neoplasm tracheobronchial obstruction: A retrospective chart review. J Bronchology Interv Pulmonol 2015; 22(4): 288-93. [http://dx.doi.org/10.1097/LBR.0000000000000203] [PMID: 26439016]

[36] Rubio E, Gupta P, Ie S, Boyd M. Cryoextraction: A novel approach to remove aspirated chewing gum. Ann Thorac Med 2013; 8(1): 58-9. [http://dx.doi.org/10.4103/1817-1737.105721] [PMID: 23440914]

[37] Nalaboff KM, Solis JL, Simon D. Endobronchial foreign body extraction: a new interventional approach. Chest 2001; 120(4): 1402-5. [http://dx.doi.org/10.1378/chest.120.4.1402] [PMID: 11591588]

[38] Duan L, Chen X, Wang H, Hu X, Jiang G. Surgical treatment of late-diagnosed bronchial foreign body aspiration: a report of 23 cases. Clin Respir J 2014; 8(3): 269-73. [http://dx.doi.org/10.1111/crj.12040] [PMID: 23848455]

[39] Flandes J, Diaz-Ajero P. Broncoscopia diagnóstica y terapeútica. Madrid: Monografias Neumomadrid 2007; Vol. X.

SUBJECT INDEX

A

Ali I. Musani (Ed.)

B

C

H

I

L

M

N

O

P

Q

R

S

T

V

W

Made in the USA
Las Vegas, NV
22 November 2025

34934088R00238